Preservation of *FERTILITY*

Preservation of FERTILITY

Edited by

Togas Tulandi MD
Department of Obstetrics and Gynecology,
McGill University, Montreal, Quebec, Canada

and

Roger G. Gosden PhD DSc
The Jones Institute for Reproductive Medicine,
Eastern Virginia Medical School, Norfolk, VA, USA

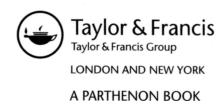

Taylor & Francis
Taylor & Francis Group

LONDON AND NEW YORK

A PARTHENON BOOK

© 2004 Taylor & Francis, an imprint of the Taylor & Francis Group

First published in the United Kingdom in 2004
by Taylor & Francis,
an imprint of the Taylor & Francis Group,
11 New Fetter Lane,
London EC4P 4EE

Tel.:   +44 (0) 20 7583 9855
Fax.:   +44 (0) 20 7842 2298
Website: www.tandf.co.uk

Although every effort has been made to ensure that all owners of copyright material have been acknowledged in this publication, we would be glad to acknowledge in subsequent reprints or editions any omissions brought to our attention.

British Library Cataloguing in Publication Data

Data available on application

Library of Congress Cataloging-in-Publication Data

Data available on application

ISBN 1-84214-242-9

Distributed in North and South America by

Taylor & Francis
2000 NW Corporate Blvd
Boca Raton, FL 33431, USA

Within Continental USA
Tel.: 800 272 7737; Fax.: 800 374 3401
Outside Continental USA
Tel.: 561 994 0555; Fax.: 561 361 6018
E-mail: orders@crcpress.com

Distributed in the rest of the world by
Thomson Publishing Services
Cheriton House
North Way
Andover, Hampshire SP10 5BE, UK
Tel.: +44 (0) 1264 332424
E-mail: salesorder.tandf@thomsonpublishingservices.co.uk

Composition by Siva Math Setters, Chennai, India
Printed and bound by Antony Rowe Ltd., Chippenham, Wiltshire, UK

Contents

List of contributors

J. Apperley
Department of Haematology
Imperial College
Hammersmith Hospital
Du Cane Road
London W12 0HS
UK

G. Bahadur
Department of Obstetrics and Gynaecology
University College London/UCL Hospital
  Trust
25 Grafton Way
London WC1E 6DB
UK

E. L. Chambers
Reproduction and Early Development
  Research Group
Department of Obstetrics and Gynaecology
Clarendon Wing
Leeds General Infirmary
Belmont Grove
Leeds LS2 9NS
UK

H. O. D. Critchley
Section of Obstetrics and Gynaecology
Department of Developmental and
  Reproductive Sciences
Centre for Reproductive Biology
University of Edinburgh
The Chancellor's Building
49 Little France Crescent
Edinburgh EH16 4SB
UK

S. L. Crockin
The Chatham Center
29 Crafts Street
Newton, MA 02460
USA

N. L. Dean
Department of Obstetrics and
  Gynecology
McGill University
Royal Victoria Hospital
687 Pine Avenue West
Montreal, Quebec
Canada H3A 1A1

J.-P. de Bruin
Division of Perinatology and
  Gynaecology
Department of Reproductive
  Medicine
University Medical Centre Utrecht
Heidelberglaan 100
3584 CX Utrecht
The Netherlands

G. Del Priore
Albert Einstein College of Medicine
Montefiore Medical Center
3332 Rochambeau Ave
New York, NY 10467
USA

J. Dor
The IVF Unit
Division of Obstetrics and
  Gynecology
Sheba Medical Center
Tel-Hashomer
Israel

K. H. Dow
School of Nursing
College of Health and Public Affairs
University of Central Florida
12479 Research Parkway
Orlando, FL 32816
USA

S. Emery
Perinatal Ultrasound
Section Maternal–Fetal Medicine
Department of Obstetrics and
    Gynecology
Cleveland Clinic Foundation
9500 Euclid Avenue
Cleveland, OH 44195
USA

T. Falcone
Department of Obstetrics and Gynecology
Cleveland Clinic Foundation
9500 Euclid Avenue
Cleveland, OH 44195
USA

R. G. Gosden
The Jones Institute for Reproductive
    Medicine
Eastern Virginia Medical School
601 Colley Avenue
Norfolk, VA 23507
USA

S. E. Harris
Reproduction and Early Development
    Research Group
Department of Obstetrics and
    Gynaecology
Clarendon Wing
Leeds General Infirmary
Belmont Grove
Leeds LS2 9NS
UK

S. Howell
Christie Hospital NHS Trust
Wilmslow Road
Withington
Manchester M20 4BX
UK

G. S. Huang
Albert Einstein College of Medicine
Montefiore Medical Center
3332 Rochambeau Ave
New York, NY 10467
USA

S. M. Kelly
Fertility Associates
Ascot Integrated Hospital
90 Greenlane Road East
Remuera
Auckland
New Zealand

S. S. Kim
Department of Obstetrics and Gynecology
Pochon CHA University School of Medicine
LA CHA Fertility Center
5455 Wiltshire Boulevard
Los Angeles, CA 90036
USA

S. P. Leibo
Department of Biological Sciences
200 CRC
University of New Orleans
New Orleans, LA 70148
USA

D. Meirow
The IVF Unit
Division of Obstetrics and
    Gynecology
Sheba Medical Center
Tel-Hashomer
Israel

M. Morshedi
The Jones Institute for Reproductive
    Medicine
Eastern Virginia Medical School
601 Colley Avenue
Norfolk, Virginia 23507
USA

M. C. Nagano
Department of Obstetrics and
    Gynecology
McGill University
Royal Victoria Hosptial
687 Pine Avenue West
Montreal, Quebec
Canada H3A 1A1

K. Oktay
Center for Reproductive Medicine
  and Infertility
Joan and Sanford I. Weill Medical
  College of Cornell University
505 East 70th St
New York, NY 10021
USA

H. M. Picton
Reproduction and Early Development
  Research Group
Department of Obstetrics and
  Gynaecology
Clarendon Wing
Leeds General Infirmary
Belmont Grove
Leeds LS2 9NS
UK

D. Rao
Department of Obstetrics and Gynecology
McGill University
Royal Victoria Hospital
687 Pine Avenue West
Montreal, Quebec
Canada H3A 1A1

N. Reddy
Department of Reproductive Medicine
Hammersmith Hospital NHS Trust
Du Cane Road
London W12 ONN
UK

N. Salooja
Department of Haematology
Imperial College
Charing Cross Hospital
Fulham Palace Road
London W6 8RF
UK

S. Shalet
Christie Hospital NHS Trust
Wilmslow Road
Withington
Manchester M20 4BX
UK

M. Sönmezer
Center for Reproductive Medicine
  and Infertility
Joan and Sanford I. Weill Medical
  College of Cornell University
505 East 70th St
New York, NY 10021
USA

S. L. Tan
Department of Obstetrics and Gynecology
McGill University
Royal Victoria Hospital
687 Pine Avenue West
Montreal, Quebec
Canada H3A 1A1

E. R. te Velde
Division of Perinatology and Gynaecology
Department of Reproductive
  Medicine
University Medical Centre Utrecht
Heidelberglaan 100
3584 CX Utrecht
The Netherlands

J. L. Tilly
Vincent Center for Reproductive
  Biology
Massachusetts General Hospital – East
149 13th Street
Charlestown, MA 02129
USA

J. M. Trasler
Montreal Children's Hospital
Research Institute
McGill University
2300 Tupper Street
Montreal, Quebec
Canada H3H 1P3

T. Tulandi
Department of Obstetrics and Gynecology
McGill University
687 Pine Avenue West
Montreal, Quebec
Canada H3A 1A1

W. H. B. Wallace
Department of Haematology/
    Oncology
Royal Hospital for Sick Children
17 Millerfield Place
Edinburgh EH9 1LW
UK

H. Yin
The Jones Institute for Reproductive
    Medicine
Eastern Virginia Medical School
601 Colley Avenue
Norfolk, VA 23507
USA

Preface

Fertility preservation has suddenly become a hot topic. Not only does it come in the wake of advances in oncology and other disciplines, it is also being spurred by the social and professional pressures on many women today to postpone having a family until their later reproductive years when they are less fertile. Advances in cancer therapy have improved the long-term survival of young patients suffering from malignancies. In fact, many childhood lymphomas and leukemias can now be cured. However, cancer treatment sometimes carries adverse side-effects, including loss of gonadal function and sterility in both sexes. Preservation of fertility in males by sperm freezing is already well established, although it is still an imperfect technology. There have been few options for young women undergoing cancer treatment, but the advent of new methods for preserving gonadal function and fertility now provides hope. Today, we can cryopreserve the embryos, oocytes and ovarian tissue of females as well as the spermatogonial stem cells and testicular tissue of males. In patients undergoing pelvic irradiation, laparoscopic lateral ovarian suspension can be considered. At last, there are better prospects for genetic parenthood, and for both child and adult patients. This book, *Preservation of Fertility*, reflects the latest advances in the field. It addresses new concepts, progress in reproductive techniques, novel treatment modalities, pregnancy after cancer treatment, patient care issues and professional responsibilities.

The contributors are physicians and researchers who are acknowledged leaders in this field with many years of experience. In the first three chapters, they discuss age and fertility, epidemiology of cancer survival and fertility, and the vulnerability of the reproductive system to radiotherapy and chemotherapy. The following five chapters are dedicated to methods for preserving fertility, including medical and surgical approaches and the use of assisted reproductive technologies. These chapters are followed by others on new developments in the laboratory for preserving gametes and gonadal tissue. The last three chapters deal with the psychosocial, legal and ethical issues of fertility preservation.

This is a book for clinical and basic researchers as well as for practicing gynecologists, students, residents and fellows. Readers will gain an understanding of alternatives for preserving fertility and learn about the development and delivery of relevant technologies. We also hope that this book will be helpful in directing new investigations and the clinical management of patients.

Togas Tulandi MD
The Milton Leong Chair in
Reproductive Medicine
Professor of Obstetrics and Gynecology
McGill University
Montreal, Quebec, Canada

and

Roger Gosden PhD DSc
The Howard and Georgeanna Jones
Professor of Reproductive Medicine
Professor of Obstetrics and Gynecology
The Jones Institute for Reproductive
Medicine, Eastern Virginia
Medical School
Norfolk, VA, USA

Foreword

'Second Law: All the acquisitions or losses wrought by nature in individuals ... are preserved by reproduction to the new individuals which arise.'

Jean Baptiste Lamark (1744–1829)

There is a renewed emphasis on the preservation of fertility in the light of rapid advances in cryopreservation, tissue transplantation and *in vitro* fertilization techniques. This scientific revolution has resulted in a reconsideration of treatment protocols for cancer. Moreover, health-care practitioners now consider gamete preservation or surgical strategies to protect the ovary or testis during cancer therapy.

Togas Tulandi and Roger Gosden have assembled an outstanding group of internationally recognized specialists to address the entire spectrum of issues regarding fertility preservation. This is an impressive text which will serve as an important resource for health-care providers. The book will be a valuable addition to the Medical Practitioner's library.

John A. Rock MD
Chancellor
The Louisiana State University Health
Sciences Center
New Orleans, LA, USA

Foreword

The importance of the technologies outlined in *Preservation of Fertility* is profound. Facing a fertility compromising situation – whether a sterilizing cancer treatment or advanced reproductive age – is daunting.

I was diagnosed with tongue cancer at age 22; as a non-smoking marathon runner it was a shocking diagnosis. Although successfully treated with aggressive radiation, one and a half year's later the cancer returned and spread. The second time around, I was less concerned with the immediate effects of my treatments. I knew I could endure the short term, so I focused on the permanent, long-term effects. I wanted to minimize anything I would have to live with forever.

Nothing stood out to me as much as infertility. It was permanent, life altering and dramatically changed my perception of the future and, therefore, my will to fight.

As illustrated in *Preservation of Fertility*, many technologies exist for men and women to preserve fertility, and advances are being made all the time. Sadly, however, this information is not well known in the oncology community and is, therefore, not presented to all eligible cancer patients.

I was lucky enough to inquire about my risks, seek out my options and successfully freeze 29 eggs prior to undergoing a potentially sterilizing chemotherapy regime. I knew egg freezing wasn't guaranteed, but any chance of success was better than the alternative. The majority of my peers in similar situations are not as fortunate.

Accordingly, I founded Fertile Hope, a national, non-profit organization dedicated to providing reproductive information, support and hope to cancer patients whose medical treatments present the risk of infertility. Fertile Hope has assumed a leadership role in the cancer survivorship movement, creating tools that help young survivors fulfill their parenthood dreams. While Fertile Hope has made great strides since its inception in 2001, there are more than 120 000 men and women in their reproductive years diagnosed with cancer each year and hundreds of thousands of cancer survivors in the USA today who need access to such information. Some of those who receive devastating blows to the prospects for genetic parenthood are children, and their parents need to know the options for their daughters and sons.

As you read *Preservation of Fertility*, I encourage you to advocate on behalf of men and women like me (and their current or future partners) so that everyone has the information they need to make educated reproductive decisions. Seek ways to disseminate this information in your community. Collaborate with health-care professionals and non-profit organizations to promote research. Optimize the opportunity to impact individual lives in a remarkable way.

Preservation of Fertility is a powerful knowledge tool for the medical community and a gift of hope to the patients it touches.

Lindsay Nohr
Founder, Executive Director
Fertile Hope – www.fertilehope.org
New York, NY
January 2004

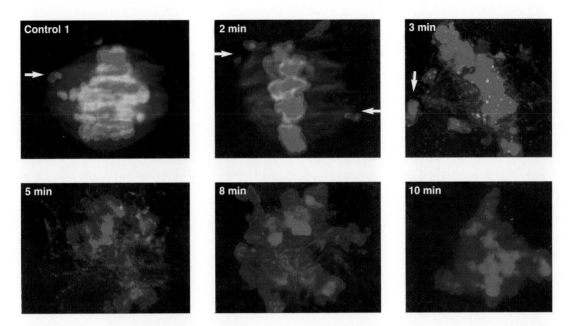

Color Plate I   Fluorescent micrographs of meiotic spindles in human oocytes that had been cooled rapidly to 0°C and held for the times indicated. The panel labeled control 1 is an untreated oocyte. The micrographs were made with an optical sectioning microscope together with deconvolution software. Chromosomes are stained red and spindles are stained green. The figure is adapted from reference 85, and is used with permission of the publisher and authors. See Chapter 11

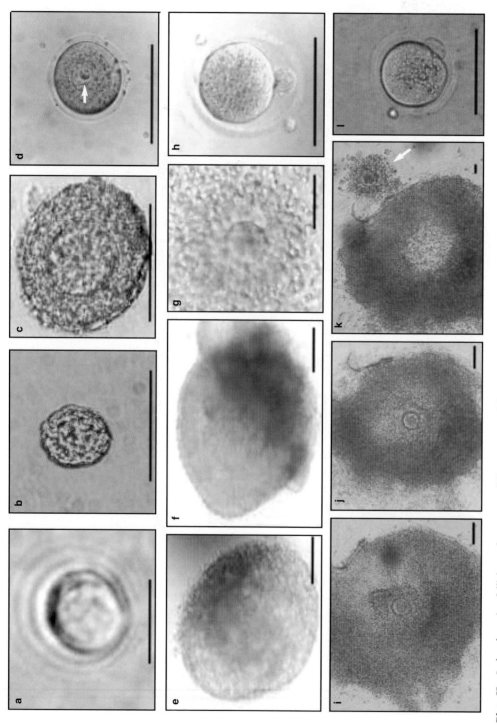

Color Plate II Isolated murine follicles and oocytes at different stages of development *in vivo* and after growth *in vitro* in an attachment culture system. Images (a)–(d) and (e)–(h) are of *in vivo*-grown follicles and oocytes: (a) primordial follicle; (b) primary follicle with 1–2 layers of granulosa cells; (c) secondary follicle with 2–3 layers of granulosa cells and one layer of theca cells; (d) immature oocyte from a secondary follicle – the germinal vesicle is visible (arrow); (e) antral follicle; (f) prevoulatory follicle; (g) *in vivo*-grown cumulus–oocyte complex; (h) denuded metaphase II oocyte grown and matured *in vivo*. Images (i)–(l) are of *in vitro*-grown follicles and oocytes derived from an attachment culture system[25]; (i) *in vitro*-grown two-dimensional follicle with antral-like cavity; (j) *in vitro*-grown two-dimensional prevoulatory follicle with antral-like cavity; (k) *in vitro*-grown follicle after ovulation of the cumulus–oocyte complex (arrow); (l) denuded metaphase II oocyte derived from a preantral follicle grown to maturity *in vitro*. Scale bars = 100 μm, except in (a) where bar = 20 μm. See Chapter 14

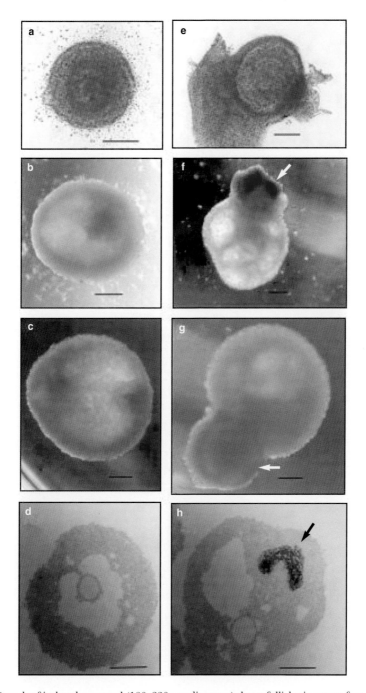

Color Plate III   Growth of isolated preantral (180–220 μm diameter) sheep follicles in serum-free culture media over 30 days *in vitro*. Theca-free follicles harvested by enzyme digestion (a) develop antral cavities *in vitro* (b and c) and show no evidence of the presence of the basement membrane at the end of culture – indicated by lack of blue staining for the presence of collagen (d). In contrast, theca-enclosed follicles collected by mechanical isolation (e) show evidence of antral cavity formation by outgrowth from the dense theca and stromal cells (arrow) (f and g) that remain concentrated within one area as indicated positive staining for collagen (blue color) (h) after extended culture. Scale bars = 50 μm. Reproduced from reference 19 with permission. See Chapter 14

Female reproductive aging: concepts and consequences

1

J.-P. de Bruin and E. R. te Velde

INTRODUCTION

At the end of the twentieth century, postponement of childbearing was one of the most striking demographic trends in Western countries. For example, the age at which women became pregnant with their first child in The Netherlands increased from 24.4 years in 1970 to 29.2 years in 2001[1]. This demographic trend reflects growing female emancipation since the early 1970s, which was the consequence of societal changes such as increasing levels of education and labor force participation, and also increased secularization, changing sexual attitudes and, above all, the introduction of oral contraceptives, which uncoupled sexuality and reproduction. For the first time, women were able to choose when to have children. As shown in Figure 1, at first women used this new freedom to have fewer children, particularly later in life. Only in the last two decades of the twentieth century did many women choose to postpone childbearing until well after completing their education or after having started a working career.

Unfortunately, sometimes women have had to pay a price for advances in social emancipation. Female fertility declines with age, and by the time the decision to start a family is made, many are facing problems of subfertility or even infertility. Consequently, an increasing number of women are seeking medical help because of involuntary childlessness[2,3]. Although the biological mechanisms of age-related fertility decline have been only partly elucidated, we know that reproductive aging is a highly variable biological

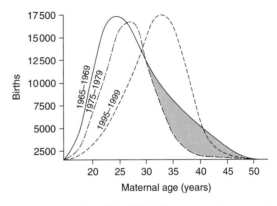

Figure 1 Relationship of birth frequency and maternal age for three time periods in The Netherlands. Curves based on data from reference 1. The gray area depicts the large proportion of women who decided not to have children later in life once oral contraceptives became available

phenomenon: the effects of aging on fertility can occur much earlier in some women than in others.

In this chapter, an overview of the age-related decline in fertility in women is presented. The following subjects are discussed:

(1) Biological concepts of female reproductive aging;

(2) Development and decline of the ovarian follicle pool;

(3) Factors that influence the rate of female reproductive aging;

(4) Endocrine changes in women with advancing reproductive age.

BIOLOGICAL CONCEPTS OF FEMALE REPRODUCTIVE AGING

Age-related decline of fertility

The age-related decline of fertility in women is a phenomenon that has been established beyond any doubt in both contemporary populations[4] and historic natural fertility populations (i.e. populations that did not have access to or were denied contraceptive measures because of religious reasons). These studies showed that a similar pattern of age-related fertility decline exists worldwide, which starts from the age of 25 and accelerates after the age of 30 years (Figure 2)[5,6]. The results of *in vitro* fertilization (IVF) treatments also reflect the effect of female reproductive aging: increasing age is significantly associated with reduced implantation, pregnancy and live-birth rates[7,8]. In natural fertility populations, the mean age at last childbirth is 41 years. This age is considered to be a proxy for the end of the effective fertile period, i.e. the period in life during which a woman is able to achieve a pregnancy that leads to a live birth. At this time the majority of women still have a regular menstrual pattern. Cycles become irregular only at a mean age of 45 years[5,9]. The menopause, the cessation of menstrual bleeding in a woman's life, occurs at a mean age of 51 years.

The ovarian concept

The prevailing concept of age-related fertility decline assumes that not only the cessation of menses but also the preceding reproductive events (onset of declining fertility, end of fertility, transition from regular to irregular cycles) are dictated by the decline in the quantity and quality of the ovarian follicle/oocyte pool. After a period of optimal fertility from age ≈18 to 30 years oocyte quality decreases, concomitant with the loss of follicle numbers. The rate of follicle loss has been studied extensively by Block[10,11], Gougeon and Chainy[12] and Richardson and colleagues[13]. Their work was mathematically modeled to a single curve by Faddy and co-workers, showing

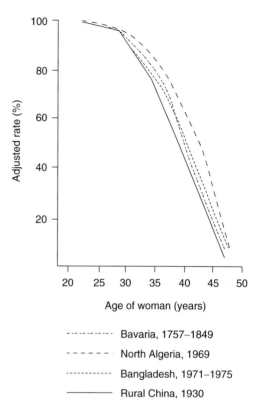

------- Bavaria, 1757–1849

- - - - - North Algeria, 1969

.... Bangladesh, 1971–1975

——— Rural China, 1930

Figure 2 Adjusted age-specific fertility rates for natural fertility populations (the adjusted rate is the rate at each age relative to the rate for the 20–24 year age group, which is taken as 100%). Reproduced with permission from reference 5

an exponential decline of follicles with age[14,15]. Faddy's curve, together with an estimation of declining oocyte quality and the timing of reproductive events, is shown in Figure 3, demonstrating the ovarian concept. Both the quantitative and qualitative decline of the ovarian follicle/oocyte pool are reviewed later in more detail.

Not the decline of the monthly probability of conception, but an increasing risk of early pregnancy loss appears to be the predominant etiologic factor in age-related fertility decline[17]. The risk of a clinically recognizable miscarriage is 10% at age 25 and 50% at age 45[18]. However, most pregnancies disappear much earlier; so early, that they remain unnoticed. Data from a natural fertility population, in which sensitive urinary pregnancy tests were used weekly from 7 days after ovulation

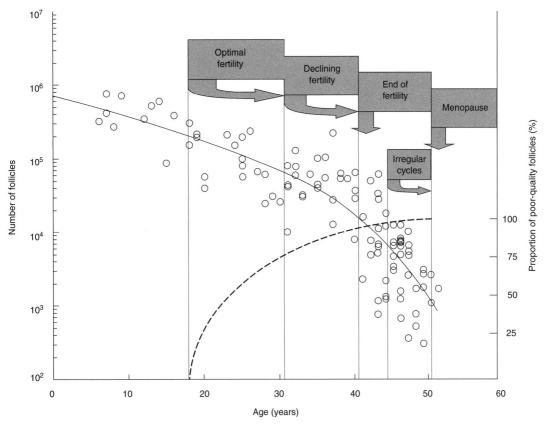

Figure 3 The quantitative and qualitative decline of the ovarian follicle/oocyte pool, which probably dictate the timing of the timing of reproductive events: onset of declining fertility, end of fertility, transition from regular to irregular cycles and the menopause. Aging is associated with a logarithmic decline in follicle numbers. The proportion of poor-quality oocytes can hardly be estimated, but probably increases rapidly and will be high in the fifth decade when most women become infertile because of age. Reproduced and adapted with permission from references 1 and 15. Data on oocyte quality derived from references 16 and 23

onwards, suggest that the monthly probability of pregnancy loss increases from 0.55 at age 20 years to 0.96 at 40 years[19]. In this and another study[20], the increasing proportion of lost pregnancies was closely paralleled by an increasing proportion of abnormal conceptuses (Figure 4). Apparently, the risk of carrying an aneuploid embryo is the predominant cause of early pregnancy loss, leading to fertility decline with aging. This assumption is confirmed by IVF studies[18,21,22]. Furthermore, oocytes from natural cycles show changes with age. After the age of 35 years, 50% of oocytes and, after the age of 40 years, 80% of oocytes

show aberrations in spindle formation and chromosome alignment at the first meiotic division, which may cause malsegregation of chromosomes and aneuploidy[16,23]. Thus, all of these observations taken together indicate that the declining quality of oocytes with age is a major factor in age-related fertility decline.

Endometrial and neuroendocrine concepts

Since some ovulated oocytes and embryos still are normal at higher ages, the aging endometrium might also play a role in age-related

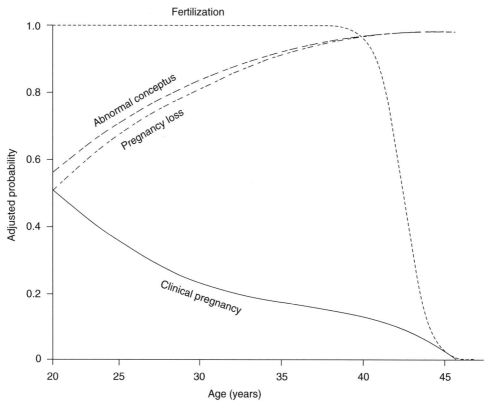

Figure 4 Probability of achieving fertilization, carrying an abnormal conceptus, experiencing pregnancy loss and achieving a clinical pregnancy in Bangladeshi women. Probabilities are adjusted to a maximum probability of fertilization of 1.0 at age 20 years. Reproduced and adapted with permission from reference 19

fertility decline. In earlier days, evidence from laboratory animals supported this line of thought: old animals receiving embryos transferred from young donor animals still had poor reproductive performance[24]. More recent and convincing evidence shows that humans behave entirely differently in this respect. Reproductive-aged patients receiving oocytes from young donors (< 35 years) show high rates of implantation and pregnancy and a reduction in the rate of miscarriage[25,26]. However, it has been suggested that the success of oocyte donation may also be attributed to the supraphysiological doses of progesterone prescribed to recipients[27]. Still, in humans the role of the endometrium in reproductive aging seems to be of minor significance.

An additional role for the hypothalamus, in which aging can lead to a dysregulation of the gonadotropin releasing hormone (GnRH) pulse generator, cannot be ruled out in humans[28]. For example, declining size of the ovarian follicle pool cannot explain why climacteric complaints may appear in women who still have regular cycles and normal estrogen levels[29]. Also, patterns of luteinizing hormone (LH) have been shown to change with age, reflecting alterations in the pulsatile release of GnRH[30]. Furthermore, the monotropic rise of follicle stimulating hormone (FSH) can be explained only partly by changes in ovarian feedback by inhibin and estradiol[31]. Aging of the hypothalamus will therefore probably contribute to the timing of the transition to irregular cycles when the precisely orchestrated hypothalamic–pituitary–gonadal axis falls out of tune. The timing of menopause in turn may be the result of the final disruption of the axis by the exhaustion of follicles and complete loss of ovarian feedback. However, most of the signs indicating hypothalamic aging occur well after initiation of the age-related decline of fertility.

Regarding the close temporal relationship between changes in the ovarian follicle pool and age-related fertility decline, the dominant pacemaker in reproductive aging must be the ovary. So, the rate of reproductive aging and the end of reproduction probably depend on the size of the follicle pool at birth and the rate of atresia, leading to the quantitative and qualitative decline of the follicle/oocyte pool thereafter.

DEVELOPMENT AND DECLINE OF THE OVARIAN FOLLICLE POOL

Development of the ovarian follicle pool before birth

The ovarian follicle pool develops during fetal life. At 6–8 weeks of gestation the gonadal ridge, which will differentiate into the ovary, is formed. Primordial germ cells migrate from the mesentery of the hindgut by amoeboid movement and arrive at the gonadal ridge at 8–10 weeks of gestation. Thereafter they start to multiply rapidly by mitosis and are called oogonia[32]. Meanwhile, pregranulosa cells, which probably derive from the mesonephros, invade the ovary through the rete ovarii. This process starts at 16 weeks of gestation. The pregranulosa cells and a delicate basal lamina surround the germ cells, forming primordial follicles, starting at 16–18 weeks of gestation. Follicle formation appears to start in the inner part of the ovary near the rete ovarii, where the pregranulosa cells invade the ovary. As the germ cells become surrounded by pregranulosa cells, they enter the first meiotic division and arrest at diplotene. At this stage they are referred to as primary oocytes. Already in fetal life a proportion of primordial follicles develop into more advanced follicle stages[32].

The numbers and distribution of follicle stages from the start of folliculogenesis until birth have been poorly investigated in humans. It is generally accepted that the number of oogonia is depleted rapidly after 20 weeks of gestation, when the peak number of about 7 million germ cells has been reached[33]. Many have mistakenly concluded that the same is true for total follicle numbers. However, strong suggestions towards rising follicle numbers in the second half of gestation are present implicitly in early reports[11,33]. Follicles form the cradles in which oocytes safely rest and grow. When oocytes are enclosed by a follicular layer, atresia strikes only a small fraction of the total number. Follicle formation takes place rapidly from 22 weeks of gestation, and by 24 weeks, only 1–2% of oocytes lack granulosa cells[34]. Recent studies have shown a large increase in the total primordial and primary follicle population from 18 to 42 weeks of gestation[35,36]. The decline of follicle numbers probably starts around the time of birth, although this conclusion is based on a limited number of cases, especially for the period from birth to puberty[10,33].

Apparently, the largest wastage of germ cells occurs in the developmental stages preceding folliculogenesis. Indeed, high atretic activity is described in oogonia during mitotic division, and also occurs at the early stages of prophase of meiosis I, especially pachytene[33,34]. The role of this wastage is not clear, but it may be a selection process to yield a population of healthy germ cells, maximizing the chance of healthy offspring (see Chapter 4).

Studies on the distribution of follicle developmental stages in fetuses are scant, but they indicate clear shifts in these stages (for definitions of follicle stages, see Figure 5). Kurilo showed a decrease in primordial follicles from 90% of the total at 20 weeks to 30% at 40 weeks. Concomitantly, primary follicles increased from 8% to 70% of all follicles, and less than 1% of follicles at 40 weeks were at more advanced stages[34]. In a recent study, a significant decline of primordial follicles was found with gestational age, while the

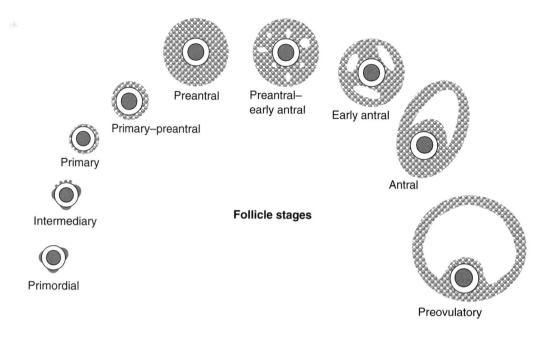

Figure 5 Schematic representation of developmental stages of ovarian follicles. Primordial: primary oocyte surrounded by flattened granulosa cells; intermediary: flattened and cuboidal granulosa cells; primary: monolayer of cuboidal granulosa cells; preantral: oocyte larger, surrounded by zona pellucida, two to seven layers of granulosa cells and theca cells; early antral: similar to preantral, but with fluid-filled spaces in granulosa layer; antral follicle: oocyte ceased growth, crescent-shaped antrum and vascularized theca; preovulatory: large fluid-filled antrum and differentiation into mural and cumulus granulosa cells

proportion of primary follicles increased. The majority of follicles were at the intermediary stage throughout gestation[36]. Therefore, in contrast to common belief, it can be concluded that at the end of gestation most follicles have already developed beyond the primordial stage.

The resting ovarian follicle pool

Why and when follicles leave the resting pool is still enigmatic. This probably explains the difficulty of making a clear distinction between non-growing/resting follicles and growing follicles. For a long time, the prevailing hypothesis has been that primordial follicles make up the resting follicle pool, and any further stages are irreversibly committed to further growth and development until atresia occurs, except for the few that eventually will ovulate. However, Gougeon and Chainy[12] cast doubt on this long-held hypothesis. Based on morphometric studies of oocytes, oocyte nuclei and follicles and granulosa cell numbers at different developmental stages, they concluded that follicles up to and including the primary stage are resting follicles. Only at the transition of the primary to the secondary stage was a clear increase in the size of the oocyte and its nucleus observed, with a rapid increase in granulosa cell numbers, marking the initiation of actual follicle growth. The transition of the primordial stage to the intermediary and subsequently primary stage is hypothesized to be a maturational process that can last up to decades[12]. The following observations support this line of reasoning:

(1) By the end of gestation, both the bovine and human fetal follicle pool consists predominantly of intermediary and primary follicles[34,36–38];

(2) In adult humans and sub-human primates, mitotic activity of granulosa cells, revealed by expression of proliferating cell nuclear antigen, is seen in only a very small proportion of primordial and intermediary follicles, but in over 50% of primary follicles[39];

(3) The earliest developmental stage at which FSH receptors appear is the primary stage[40].

Considering this last observation, although initiation of follicle growth independent of gonadotropins is possible, there is mounting evidence that FSH may facilitate the initiation of follicle growth or stimulate early follicular development in a complex cooperation with other growth factors[41]. Recently, a number of such factors have been identified, e.g. stem cell factor, growth differentiation factor-9, transforming growth factor-β and KIT ligand, which all may play a part in the initiation of growth, possibly counterbalanced by inhibitory factors, such as bone morphogenetic protein-15 and anti-Müllerian hormone (AMH)[42–44]. Once we understand the mechanisms by which these different factors determine the fate of the follicle, we will probably be able to accurately determine which follicle stages are growing or non-growing, and possibly also be able to explain the variability between the rate of ovarian depletion in women or influence the rate at which follicles leave the resting pool.

Quantitative and qualitative decline of the ovarian follicle pool

As previously stated, follicle numbers decline after birth. This process of follicular decay is generally referred to as atresia. The first report of total follicle numbers in the ovaries of an 18-year-old woman by Henle was published in 1866[45]. It was not until 86 years later that Block presented data on total numbers of primordial and growing follicles in a group of 43 women aged 7 to 44 years[10]. He also quantified follicle numbers in ten neonates of gestational age 7–9 months[11]. Based on the combined data, Block constructed a diagram showing that the average number of primordial follicles declined from 730 000 at birth to zero at 44 years. Some 10 years later Baker published his findings from 46 fetuses, five neonates and 15 prepubertal girls[33]. Unfortunately, he did not mention follicle numbers, but presented total germ cell numbers in a subset. Total germ cells rose from 600 000 at 8 weeks of gestation to a maximum of 7 million at 20 weeks of gestation and declined to 2 million at birth. This decline continued after birth. However, his postnatal data were based on a very small number of cases. Further data on adult women were provided by Gougeon and Chainy[12]. They studied whole ovaries and large ovarian resections from 49 women aged 19–49 years. Their findings were in line with Block's model, with follicle numbers decreasing from 80 000 in the 19–30 year age group to 3000 in the group older than 46 years.

Richardson and associates investigated the size of the follicle pool in the perimenopause. They clearly showed that resting follicle numbers are ten times higher in women who still have regular cycles compared to those with irregular cycles, and that resting follicles are virtually absent in postmenopausal women, irrespective of age. This indicates that the exhaustion of the follicle pool causes the cessation of menses[13]. As mentioned on p. 2, the data on follicle numbers from the various authors were combined in a single curve by Faddy and co-workers (Figure 3).

During the past 10 years we have acquired some understanding of the qualitative decline of the follicle pool. Prevailing theories about the decline in quality are based on three hypotheses, which do not necessarily exclude each other. According to the first hypothesis, posed by Henderson and Edwards in 1968 and known as the production line hypothesis, follicle quality is determined at the time of folliculogenesis[46]. Oocytes of follicles that are formed first in gestation are of the best quality; oocytes of follicles that are formed last are poorest in quality. In this hypothesis quality decline is reflected by a reduction in the frequency of chiasmata, leading to recombination errors during meiosis and aneuploidy. During reproductive life resting follicles are recruited for growth, and ultimately ovulation, in the order in which they were produced. Accordingly, the best follicles are recruited early and the worst follicles last in reproductive life. This results in an increasing proportion of poor-quality oocytes with age, explaining the aging-related increasing incidence of miscarriage and offspring with chromosomal abnormalities. Cytological evidence for this hypothesis has been supplied in a rat model by Hirshfield[47].

The second hypothesis, for which the arguments were summarized by Gosden, explains the decline in quality with age by the accumulation of damage in the oocytes resting for decades in the ovary, suspended at diplotene[48,49]. Underlying mechanisms would be increasing oxidative stress, deteriorating follicular conditions because of changing hormone profiles, and prolonged exposure to toxic agents such as nicotine, medications and environmental pollutants[50,51].

The third hypothesis states that aging compromises the vascularization of the leading follicles[52]. Accordingly, follicles are exposed to a hypoxic milieu, affecting their developmental competence in a manner that leads to disturbed chromosomal segregation. Indeed, ultrasonographic Doppler studies show reduced perifollicular flow with aging and increases in the follicular fluid levels of angiogenic factors such as vascular endothelial growth factor[53,54]. Interesting in this respect is the recent finding that Factor V Leiden mutation, a clotting disorder that causes thrombophilia, is related to earlier menopause[55].

It is not clear whether resting follicles in young women enter the atretic process directly, or only after they have been recruited for follicle growth. From mathematical modeling on follicle dynamics, Faddy and Gosden concluded that until the age of 37 the loss of resting follicles is due to progression to further developmental stages and subsequent atresia, and not to direct atresia of resting follicles. After that age follicle decline increases and a significant proportion of resting follicles become atretic before further growth, explaining the exhaustion of the follicle pool at midlife[56]. In contrast, using similar modeling, Gougeon and colleagues concluded that the loss of resting follicles is mainly due to direct atresia. The acceleration of the decline in follicle numbers after the age of 37 could be largely explained by a greater proportion entering the growth phase[57]. However, this contrasting conclusion may result from another definition used for resting follicles[58].

Whether or not atresia occurs in resting follicles is not the only subject of debate. In addition, opinions differ about the nature of the atretic process itself, which can be either necrosis or apoptosis. Whereas the involvement of apoptosis in atresia of oogonia and growing follicles is firmly established[59-61], studies on apoptosis in resting follicles remain inconclusive. Apoptosis was demonstrated in primordial follicles of chicken and pig ovaries[59], whereas in sheep, in which resting follicles are known to undergo direct atresia, apoptosis in primordial follicles was never noted[62]. A study on human ovaries showed signs of apoptosis only beyond the primary stage[60].

In ultrastructure studies of human resting follicles, atresia was limited to a small proportion and carried morphological sequelae generally ascribed to necrosis and not apoptosis[63]. When these data were compared to similar data from women of advanced reproductive age, atresia in resting follicles did not increase with age. However, significant age-related changes in mitochondria and other cell organelles of oocytes and granulosa cells occurred, which may reflect accumulation of damage[64]. Changes in mitochondrial morphology with age have also been demonstrated in oocytes from antral follicles, and have been related to increases in oxidative stress[65]. It can be postulated that these qualitative changes in cell organelles reflect impaired metabolic and synthetic capacity of the oocyte. As long as the follicle is resting, the oocyte has a low metabolic rate and reduced metabolic capacity will have little consequence for follicle and oocyte survival. However, when follicle growth is initiated, metabolic activity increases, as reflected by a sharp increase in the number of mitochondria[66].

Meiotic competence (the ability to resume meiosis up to and including the second meiotic metaphase) is acquired during the later stages of follicle development[23]. This involves maturation of the cytoplasm along with associated synthesis of proteins, fatty acids and microtubular structures. If the organelles fail to answer this high demand, errors at meiosis, which is an energy-expensive process, might occur[67]. From mouse models, Eichenlaub-Ritter concluded that protein synthesis and mitochondrial function are compromised with increased age, with adverse effects on the kinetics of maturation and spindle formation that lead to an untimely segregation and malsegregation of chromosomes, in turn resulting in aneuploidy[68]. Similar segregation errors have been found to occur more frequently with increasing age in human oocytes[23].

Mitochondrial deterioration with age may play a central role in the decline of oocyte quality. MtDNA, which is inherited maternally, deteriorates by point and deletion mutations far more rapidly than nuclear DNA. Owing to their long lifespan, oocytes are suspended at diplotene of first meiosis for several decades, theoretically providing plenty of time for the mtDNA to deteriorate. This reveals a potential vulnerability of human reproduction to mitochondrial pathology. Indeed, mtDNA rearrangements can be found in 50% of oocytes[69]. However, data on the presence of age-related changes in mtDNA in ovarian tissues and oocytes are conflicting. A significant relation between mtDNA deletions and age was reported in women of reproductive age in one study[70]; a particularly rapid accumulation of deleted mtDNA in the postmenopause in another[71]. However, two more recent studies failed to detect a significant relationship between the proportion of oocytes carrying various mtDNA rearrangements and age[72,73]. Furthermore, women with mitochondrial diseases, carrying severe mtDNA mutations, generally can achieve pregnancies[74]. But, to our knowledge, no published data exist on the incidence of subfertility or premature ovarian failure in this group.

By which mechanisms is the transmission of healthy mitochondria promoted? First, only a few mitochondrial genome replicas are inherited by the embryo, this tight restriction event being referred to as 'the mitochondrial bottleneck'. One of the aspects of the bottleneck is that, during the reduction of the thousands of mitochondria residing in the ooplasm to a very small number (~10), most mutant mtDNA that accumulates in oocytes will probably have been eliminated, thus ensuring healthy transmission to the next generation. However, should any mtDNA that is passed on contain non-lethal mutations, for which the chances possibly increase with age, this will substantially increase the proportion of mitochondria with mutated mtDNA once replication is resumed after fertilization[75]. Second, follicle atresia may be another mechanism to eliminate oocytes with defective mitochondria. In fact, evidence is mounting that mitochondrial death or dysfunction is a central component of the pathways leading to apoptosis, the common process causing death in growing follicles[76]. This background is the rationale for attempts to improve embryo development and implantation rates by cytoplasmic transfer from young to aged oocytes[72]. However, more research is needed to verify this concept.

One further important question about the demise of the ovarian follicle pool remains.

Are the declines in quantity of follicles and quality of oocytes causally correlated, or are we dealing with two independent processes, each being responsible for different events in reproductive aging? In favor of the 'independent model' is the observation that follicle numbers at the age of 25 years are half those at the age of 20, yet fertility does not show an appreciable decrease in the same period[4,14]. Apparently, quality is maintained despite a dramatic fall in quantity. Further support comes from an IVF study in which young women with elevated FSH levels were compared with older women with normal FSH levels. According to what was expected, the young women with elevated FSH showed signs of diminished ovarian reserve, experiencing IVF-cycle cancelations more often than the older women, because of small numbers of growing follicles after ovarian hyperstimulation. However, these young women performed better than the older women in terms of implantation rate per embryo, which is likely to reflect better oocyte quality[77].

On the other hand, a causal relation between follicle quantity and oocyte quality emerges in animal models, in which inbred mice or rats were unilaterally ovariectomized. Follicle dynamics changed significantly after total follicle numbers were halved[47,78]. Moreover, increased numbers of chromosomally abnormal embryos were found when comparing hemi-ovariectomized mice to intact controls[79]. Also in humans, a link between a reduced quantity and changes in follicle dynamics and growth patterns seems likely. In older women, follicle recruitment seems to be advanced, already starting in the luteal phase of the preceding cycle[80]. This loss of the normal synchrony of endocrine and developmental events may lead to a less favorable environment for oocytes to develop. The resumption of meiosis, occurring in the later stages of the follicular phase, possibly has to take place at an increased pace, as has been shown in mouse models. In these circumstances, the oocyte may be more prone to aneuploidy because cell cycle checkpoints appear to have less integrity than in somatic cells or male meiotic cells[68]. More directly, it has been shown that women who give birth to a child with Down's syndrome or with the loss of an aneuploid fetus early in pregnancy show signs of a reduced ovarian follicle pool[81,82].

If the quality of oocytes and the remaining number of follicles are indeed causally associated, what mechanism could be responsible? Obviously, deteriorating oocyte quality can eventually lead to follicle atresia and elimination. Conversely, quantitative decline may drive a decline in quality. As the follicle pool becomes smaller, ovarian feedback to the pituitary changes and the ability to sustain normal endocrine functions may be gradually lost. Maturational problems may be aggravated further when the paracrine milieu is disturbed by the loss of neighboring cells, as follicle density declines. Finally, the so-called 'limited oocyte model' has been suggested by Warburton and associates as a mechanism explaining quality decline with age[20]. They argue that it becomes less likely that a follicle will appear at the most optimal time in the FSH window (the intercycle rise of FSH by which small antral follicles are recruited for further growth and development) as the number of recruitable follicles becomes limited. Consequently, upregulation of the number of FSH receptors on the follicle may be suboptimal, hampering the ability to develop into a Graafian follicle of optimal quality.

On the basis of both the available literature and biological plausibility, it is most likely that oocyte quality and follicle quantity decline go hand in hand. Explanations for their relationship are still hypothetical. Quality decline probably determines a woman's fertility, since the median age of last childbirth (at 41 years) coincides with a proportion of over 80% of chromosomally abberrant ovulated oocytes[16]. On the other hand, the decline in numbers of follicles below a critical threshold is responsible for the onset of cycle irregularity and of the menopause (Figure 6)[13].

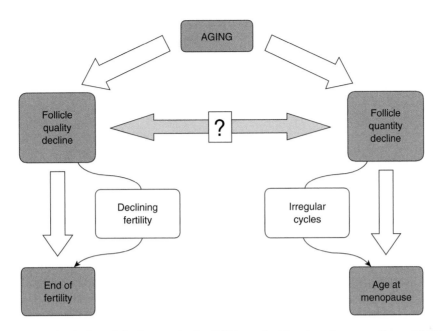

Figure 6 Model of the decline of the human ovarian follicle pool with aging. Oocyte quality and follicle quantity decline are probably causally related, although the interacting mechanisms have not yet been fully ascertained

FACTORS THAT INFLUENCE THE RATE OF FEMALE REPRODUCTIVE AGING

Menopause, the final reproductive event, marks the exhaustion of the resting follicle pool (Figure 3). Age at menopause shows a remarkably large variation, with a 95% confidence interval of 45–54 around a median age of 51 years[9]. If we assume that reproductive aging is determined by the decline of quantity and quality of the follicle/oocyte pool, it is plausible that the preceding reproductive events show similar age variations as age at menopause. Accordingly, earlier menopause is associated with earlier onset of subfertility, sterility and transition to cycle irregularity. This temporal relationship between the various reproductive events is shown in Figure 7. Curve D shows the cumulative distribution of age at menopause and is based on data by Treloar[9]. Curve C depicts the cumulative distribution of age at the transition to cycle irregularity. It has been confirmed that the difference between the age at onset of cycle irregularity and age at menopause appears to be 6–7 years irrespective of whether menopause comes early or late[83]. Curve B demonstrates the cumulative distribution of age at the onset of sterility in a natural nineteenth century population, which appeared to be almost the same as that of menopausal age, but 10 years earlier[84]. Curve A is hypothetical, but it is plausible that the start of the fertility decline also depends on the size and quality of the follicle/oocyte pool. Thus, women differ significantly with respect to the age at which they experience the effects of age-related fertility decline. The age at menopause is the only clear and unambiguous event, and is therefore a biomarker of reproductive aging. Accordingly, it is not the chronological age of a woman *per se*, but the period of time elapsing before menopause ensues, that would define her reproductive age.

If this concept holds, it is reasonable to assume that the factors determining the timing of menopause also determine the rate of fertility decline and the timing of the preceding reproductive events. These factors may

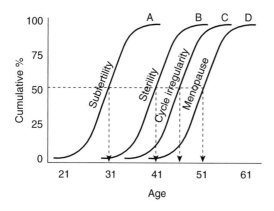

Figure 7 The age variations of the main reproductive events in women probably show parallel distributions. Reproduced with permission from reference 1

exert their influence on the development of the follicle pool during fetal life, or affect follicle decline by atresia postnatally. Identification of such factors could help to identify women at risk of early reproductive failure.

Factors influencing follicle pool development

After birth, folliculogenesis is believed to cease irreversibly, and the pool of follicles laid down during fetal life forms the lifetime reserve. Accordingly, a small follicle pool will lead to early exhaustion of the follicle pool and early reproductive failure. The variation in the size of the follicle pool is partly the result of stochastic processes[85], as is illustrated by the variation noted within inbred laboratory animal strains[86]. In addition, environmental factors, such as toxins present in tobacco smoke and urban atmosphere, might influence follicle numbers or oocyte quality[85]. For example, prenatal exposure to smoking has been shown to correlate with reduced fecundity[87].

Another possible factor disturbing folliculogenesis is the effect of a restriction of oxygen and nutrients in the case of fetuses with intrauterine growth restriction (IUGR). According to the 'fetal origins hypothesis of adult diseases', disturbed fetal organogenesis in IUGR is due to nutritional deprivation[88]. Several studies have embarked upon linking

postnatal parameters for fertility with fetal growth, to evaluate whether the ovaries can also be affected by IUGR, but the results remain inconclusive. An association between early menopause and shortness at birth was reported[89]. In contrast, in a recent study no association between low birth weight and earlier menopause was found[90]. More directly, a histological study on fetal ovarian development failed to show significant differences between the ovaries of normal and growth-restricted human fetuses[36]. In conclusion, IUGR does not appear to significantly influence fetal ovarian development in humans. However, data from the 1944 Dutch famine indicate that severe malnutrition, experienced in early childhood, can advance age at menopause by almost 2 years[91].

Factors influencing follicle decline

After birth, there are obvious factors that can lead to a reduction of follicle numbers, such as surgical removal of ovarian tissue or loss of follicles due to radio- or chemotherapy for malignancies. Oxidative stress, to which tissues become increasingly vulnerable with age, might also variably affect the follicle pool[85]. Whether high levels of FSH (induced by hypothalamic aging[28]) are primarily responsible for accelerated follicle decline, or are secondary to follicle decline, is still subject to debate[41,57]. Various factors related to lifestyle, environment and fecundity have been shown to have a significant influence on the age at natural menopause. For example, parity is positively correlated and smoking is negatively correlated with age at natural menopause[92]. A recent study even provides direct evidence for an association between current or past smoking and follicle density in the ovary[93]. Higher socioeconomic class is also correlated with a later menopause in various studies, implying the effects of other lifestyle factors that not yet have been identified[92,94]. However, all these factors can explain only less than 5% of the total variation in menopausal age[92].

Cramer and colleagues reported an association between the menopausal ages of mothers and daughters, and suggested a role for genetic factors in controlling age at menopause[95]. Data from British and Australian twin registries have confirmed this suggestion, with heritability estimates for age at natural menopause of between 31% and 63%[96,97]. Also, in a random population sample of full sisters and twin sisters, a high estimate (85%) for the heritability of age at natural menopause was noted[98]. Therefore, it seems that the age at natural menopause, and consequently the rate of decline of the ovarian follicle pool, is largely under genetic control.

An exciting future perspective is to identify the genes responsible for age at menopause. Since menopause is a continuously varying trait, it can be assumed that it is a so-called complex genetic trait, with several to many genes, and polymorphism of these genes, contributing independently to the variation. Genetic research should be aimed at determining the number and genetic variation of the genes involved by gene mapping, followed by DNA sequence analysis of candidate genes to identify the specific variation responsible for modulating the age of menopause[99]. Some candidate genes are likely to be located on the X chromosome, given the propensity of this chromosome to exhibit long-arm deletions in some cases of premature ovarian failure. However, it should be noted that the etiology of premature ovarian failure is different from the normal variation of menopause: in familial situations it invariably exhibits Mendelian (single gene) segregation and not the polygenic segregation exhibited by age of normal menopause. Nevertheless, the same genes that cause premature ovarian failure may also be involved in normal menopause[84]. In general, it might be assumed that genes involved in ovarian apoptosis or ovarian metabolic maintenance pathways will be involved in determining the rate of decline of the follicular pool and the age at which menopause commences. In fact, recent genetic data from sister pairs discordant and concordant for age at menopause showed suggestive linkage located on chromosome 9, region 9q21.3. One of the genes in this region

encodes for the BCL2 family, which is involved in apoptosis[100].

Once the genes and the variation that determine either early or late onset of menopause are identified, we should be able not only to predict the age at which menopause occurs but also determine the risk of early reproductive failure in individuals from their genetic profile. These women could be candidates for fertility preservation.

ENDOCRINE CHANGES IN WOMEN WITH ADVANCING REPRODUCTIVE AGE

The best-known endocrine change with aging in women is the monotropic rise of FSH[101]. Generally, FSH rises from age 35–40 years onwards and continues to increase up to the high levels found in postmenopausal women. Single serum FSH measurements on day 2–4 of the menstrual cycle ('basal FSH') are widely used as a clinical diagnostic test for assessment of the ovarian reserve or the prediction of ovarian response in IVF. However, a large variation in FSH levels with aging exists, and the levels in aged women overlap levels at younger ages[80,102]. Moreover, considerable cycle-to-cycle variation is present[103]. Only very high FSH levels unambiguously indicate a largely exhausted ovarian reserve. Accordingly, the results from a recent meta-analysis showed that basal FSH measurements are of limited value as a prognostic test for poor ovarian response or non-pregnancy in IVF. Only at a high cutoff level for FSH is there clinical value for a few patients only[104].

Rising levels of LH also occur with age, but are less pronounced and occur considerably later than the rise in FSH[105]. Studies of estradiol and progesterone levels with age have produced conflicting results. Overall, it appears that the concentrations of these hormones do not change appreciably until cycle regularity is lost[101,106,107].

Inhibin is a glycoprotein heterodimer that inhibits FSH synthesis and secretion. Inhibin A (composed of inhibin α and β_A subunits) is secreted by granulosa cells from the dominant follicle and corpus luteum. Inhibin B (composed of inhibin α and β$_B$ subunits) is produced by the granulosa cells of smaller antral follicles. Activin counteracts the effect of inhibin on FSH, and both share follistatin as a potent binding protein that inhibits their bioavailability[108]. The inverse correlation between inhibin B and FSH with age probably reflects the dwindling size and function of the antral follicle cohort and partly explains the concurrent fall in negative feedback to the pituitary[109,110]. Inhibin B is a more direct marker of ovarian reserve than FSH, although not necessarily a better predictive test than basal FSH. In fact, all the aforementioned basal endocrine markers for ovarian reserve in normal women and infertility patients are surpassed in prognostic power by the antral follicle count as determined by transvaginal ultrasonography[111,112].

Recently, AMH has gained a lot of interest. AMH is a dimeric glycoprotein and a member of the transforming growth factor-β superfamily. It is produced by granulosa cells of primary to preantral follicles from late in pregnancy until the menopause, and binds to the AMH type II receptor in the ovary. Studies on female AMH knockout (AMHKO) mice revealed an increased rate of loss of the resting follicle pool with age and an increased number of growing follicles compared with controls. The reproductive lifespan was correspondingly reduced in AMKO females, but not in males[44]. Thus, AMH is an inhibitory factor for the initiation of follicle growth and the early stages of follicle development. Furthermore, it reduces FSH-induced granulosa cell proliferation, which may affect the cyclic recruitment of early antral follicles.

In women, serum AMH levels were found to change significantly with age. In two longitudinal studies in healthy volunteers, assessed after a mean interval of 2.6 and 3.9 years respectively, a highly significant decrease in levels was found. This decrease also had a strong correlation with age at an individual level. Changes occurred at an earlier age in AMH than in other hormonal markers[113,114]. In IVF patients, serum AMH concentrations were highly correlated with the number of retrieved oocytes. Low concentrations were predictive of poor response to ovarian hyperstimulation[115].

Endocrine markers, except AMH, mainly reflect the function of the granulosa cell compartment of the antral follicle cohort only, as they are either produced by this cohort (inhibin B and estradiol) or under the influence of this cohort by means of its negative feedback on the pituitary (FSH). Most of these markers show relatively limited changes with aging, as long as menstrual cycles are regular. Granulosa cell function, therefore, seems rather robust and the ability of follicles to develop to ovulation remains intact well after the time when women have become infertile[80]. Therefore, assessing reproductive aging using these markers has only limited value. AMH levels, which mirror the function of small growing follicles, are more promising for detecting the early stages of ovarian aging, but their clinical usefulness still has to be proven.

CONCLUDING REMARKS AND FUTURE PERSPECTIVES

In this era of female emancipation and delayed childbearing to ages at which women are less fertile, reproductive aging is an important issue with consequences for medical practice. At present, many women and their family doctors still believe that as long as regular menstrual cycles are present, there is nothing to worry about. Moreover, many believe that assisted reproductive techniques are a good solution for age-related infertility[116]. We should make them aware that these assumptions are incorrect. Women should be informed at a young age that the optimal time to achieve pregnancy is before age 35, preferably before the age of 30 years. Furthermore, women should know of the harmful effects of tobacco on their follicle/oocyte pool[93]. A healthy lifestyle is helpful for preserving fertility potential, as is also indicated by later menopausal ages observed in higher socioeconomic classes[92,94].

In addition, gynecologists should be aware of the delicacy of the ovarian reserve. For example, even a laparoscopic cyst extirpation may affect the follicle pool[117]. Accordingly, translucent (serous) ovarian cysts, which are detected frequently with ultrasound in pre-menopausal women and rarely prove to be malignant (< 1%)[118], should be managed conservatively as a rule. If surgery becomes necessary, the gynecologist should treat the ovary with respect and try to preserve as much healthy tissue as possible. Moreover, whenever possible, oncologists should aim to shield the ovaries from the devastating effects of chemo- or radiotherapy, either by moving the ovary away from the radiation field (oophoropexy) or by considering the banking of ovarian tissue (see Chapters 12 and 13).

A major practical challenge in reproductive biology will be to preserve female fertility by optimizing these ovarian banking strategies and, ultimately, to develop treatments that reversibly arrest follicles from leaving the resting follicle pool. For this latter purpose we need to unravel further the complex interactions of growth factors and hormonal stimuli that control the initiation of early follicle growth.

References

1. Central Bureau of Statistics, the Netherlands. http://statline.cbs.nl/statweb/
2. te Velde ER, Dorland M, Broekmans FJ. Age at menopause as a marker for reproductive ageing. Maturitas 1998;30:119–25
3. Stephen EH. Postponement of childbearing and its effect on the prevalence of subfecundity. In te Velde ER, Pearson PL, Broekmans FJ, eds. Female Reproductive Aging. Carnforth, UK: Parthenon Publishing Group, 2000:59–70
4. van Noord-Zaadstra BM, Looman CWN, Alsbach H, et al. Delaying childbearing: effect of age on fecundity and outcome of pregnancy. Br Med J 1991;302:1361–5
5. Wood JW. Fecundity and natural fertility in humans. Oxford Rev Reprod Biol 1989;11: 61–109
6. Menken J, Trussell J, Larsen U. Age and infertility. Science 1986;233:1389–93
7. Templeton A, Morris JK, Parslow W. Factors that affect outcome of in vitro fertilisation treatment. Lancet 1996;348:1402–6
8. Chuang CC, Chen CD, Chao KH, et al. Age is a better predictor of pregnancy potential than basal follicle-stimulating hormone levels in women undergoing in vitro fertilization. Fertil Steril 2003;79:63–8
9. Treloar AE. Menstrual cyclicity and the pre-menopause. Maturitas 1981;3:49–64
10. Block E. Quantitative morphological investigations of the follicular system in women; variations at different ages. Acta Anat 1952;14: 108–23
11. Block E. A quantitative morphological investigation of the follicular system in newborn female infants. Acta Anat 1953;17:201–6
12. Gougeon A, Chainy GBN. Morphometric studies of small follicles in ovaries of women at different ages. J Reprod Fertil 1987;81:433–42
13. Richardson SJ, Senikas V, Nelson JF. Follicular depletion during the menopausal transition: evidence for accelerated loss and ultimate exhaustion. J Clin Endocrinol Metab 1987;65: 1231–7
14. Faddy MJ, Gosden RG, Gougeon A, et al. Accelerated disappearance of ovarian follicles in mid-life: implications for forecasting menopause. Hum Reprod 1992;7:1342–6
15. Faddy MJ. Follicle dynamics during ovarian ageing. Mol Cell Endocrinol 2000;163:43–8
16. Battaglia DE, Goodin P, Klein NA, et al. Influence of maternal age on meiotic spindle assembly. Hum Reprod 1996;11:2217–22
17. O'Connor KA, Holman DJ, Wood JW. Declining fecundity and ovarian ageing in natural fertility populations. Maturitas 1998;30:127–36
18. Sauer MV. The impact of age on reproductive potential: lessons learned from oocyte donation. Maturitas 1998;30:221–5
19. Holman DJ, Wood JW, Campbell KL. Age-dependent decline of fecundity is caused by early fetal loss. In te Velde ER, Pearson PL, Broekmans FJ, eds. Female Reproductive Aging. New York: Parthenon Publishing Group, 2000:123–36
20. Warburton D, Kline J, Stein Z, et al. Cytogenetic abnormalities in spontaneous abortions of recognised conceptions. In Porter JH, Wiley A, eds. Perinatal Genetics: Diagnosis and Treatment. New York: Academic Press, 1986:133–40

21. Hassold T, Chiu D. Maternal age-specific rates of numerical chromosome abnormalities with special reference to trisomy. *Hum Genet* 1985; 70:11–17

22. Munne S, Grifo JA, Cohen J, *et al*. Chromosome abnormalities in human arrested embryos: a multiple-probe FISH study. *Am J Hum Genet* 1994;55:150–9

23. Volarcik K, Sheean L, Goldfarb J, *et al*. The meiotic competence of *in vitro* matured oocytes is influenced by donor age: evidence that folliculogenesis is compromised in the reproductively aged ovary. *Hum Reprod* 1998; 13:154–60

24. Harman SM, Talbert GB. The effect of maternal age on ovulation, corpora lutea of pregnancy and implantation failure in mice. *J Reprod Fertil* 1970;23:33–9

25. Sauer MV, Paulson RJ, Ary BA, *et al*. Three hundred cycles of oocyte donation at the University of Southern California: assessing the effect of age and diagnosis on pregnancy and implantation rates. *J Assist Reprod Genet* 1994;11:92–6

26. Navot D, Bergh PA, Williams MA, *et al*. Poor oocyte quality rather than implantation failure as a cause of age-related decline in female fertility. *Lancet* 1991;337:1375–7

27. Meldrum DR. Female reproductive aging – ovarian and uterine factors. *Fertil Steril* 1993; 59:1–5

28. Wise PM. Neuroendocrine modulation of the 'menopause': insights into the aging brain. *Am J Physiol* 1999;277:965–70

29. Oldenhave A, Jaszmann LJ, Haspels AA, *et al*. Impact of climacteric on well-being. A survey based on 5213 women 39 to 60 years old. *Am J Obstet Gynecol* 1993;168:772–80

30. Matt DW, Kauma SW, Pincus SM, *et al*. Characteristics of luteinizing hormone secretion in younger versus older premenopausal women. *Am J Obstet Gynecol* 1998;178:504–10

31. Scheffer GJ. *Assessment of reproductive aging in normal women*. Thesis, Utrecht University, 2000

32. Byskov AG. Differentiation of mammalian embryonic gonad. *Physiol Rev* 1986;66:71–117

33. Baker TG. A quantitative and cytological study of germ cells in human ovaries. *Proc R Soc Lond B Biol Sci* 1963;158:417–33

34. Kurilo LF. Oogenesis in antenatal development in man. *Hum Genet* 1981;57:86–92

35. Sforza C, Ferrario VF, De Pol A, *et al*. Morphometric study of the human ovary during compartmentalization. *Anat Rec* 1993; 236:626–34

36. De Bruin JP, Nikkels PGJ, Bruinse HW, *et al*. Morphometry of human ovaries in normal and growth restricted fetuses. *Early Hum Dev* 2001;60:179–92

37. Lintern-Moore S, Peters H, Moore GP, Faber M. Follicular development in the infant human ovary. *J Reprod Fertil* 1974;39:53–64

38. van Wezel I, Rodgers RJ. Morphological characterization of bovine primordial follicles in their environment *in vivo. Biol Reprod* 1996; 55:1003–11

39. Gougeon A, Busso D. Morphologic and functional determinants of primordial and primary follicles in the monkey ovary. *Mol Cell Endocrinol* 2000;163:33–41

40. Oktay K, Briggs D, Gosden RG. Ontogeny of follicle-stimulating hormone receptor gene expression in isolated human ovarian follicles. *J Clin Endocrinol Metab* 1997;82:3748–51

41. te Velde ER, Scheffer GJ, Dorland M, *et al*. Developmental and endocrine aspects of normal ovarian aging. *Mol Cell Endocrinol* 1998;145:67–73

42. Driancourt MA, Reynaud K, Cortvrindt R, *et al*. Roles of KIT and KIT LIGAND in ovarian function. *Rev Reprod* 2000;5:143–52

43. Findlay JK, Drummond AE, Dyson ML, *et al*. Recruitment and development of the follicle; the roles of the transforming growth factor-β superfamily. *Mol Cell Endocrinol* 2002;191: 35–43

44. Durlinger ALL, Visser JA, Themmen APN. Regulation of ovarian function: the role of anti-Müllerian hormone. *Reproduction* 2002; 124:601–9

45. Henle J. *Handbuch der systemicher Anatomie den Menschen*. Band 2: *Eingeweidelehre*. Braunschweig: 1866

46. Henderson SA, Edwards RG. Chiasma frequency and maternal age in mammals. *Nature* 1968;218:22–8

47. Hirshfield AN. Relationship between the supply of primordial follicles and the onset of follicular growth in rats. *Biol Reprod* 1994;50: 421–8

48. Gosden RG. Maternal age: a major factor affecting the prospects and outcome of pregnancy. *Ann N Y Acad Sci* 1985;442:45–57

49. Gosden RG. Oocyte development throughout life. In Grudzinskas JG, Yovich JL, eds. *Cambridge Reviews in Human Reproduction, Gametes – The Oocyte*. Cambridge: Cambridge University Press, 1995:119–49

50. Zenzes MT. Smoking and reproduction: gene damage to human gametes and embryos. *Hum Reprod Update* 2000;6:122–31

51. Hunt PA, Koehler KE, Susiarjo M, *et al*. Bisphenol a exposure causes meiotic aneuploidy in the female mouse. *Curr Biol* 2003;13: 546–53

52. Gaulden ME. Maternal age effect: the enigma of Down syndrome and other trisomic conditions. *Mutat Res* 1992;296:69–88

53. Van Blerkom J, Antczak M, Schrader R. The developmental potential of the human oocyte is related to the dissolved oxygen content of follicular fluid: association with vascular endothelial growth factor levels and perifollicular blood flow characteristics. *Hum Reprod* 1997;12:1047–55

54. Manau D, Balasch J, Jimenez W, *et al.* Follicular fluid concentrations of adrenomedullin, vascular endothelial growth factor and nitric oxide in IVF cycles: relationship to ovarian response. *Hum Reprod* 2000;15: 1295–9

55. van Asselt KM, Kok HS, Peeters PH, *et al.* Factor V Leiden mutation accelerates the onset of natural menopause. *Menopause* 2003;10: 477–81

56. Faddy MJ, Gosden RG. A mathematical model of follicle dynamics in the human. *Hum Reprod* 1995;10:770–5

57. Gougeon A, Ecochard R, Thalabard JC. Age-related changes of the population of human ovarian follicles: increase in the disappearance rate of non-growing and early-growing follicles in aging women. *Biol Reprod* 1994;50: 653–63

58. Gougeon A. Regulation of ovarian follicular development in primates: facts and hypotheses. *Endocr Rev* 1996;17:121–55

59. Tilly JL, Kowalsky KI, Johnson AL, *et al.* Involvement of apoptosis in ovarian follicular atresia and postovulatory regression. *Endocrinology* 1991;129:2799–801

60. Yuan W, Giudice LC. Programmed cell death in human ovary is a function of follicle and corpus luteum status. *J Clin Endocrinol Metab* 1997;82:3148–55

61. de Pol A, Marzona L, Vaccina F, *et al.* Apoptosis in different stages of human oogenesis. *Anticancer Res* 1998;18:3457–61

62. Reynaud K, Driancourt MA. Oocyte attrition. *Mol Cell Endocrinol* 2000;163:101–8

63. de Bruin JP, Dorland M, Spek ER, *et al.* Ultrastructure of the resting ovarian follicle pool in healthy young females. *Biol Reprod* 2002;66:1151–60

64. de Bruin JP, Dorland M, Spek ER, *et al.* Age-related changes in the ultrastructure of the resting follicle pool in human ovaries. *Biol Reprod* 2004;70:419–24

65. Muller-Hocker J, Schafer S, Weis S, *et al.* Morphological–cytochemical and molecular genetic analysis of mitochondria in isolated human oocytes in the reproductive age. *Mol Hum Reprod* 1996;2:951–8

66. Gosden RG, Bownes M. Molecular and cellular aspects of oocyte development. In Grudzinskas JG, Yovich JL, eds. *Cambridge Reviews in Human Reproduction, Gametes – The Oocyte.* Cambridge: Cambridge University Press, 1995

67. Van Blerkom J, Sinclair J, Davis P. Mitochondrial transfer between oocytes: potential applications of mitochondrial donation and the issue of heteroplasmy. *Hum Reprod* 1998; 13:2857–68

68. Eichenlaub-Ritter U. Genetics of oocyte ageing. *Maturitas* 1998;30:143–69

69. Barritt JA, Brenner CA, Cohen J, *et al.* Mitochondrial DNA rearrangements in human oocytes and embryos. *Mol Hum Reprod* 1999;10:927–33

70. Kitagawa T, Suganuma N, Nawa A, *et al.* Rapid accumulation of deleted mitochondrial deoxyribonucleic acid in postmenopausal ovaries. *Biol Reprod* 1993;49:730–6

71. Keefe DL, Niven-Fairchild T, Powell S, *et al.* Mitochondrial deoxyribonucleic acid deletions in oocytes and reproductive aging in women. *Fertil Steril* 1995;64:577–83

72. Barritt JA, Brenner CA, Willadsen S, *et al.* Spontaneous and artificial changes in human ooplasmic mitochondria. *Hum Reprod* 2000;15 (Suppl 2):207–17

73. Yesodi V, Yaron Y, Lessing JB, *et al.* The mitochondrial DNA mutation (delta mtDNA5286) in human oocytes: correlation with age and IVF outcome. *J Assist Reprod Genet* 2002;19:60–6

74. Zeviani M, Antozzi C. Defects of mitochondrial DNA. *Brain Pathol* 1992;2:121–32

75. Jansen RP, de Boer K. The bottleneck: mitochondrial imperatives in oogenesis and ovarian follicular fate. *Mol Cell Endocrinol* 1998;145:81–8

76. Cummins JM. Mitochondrial dysfunction and ovarian aging. In te Velde ER, Pearson PL, Broekmans FJ, eds. *Female Reproductive Aging.* Carnforth, UK: Parthenon Publishing Group, 2000:207–24

77. van Rooij IAJ, Bancsi LFJMM, Broekmans FJM, *et al.* Women older than 40 years of age and those with elevated follicle-stimulating hormone levels differ in poor response rate and embryo quality in *in vitro* fertilization. *Fertil Steril* 2003;79:482–8

78. Gosden RG, Telfer E, Faddy MF, *et al.* Ovarian cyclicity and follicular recruitment in unilaterally ovariectomized mice. *J Reprod Fertil* 1989; 87:257–64

79. Brook JD, Gosden RG, Chandley AC. Maternal ageing and aneuploid embryos – evidence from the mouse that biological and not chronological age is the important influence. *Hum Genet* 1984; 66:41–5

80. van Zonneveld P, Scheffer GJ, Broekmans FJ, *et al*. Do cycle disturbances explain the age-related decline of female fertility? Cycle characteristics of women aged over 40 years compared with a reference population of young women. *Hum Reprod* 2003;18:495–501
81. van Montfrans JM, van Hooff MH, Martens F, *et al*. Basal FSH, estradiol and inhibin B concentrations in women with a previous Down's syndrome affected pregnancy. *Hum Reprod* 2002;17:44–7
82. Nasseri A, Mukherjee T, Grifo JA, *et al*. Elevated day 3 serum follicle stimulating hormone and/or estradiol may predict fetal aneuploidy. *Fertil Steril* 1999;71:715–18
83. den Tonkelaar I, te Velde ER, Looman CW. Menstrual cycle length preceding menopause in relation to age at menopause. *Maturitas* 1998;29:115–23
84. te Velde ER, Pearson PL. The variability of female reproductive ageing. *Hum Reprod Update* 2002;8:141–54
85. Gosden RG, Finch CE. Definition and character of reproductive aging and senescence. In te Velde ER, Pearson PL, Broekmans FJ, eds. *Female Reproductive Aging*. Carnforth, UK: Parthenon Publishing Group, 2000:11–26
86. Jones EC, Krohn PL. The relationship between age, numbers of oocytes and fertility in virgin and multiparous mice. *J Endocrinol* 1961;21:469–96
87. Weinberg CR, Wilcox AJ, Baird DD. Reduced fecundability in women with prenatal exposure to cigarette smoking. *Am J Epidemiol* 1989;129:1072–8
88. Barker DJP. *Mothers, Babies, and Diseases Later in Life*. London: BMJ Publishing, 1994
89. Cresswell JL, Egger P, Fall CHD, *et al*. Is the age of menopause determined *in utero*? *Early Hum Dev* 1997;49:143–8
90. Treloar SA, Sardzadeh S, Do KA, *et al*. Birthweight and age at menopause in Australian female twin pairs: exploration of the fetal origin hypothesis. *Hum Reprod* 2000;15:55–9
91. Elias SG, van Noord PA, Peeters PH, *et al*. Caloric restriction reduces age at menopause: the effect of the 1944–1945 Dutch famine. *Menopause* 2003;10:399–405
92. van Noord PAH, Dubas JS, Dorland M, *et al*. Age at natural menopause in a population-based screening cohort: the role of menarche, fecundity, and lifestyle factors. *Fertil Steril* 1997;68:95–102
93. Westhoff C, Murphy P, Heller D. Predictors of ovarian follicle number. *Fertil Steril* 2000;74:24–8
94. Torgerson DJ, Avenell A, Russell IT, *et al*. Factors associated with onset of menopause in women aged 45–49. *Maturitas* 1994;19:83–92
95. Cramer DW, Xu H, Harlow BL. Family history as a predictor of early menopause. *Fertil Steril* 1995;64:740–5
96. Snieder H, MacGregor AJ, Spector TD. Genes control the cessation of a woman's reproductive life: a twin study of hysterectomy and age at menopause. *J Clin Endocrinol Metab* 1998;83:1875–80
97. Treloar SA, Do KA, Martin NG. Genetic influences on the age at menopause. *Lancet* 1998;352:1084–5
98. de Bruin JP, Bovenhuis H, van Noord PAH, *et al*. The role of genetic factors in age at natural menopause. *Hum Reprod* 2001;16:2014–8
99. Pearson PL. Genetic parameters of oocyte ageing. In te Velde ER, Pearson PL, Broekmans FJ, eds. *Female Reproductive Aging*. Carnforth, UK: Parthenon Publishing Group, 2000:137–48
100. van Asselt KM, Kok HS, Putter H, *et al*. Linkage analysis of extremely discordant and concordant sibling pairs identifies quantitative trait loci influencing variation in human menopausal age. In van Asselt KM, Kok HS. *Age at Menopause; A Genetic–Epidemiologic Study*. Utrecht: University Utrecht, 2003
101. Klein NA, Battaglia DE, Fujimoto VY, *et al*. Reproductive aging: accelerated ovarian follicular development associated with a monotrophic follicle-stimulating hormone rise in normal older women. *J Clin Endocrinol Metab* 1996;81:1038–45
102. Schipper I, de Jong FJ, Fauser BCJM. Lack of correlation between maximum early follicular phase serum follicle stimulating hormone concentrations and menstrual cycle characteristics in women under the age of 35 years. *Hum Reprod* 1998;13:1442–8
103. Brown JR, Liu JC, Sewitch KF, *et al*. Variability of day 3 follicle-stimulating hormone levels in eumenorrhoic women. *J Reprod Med* 1998;40:620–4
104. Bancsi LFJMM, Broekmans FJM, Mol BWJ, *et al*. Performance of basal follicle-stimulating hormone in the prediction of poor ovarian response and failure to become pregnant after *in vitro* fertilization: a meta-analysis. *Fertil Steril* 2003;79:1091–100
105. Ahmed Ebbiary NA, Lenton EA, Cooke ID. Hypothalamic–pituitary aging: progressive increase in FSH and LH concentrations throughout the reproductive lifespan in regularly cycling women. *Clin Endocrinol* 1994;41:199–206
106. Sherman BM, West JH, Korenman SG. The menopausal transition: analysis of LH, FSH,

estradiol and progesterone concentrations during menstrual cycles of older women. *J Clin Endocrinol Metab* 1976;42:629–36

107. Lee SJ, Lenton EA, Sexton L, *et al*. The effect of age on cyclical patterns of plasma LH, FSH, oestradiol and progesterone in women with regular menstrual cycles. *Hum Reprod* 1988;3:851–5

108. Krummen L, Woodruff T, de Guzman G. Identification and characterization of binding proteins for inhibin in human serum and follicular fluids. *Endocrinology* 1993;132: 431–43

109. Groome NP, Illingworth PJ, O'Brien M, *et al*. Measurement of dimeric inhibin B throughout the human menstrual cycle. *J Clin Endocrinol Metab* 1996;81:1401–5

110. Klein NA, Illingworth PJ, Groome NP, *et al*. Decreased inhibin B secretion is associated with the monotropic FSH rise in older ovulatory women: a study of serum and follicular fluid levels of dimeric inhibin A and B in spontaneous menstrual cycles. *J Clin Endocrinol Metab* 1996;81:2742–5

111. Bancsi LFJMM, Broekmans FJM, Eijkemans MJC, *et al*. Predictors of poor ovarian response in *in vitro* fertilization: a prospective study comparing basal markers of ovarian reserve. *Fertil Steril* 2002;77:328–36

112. Scheffer GJ, Broekmans FJ, Looman CW, *et al*. The number of antral follicles in normal women with proven fertility is the best reflection of reproductive age. *Hum Reprod* 2003;18:700–6

113. de Vet A, Laven JS, de Jong FH, *et al*. Antimullerian hormone serum levels : a putative marker for ovarian aging. *Fertil Steril* 2002;77:357–62

114. van Rooij IAJ, Broekmans FJM, Scheffer GJ, *et al*. Serum anti-Müllerian hormone levels best reflect the reproductive decline with age of normal women with proven fertility; a longitudinal study. In van Rooij IAJ. *Comparison of anti-Müllerian Hormone Serum Levels with Currently Used Ovarian Reserve Tests in Normal and Subfertile Women*. Utrecht: Utrecht University, 2003

115. Van Rooij IAJ, Broekmans FJM, te Velde ER, *et al*. Serum anti-Müllerian hormone levels: a novel measure of ovarian reserve. *Hum Reprod* 2002;17:3065–71

116. Hewlett SA. *Baby Hunger. The New Battle for Motherhood*. London: Atlantic Books, 2002:184

117. Somigliana E, Ragni G, Benedetti F, *et al*. Does laparoscopic excision of endometriotic ovarian cysts significantly affect ovarian reserve? Insights from IVF cycles. *Hum Reprod* 2003;18:2450–3

118. Osmers RGW, Osmers M, von Maydell B, *et al*. Preoperative evaluation of ovarian tumours in the premenopause by transvaginosonography. *Am J Obst Gynecol* 1996; 175:428–34

Epidemiology and infertility in cancer patients

2

D. Meirow and J. Dor

INTRODUCTION

Cancer is a common disease and its incidence varies according to many factors. For childhood cancer, prognosis has been dramatically improved and today more than 70% of all patients are likely to be cured. Thus it has been estimated that, in the year 2000, one out of 700 young adults had survived cancer in childhood. Cancer is also common after puberty during the reproductive lifespan of men and women, and many of these patients will be cured following the use of different treatment modalities. Thus, the number of young adults who desire parenthood after cancer treatment and cure has increased significantly. However, cancer treatments and, in some circumstances, cancer itself may jeopardize the prospects of these young adults for fertility and the ability to have a normal healthy child. To investigate, consult and treat these patients successfully, specialists in oncology, hematology and reproductive medicine should be aware of the incidence and long-term survival rates, and of effects of the disease and treatment on future fertility. This is especially true because there are certain treatment options before and after chemotherapy that increase the chances of fertility and parenthood. On the other hand, it is important for patients and staff involved in cancer treatment to know when there is no need for intervention, since some fertility treatments are invasive, expensive, experimental and are performed on sick patients, and also because treatments for fertility preservation can delay cancer treatment.

Knowledge of the risks and probabilities of gonadal failure caused by treatment is crucial for patients and physicians to enable them to make informed choices that will best serve patients' interests. This chapter brings together epidemiological information about cancer incidence and the cure rates of common cancers in men and women. It then presents data on testicular and ovarian damage and failure following exposure to radiotherapy, chemotherapy and ablative therapy. The risk is evaluated from the published literature according to a patient's age, treatment protocol and also according to the diagnosis of some common malignancies. Men can suffer temporarily or over a longer term from testicular damage that results in reversible infertility, while many treated women are not sterilized immediately by treatment but will eventually suffer from premature menopause.

CANCER EPIDEMIOLOGY

The incidence of different cancers differs according to age, gender, geographical location and race. Incidence rates for common cancers in prepubertal boys and girls and in men and women less than 50 years of age are presented in Appendix 1[1].

Looking at survival data is very helpful for auditing the effects of cancer treatment over the last 25 years. Whereas earlier diagnosis, for instance via a screening program, can have an impact on survival figures for some cancers, the continued refinements in high-dose chemotherapy and radiotherapy have significantly improved the cure rates of many young patients with some types of hematological malignancies and solid tumors[2].

Data presented by McVie based on cancer registries throughout England and Wales describe survival rates for 3 million patients[3]. The cancer registries indicate that the treatment of leukemia in children is a success story. Five-year survival rate in the period 1971–1975 was 33% for all leukemias diagnosed in children and is now approaching 80%. Hodgkin's disease now has a 5-year survival rate above 90%, and the corresponding figure for acute lymphocytic leukemia (ALL) and non-Hodgkin's lymphoma is around 75%. The treatment of solid tumors, such as Wilms' tumor and hepatoblastoma, has resulted in increased survival rates, from 61 to 84% and from 15 to 43%, respectively. Equally spectacular improvements have been noted for sarcomas from 17 to 51% for osteosarcoma, from 33 to 61% for Ewing's sarcoma and from 41 to 66% for soft tissue sarcoma. As for adult cancers, the overall increase in relative survival, comparing adults diagnosed in 1971–1975 to those diagnosed in 1986–1990, indicates that the increase in 5-year survival rate is clearly due to improved treatment for cancers such as those of the testes, bone, bladder, and colon, and leukemia and Hodgkin's disease (Table 1).

CANCER AND MALE FERTILITY

The impact of cancer on fertility

Several forms of cancer may influence fertility due to the adverse effects of these malignancies *per se* (even before treatment) on the testis or other endocrine glands. In fact, in many cases infertility may be the first symptom of these cancers.

Hodgkin's disease

Hodgkin's disease is the most common lymphoma during the reproductive years. The condition is almost twice as common in males as in females. As in several other malignancies, decreased fertility exists in males suffering from Hodgkin's disease before treatment or diagnosis[4,5]. Semen analysis performed prior to therapy for male patients with Hodgkin's disease showed that up to 70% of them had a decreased chance of fertility, i.e. azoospermia and astheno- or teratospermia, while levels of follicle stimulating hormone (FSH), luteinizing hormone (LH) and testosterone were all within normal limits in most cases. Also, gonadal dysfunction was not correlated with the stage of the disease – patients in stages I and II were as much affected as those in stages III and IV[6].

The effect of Hodgkin's disease on the testes does not appear to involve a local tumor effect or metastatic cells. These patients demonstrate significant damage to the spermatogenic stem cells, manifested as germinal epithelial hypoplasia. Structural abnormalities in the form of tubular hyalinization have been identified on testicular biopsy[4]. It is hypothesized that these abnormalities reflect changes in the cellular regulation of spermatogenesis. Barr and associates[7] suggested that these abnormalities are an immune-mediated disorder, which reflects alterations in the balance between distinct subpopulations of lymphocytes that normally either inhibit or stimulate the production of sperm. The cause of testicular dysfunction in Hodgkin's disease should be investigated further. The immune-mediated hypothesis in particular should be challenged because endocrine function is normal, no cancerous cells are found in the testes and disease stage does not correlate with dyspermia.

Testicular cancer

Testicular cancer is a common malignancy among men in their third or fourth decade. Patients who suffer from testicular cancer show semen abnormalities at diagnosis, before initiation of treatment. Several studies have indicated (Table 2) that most of these patients (mean 52%, range 17–77%) already have oligospermia prior to treatment initiation. Analysis of 170 men with testicular germ cell cancers who underwent chemotherapy showed pretreatment azoospermia in 40 patients (24%), with a further 41 (24%) being oligospermic[17]. Semen alterations can be related to neoplasm itself, since most patients fathered children

Table 1 Cure rates of common cancers that occur in young patients, according to calendar year of diagnosis. Adapted from references 2 and 3

Disease	1960–63	1970–73	1977–79	1986–90
Acute lymphocytic leukemia*	4	34	67	72
Acute myeloid leukemia*	3	5	27	31
Sarcoma (osteosarcoma, Ewing's sarcoma, soft tissue sarcoma)	16–40	—	—	50–66
Hodgkin's disease	52	90	83	> 90
Non-Hodgkin's lymphoma	18	26	50	75
Testicular cancer	63	72	88	93
Breast cancer	63	72	75	81

*Children below 15 years of age

Table 2 The occurrence of oligospermia in patients diagnosed with testicular cancer

Study	n	Patients with oligospermia (%)
Thachil et al., 1981[8]	42	52*
Fossa et al., 1982[9]	35	57*
Hendry et al., 1983[10]	208	73*
Drasga et al., 1983[11]	30	77*
Jewett et al., 1983[12]	86	27
Fossa et al., 1985[13]	30	62
Fritz and Weissbach, 1985[14]	36	17
Horwich et al., 1988[15]	97	47
Fossa et al., 1989[16]	147	69
Lampe et al., 1997[17]	170	48*

*Sperm count < 10 million/ml

prior to the onset of the disease[18]. Infertility can be the presenting symptom of testicular cancer. There is a high incidence of carcinoma in situ in infertile men, and infertility ranges from 0.4 to 1.1%. Moreover, infertility is at least three times more common in men with germ cell tumors than in the general population[19–22].

Among the common etiologies proposed to explain semen abnormalities and infertility in testicular cancer are:

(1) Local pathological changes. Biopsy of the contralateral testis after radical orchiectomy has shown significant fibrosis of the seminiferous tubules in 24–60% of patients, Sertoli cell only in 8% of patients and carcinoma in situ in 5–8% of patients[23].

(2) Sperm autoimmunity mechanism. Before orchiectomy 21–77% of patients with testicular cancer showed sperm antibodies, compared with 10% in the general population[24,25]. The percentage with sperm antibodies is higher in patients with dvanced disease and lower following therapy. Local tumor effects, such as elevation of scrotal temperature with alteration in blood flow or disruption of the blood–testis barrier, can stimulate an autoimmune response resulting in the production of antisperm antibodies. In a group of 30 patients with testicular cancer, Saint and colleagues recently found a relationship between tumor size and inflammatory dendritic cells. The latter are considered to trigger the antitumoral immune response against tumors such as germ cell tumors, which can be associated with male infertility and necrospermia due to endocrine or immunological factors[26].

(3) Endocrine factors. Testicular cancer can be hormonally active, the common hormonal abnormalities being elevated levels of β human chorionic gonadotropin, α-fetoprotein, estradiol and LH, and depressed testosterone level[23].

Fertility following cancer treatment

Among the most common long-term consequences of cancer treatment in men is testicular dysfunction. Infertility in these patients can be due to chemotherapy, radiotherapy, surgery or a combination of these treatment modalities.

Surgery

Pelvic or groin surgery can impair fertility. Extensive dissection of lymph nodes during surgery for testicular cancer can cause neurogenic dysfunction, ejaculation failure or retrograde ejaculation[13,14,27,28]. Treatment options include sympathomimetic medication, to which approximately 30% of men respond with some antegrade ejaculation. Alternatively, electro ejaculation can be used in combination with *in vitro* fertilization[29]. Since electroejaculates typically have normal sperm numbers but poor motility, morphology and functional deficiencies, intracytoplasmic sperm injection is required for high fertilization efficiency[30].

In patients with testicular cancer, removal of one gonad causes oligospermia in 50% of cases[31]. Mild Leydig cell dysfunction, as indicated by raised LH levels in the presence of a normal testosterone level, was found in 6 to 45% of patients following orchiectomy alone[32]. Unilateral orchiectomy in patients with bilateral testicular germ cell malignancy results in higher serum levels of FSH and LH than in controls, along with a lower sperm count. Thus, the paternity rate is lower and there is an increased need for assisted reproductive technologies[33].

Radiotherapy

Radiotherapy is used to treat a number of malignancies, either alone or with chemotherapy. Ionizing radiation directed at or scattered toward the male reproductive organs inflicts potentially irreversible damage to cellular DNA. The germinal epithelium is very sensitive to radiation-induced damage. Dose–injury curves of ionizing irradiation on testicular tissues show temporary oligospermia occurring at a measured dose of 0.1–0.3 Gy and irreversible azoospermia due to permanent damage to spermatogonia at exposures of 2 Gy[34,35]. In addition, testicular endocrine function has been shown to be impaired after testicular irradiation with 14–20 Gy. With minor irradiation doses, a little impairment – probably without clinical significance – is seen in Leydig cell function[36-38]. Following bone marrow transplantation (BMT) (induction included total body irradiation (TBI) and cyclophosphamide), Leydig cell insufficiency, diminished libido, erectile dysfunction and gynecomastia have been reported. Endocrine evaluation showed severe hypogonadism, very low testosterone levels and marked hyperprolactinemia. These impairments responded well to testosterone replacement therapy[39].

Studies on animals and humans have shown that radiation has direct mutagenic effects on germ cells in relation to dose. Sperm samples taken 3 years after radiotherapy had an increased frequency of chromosomal abnormalities (both numerical and structural) in 20.9% of spermatozoa, compared to a control rate of 8.5%[40,41]. The data suggest that these patients have a permanent or at least long-lasting DNA fragmentation in their spermatozoa[42]. These studies have also found a greater frequency of hypohaploidy relative to hyperhaploidy, suggesting that radiotherapy causes chromosomal loss rather than non-disjunction. These effects seem to be dose-related, with an apparent threshold[43,44].

Factors contributing to the adverse effects of ionizing radiation include radiation field, shielding of the testes and radiation doses. In addition, testicular function and patient's age prior to therapy are important prognostic factors. Radiotherapy combined with chemotherapy has the worst prognosis. In a group of 55 men treated for different malignancies in childhood, the risk of azoospermia in those who had received testicular radiation was 8.2 fold that of others[45]. In 595 male survivors of childhood or adolescent cancer, relative fertility was 0.89 following radiation above the diaphragm and 0.74 following radiation below the diaphragm[46].

Chemotherapy

The male gonads are highly susceptible to the toxic effects of chemotherapy and testicular dysfunction is the most common long-term side-effect of chemotherapy. The first description in humans of testicular damage from cytotoxic drugs was in 1948, when Spitz reported azoospermia in 27 of 30 men following treatment with nitrogen mustard[47]. In general, only 20 to 50% of cancer patients resume spermatogenesis 2 to 3 years after completion of treatment[48–51]. However, the recovery of fertility in patients is dependent on the site of malignancy, with testicular cancer having the worst recovery rates[50]. Fertility recovery depends on sperm quality prior to treatment and also on chemotherapy doses and treatment cycles[52,53].

Alkylating agents are toxic to male gonads. Most clinical studies have focused on cyclophosphamide given as part of a combination chemotherapy protocol or as a single agent. Of 116 males who had been treated with cyclophosphamide alone, 52 patients (45%) had evidence of testicular dysfunction following treatment. The incidence of gonadal dysfunction was correlated with the total dose of cyclophosphamide (being 80% in patients who received more than 300 mg/kg)[54].

Testicular function following chemotherapy for the treatment of lymphomas, especially Hodgkin's disease, has been widely reported. Several studies have reported azoospermia with raised FSH levels in over 90% of men following cyclical chemotherapy with MVPP (mechlorethamine, vinblastine, procarbazine and prednisolone)[55,56]. Similar results were also reported with the MOPP protocol (similar to MVPP but with vinblastine replaced by vincristine). Other chemotherapy regimens for the treatment of lymphomas are COPP (cyclophosphamide, vincristine, procarbazine and prednisolone) and COPP/ABVD (COPP alternating with doxorubicin, bleomycin, vinblastine and dacarbazine), and are associated with marked permanent germinal epithelial failure. Azoospermia was reported in 86% of men after the COPP/ABVD regimen[57,58]. A significantly less toxic protocol is used for the treatment of patients with low-stage Hodgkin's disease. The ABVD protocol does not use alkylating agents and

procarbazine. Viviani and colleagues reported a normal sperm count in 11 of 24 patients and oligospermia in a further five[59].

Chemotherapy protocols for the treatment of non-Hodgkin's lymphoma usually use alkylating agents. However, since low doses are used, these regimens are less toxic to male gonads. A study of 71 patients treated with the CHOP protocol (cyclophosphamide, doxorubicin, vincristine and prednisolone) revealed that 67% had recovered to normospermic levels, with a further 5% oligospermic, at 5 years post-treatment[60]. Also, the majority of male patients treated with the VACOP-B protocol (vinblastine, doxorubicin, cyclophosphamide, vincristine, prednisolone and bleomycin) reported normal post-treatment fertility[61].

Soft tissue sarcoma and bone sarcoma are relatively common in young adults. In recent years the treatment of choice has been limited surgery, causing minimal functional damage, combined with high-dose chemotherapy that commonly includes alkylating agents. A recent study reported sperm analysis of 26 male patients who received chemotherapy for localized bone osteosarcoma of the extremities. Four drugs were administered (doxorubicin, cisplatin, methotrexate, ifosfamide) according to six different protocols. Of this group, 20 patients showed oligo- or azoospermia. High-dose ifosfamide was positively correlated with a higher incidence of azoospermia[62]. Semen analyses on patients with Ewing's and soft tissue sarcomas showed that recovery of spermatogenesis with the CYADIC (cyclophosphamide, doxorubicin and dacarbazine) protocol, with or without vincristine, is related to cyclophosphamide dose – when the cumulative dose was greater than 7.5 g/m^2 only 10% of patients recovered spermatogenesis[63].

Assessment of the effects of cytotoxic chemotherapy on sperm production in patients treated for testicular cancer needs to take into account pretreatment sperm production and quality as well as the impact of any orchiectomy. Of 170 patients with testicular germ cell cancers, Lampe and associates showed that 24% were azoospermic before treatment and a further 24% oligospermic[17].

Recovery of a normal sperm count was related to normal pretreatment sperm count and the use of cisplatin, rather than carboplatin therapy[64].

The majority of patients treated for leukemia do not have persistent gonadal dysfunction. In patients treated during childhood for ALL, only 17% of males had gonadal dysfunction[65]. However, a considerable fraction of patients suffering from leukemia will be treated further by BMT.

BMT has been used widely in recent decades. One of the commonest indications for such treatments is oncohematological malignancy, for which a clear dose–response relationship with chemotherapy exists. In this population BMT is usually performed on children or young patients mainly during the reproductive years. The conditioning regimens used for BMT include high-dose chemotherapy, with or without body irradiation. There is a very high risk of gonadal failure among children and adult patients cured by BMT. However, most patients receive chemotherapy prior to BMT in order to achieve remission, and thus it is difficult to assess the net effects of BMT on spermatogenesis. As previously stated, recovery of fertility after TBI is a rare occurrence. Sanders and co-workers[66] reported findings in 155 men conditioned prior to BMT with chemotherapy-only protocols – cyclophosphamide (200 mg/kg) or busulfan and cyclophosphamide (busulfan 16 mg/kg, cyclophosphamide 200 mg/kg). At 2 to 3 years post-transplant, 61% of patients who received cyclophosphamide and only 17% of patients treated with busulfan and cyclophosphamide had recovery of testicular function. Jacob and colleagues reported that only four out of 25 patients recovered sperm counts after transplant[67].

Table 3 indicates the prognosis for long-term sperm recovery following treatment with different chemotherapeutic agents.

Impact of age and pubertal status

It has been suggested that prepubertal boys are less susceptible to the effects of

Table 3 Long-term recovery of spermatogenesis following treatment with different chemotherapeutic agents and combinations

Good	Moderate	Poor
Methotrexate	vincristine	cyclophosphamide
Prednisone	cisplatin	chlorambucil
Androgens	BEP	mechlorethamine
Estrogens	ABVD	procarbazine
Mercaptopurine	CHOP	ifosfamide
Thioguanin	VACOP-B	carboplatin
Doxorubicin		MOPP
		MVPP
		COPP
		COPP/ABVD
		CYADIC
		BMT

BEP, bleomycin, etoposide and cisplatin; ABVD, doxorubicin, bleomycin, vinblastine and dacarbazine; CHOP, cyclophosphamide, doxorubicin, vincristine and prednisone; VACOP-B, vinblastine, doxorubicin, cyclophosphamide, vincristine, prednisone and bleomycin; MOPP, mechlorethamine, vincristine, procarbazine and prednisone; MVPP, mechlorethamine, vinblastine, procarbazine and prednisone; COPP, cyclophosphamide, vincristine, procarbazine and prednisone; COPP/ABVD, alternating cycles of COPP and ABVD; CYADIC, cyclophosphamide, doxorubicin and dacarbazine; BMT, bone marrow transplantation

chemotherapy than adult men. There is, however, no convincing evidence to support this hypothesis. Testicular dysfunction with raised FSH and LH levels can occur following chemotherapy but rarely prevents normal progress through puberty. Overt hypogonadism causing fatigue, sexual dysfunction and altered mood can occur more commonly in patients following cytotoxic chemotherapy, and testosterone replacement may therefore be beneficial[68]. However, in most cases Leydig cell dysfunction following chemotherapy is subtle and its clinical significance questionable.

CANCER AND FEMALE FERTILITY

The effects of radiotherapy and chemotherapy

Ovarian damage and failure are important and unfortunately common long-term side-effects of radiotherapy and curative chemotherapy.

Sterilization and early menopause in a young female adult have high impact on the patient's self-esteem and quality of life. Also, patients who recover menses after chemotherapy face the likelihood of premature menopause as the result of a depleted follicular store. This represents a serious problem for these cured patients, because many of them are relatively young and have expectations of a normal reproductive life.

The prospect of ovarian failure and impaired fertility after therapy are difficult topics for patients and clinicians to deal with, because of the lack of good prognostic information on an individual basis. To clarify and quantify the risk of ovarian failure after cancer treatment, this section provides relevant information that will assist consultation and can advocate when fertility preservation procedures should be considered.

Radiotherapy

Ionizing radiation has adverse effects on the ovaries at all ages. The degree and persistence of the damage depend on the dose, irradiation field and patient's age, with older women being at greater risk of damage. The ovaries are exposed to significant doses of radiation when radiotherapy is used to treat pelvic and abdominal disease such as cervical and rectal cancer, and with craniospinal radiotherapy for malignancies of the central nervous system. Also, the ovaries are exposed when pelvic lymph nodes are irradiated for hematological malignancies such as Hodgkin's disease and with TBI as part of the conditioning regimen prior to BMT. In many of these cases the patients are young. Shielding of the gonads is used where possible, or the radiation field is restricted to avoid direct irradiation of the ovaries, but in some cases this cannot be achieved.

The estimated dose at which half of the follicles are lost in humans (LD_{50}) is 4 Gy[69]. Lushbaugh and Casarett have indicated that women younger than 40 years of age are less sensitive to radiation-induced ovarian damage, with an estimated dose of 20 Gy required to

produce permanent ovarian failure compared with 6 Gy in older women[70]. Bath and associates studied the effect of TBI (14.4 Gy) on ovarian function in childhood and adolescence. Six of eight women treated with TBI had ovarian failure. Biochemical evidence of incipient ovarian failure was seen in two girls treated before puberty[71]. Thibaud and co-workers[72] showed that TBI of 10 Gy or less given in a single dose before puberty causes a high rate of ovarian failure (55–80%). However, fractionated TBI is less toxic to the ovaries, even in higher doses. A fractionated TBI dose of 15 Gy or more is required to cause ovarian failure in all cases. TBI is more toxic to the ovaries after women reach the age of 25.

Young women who are not sterilized by radiotherapy treatment have an increased risk of infertility and early menopause. Byrne and colleagues found a relative fertility of 0.78 in women who received radiation below the diaphragm[46]. In their study Chiarelli and associates[73] evaluated female childhood cancer survivors who had received abdominal pelvic irradiation and/or chemotherapy with alkylating agents, comparing their risk of premature menopause and infertility with that of survivors who had been treated by non-sterilizing surgery only. The results indicated that the risk of premature ovarian failure increased significantly with increasing dose of abdominal pelvic irradiation. At doses below 20 Gy the relative risk was only 1.02, with irradiation of 20–35 Gy the relative risk increased to 1.37, and with doses above 35 Gy the relative risk of premature ovarian failure was 3.27. Infertility was also correlated with increasing dose of abdominal pelvic irradiation – treatment doses of 20–35 Gy caused infertility in 22% of cases and doses above 35 Gy caused infertility in 32%[73]. A modality that commonly causes early menopause in young women as a result of ovarian exposure to radiation is the inverted Y irradiation used in the treatment of Hodgkin's disease with pelvic lymph node involvement.

Radiation reduces the total number of surviving primordial follicles in a dose-related manner[74]. This explains why sterilization with total depletion of the primordial follicle reserve results following exposure to high doses of radiotherapy, while doses of lower intensity, which cause only partial depletion of the primordial follicle reserve, result in premature ovarian failure.

Chemotherapy

Cytotoxic agents can be grouped into five classes of drug based on their mode of action: alkylating agents, cytoskeleton inhibitors, topoisomerase II inhibitors, antimetabolites and radiomimetics. Frequently, chemotherapeutic agents are used in combination to increase their antitumor effects, but on many occasions their adverse effects are increased as well. Late complications associated with chemotherapy, such as secondary malignancies and adverse effects on the female gonads, assume greater significance. Unfortunately, ovarian damage and failure are common long-term side-effects of curative chemotherapy. The risk is influenced by the patient's age at treatment and the chemotherapy regimen.

Effect of age

Clinical studies have stressed the importance of age as a significant factor in determining the effects of chemotherapy on subsequent ovarian function. Older women have a much higher incidence of complete ovarian failure and permanent infertility than do younger women[75–77]. Of 44 adult females suffering from Hodgkin's disease who had previously received chemotherapy with the MVPP protocol, 17 patients (median age 22 years) maintained regular menses while 17 patients whose median age was 30 stopped menstruating[55]. Also, chemotherapy treatments for breast cancer during the reproductive years result in ovarian failure in more than 50% of patients, but in those under the age of 35 the ovarian failure rate is less than 30%[78].

In a prospective study of 168 patients with cancer (mean age 29.9 years) who were treated with conventional chemotherapy[79], it was shown that the ovarian failure rate for the

Table 4 Influence of age at chemotherapy on treatment-induced ovarian failure

| | Ovarian function | | | |
	Lost	Normal	Total	p Value
n	57	109	168	—
Mean age ± SD (years)	34.7 ± 8.0	27.4 ± 8.3	29.9 ± 8.9	< 0.0001
Range (years)	14–44	11–43	11–44	—

entire group was 34% and that the risk of sterilization was significantly affected by age – the older the patient, the higher the chances of ovarian failure ($p = 0.0001$; Table 4). While young girls and adolescents can also be affected by chemotherapy, they are more resistant most probably because of larger follicle stores prior to treatment[76].

Effect of treatment protocol

Few treatment protocols are accepted for each cancer and when a diagnosis is established, one of the protocols is administered. Lower and co-workers determined the prevalence and timing of menstrual abnormalities in 109 premenopausal, early-stage breast cancer patients undergoing adjuvant treatment with a methotrexate- or anthracycline-based combination chemotherapy protocol. In both groups, cyclophosphamide was administered as part of the treatment protocol. Amenorrhea occurred in about a third of patients during chemotherapy (methotrexate group 31%, anthracycline group 33%), and a higher proportion were amenorrheic 1 year after chemotherapy was completed (methotrexate group 45%, anthracycline group 46%)[78]. Bines and colleagues reviewed reports on ovarian failure after adjuvant chemotherapy in premenopausal breast cancer survivors and reported that for regimens based on cyclophosphamide, methotrexate and fluorouracil (CMF) the average chemotherapy-related amenorrhea rate was as high as 68%[80]. Following a CMF protocol, Jonat found that 60% of patients suffered from amenorrhea and the rate gradually increased to 90% at 5 years post-chemotherapy[81] (Table 5).

Table 5 Ovarian failure rates following treatments for breast cancer

Study	Age (years)		Ovarian failure rate (%)
Lower et al., 1999[78]	premenopause		45
	< 35		28
Bines et al., 1996[80]	premenopause		68
Meirow, 1999[79]	< 44		50
Goodwin et al., 1999[82]	CMF	43.7 ± 5.2	65
Burstein et al., 2000[83]	CMF	> 30	19
		30–39	30–40
	CAF	> 30	0
		30–39	10–25
	AC	> 30	—
		30–39	13
Jonat, 2001[81]	premenopause		60

CMF, cyclophosphamide, methotrexate and fluorouracil; CAF, cyclophosphamide, doxorubicin and fluorouracil; AC, doxorubicin and cyclophosphamide

Table 6 Ovarian failure rates following treatments for Hodgkin's disease

Study	Treatment		Ovarian failure rate (%)
Howell and Shalet, 1998[35]	aggressive treatment		38–57
Meirow, 1999[79]	relapse post 1st treatment		32
Bokemeyer et al., 1994[86]	infra diaphragmatic irradiation		50
Brusamolino et al., 2000[84]	ovarian sparing	< 25 years	0
	protocol	< 45 years	30

Several protocols are accepted for the treatment of Hodgkin's disease. Howell and Shalet have reviewed the risk of ovarian damage among women with Hodgkin's disease following aggressive treatment with combination cytotoxic chemotherapy and radiotherapy. Treatment with MVPP, COPP and ChlVPP (chlorambucil, vinblastine, procarbazine and prednisolone) resulted in ovarian failure in 38–57% of patients[35]. The use of combined modality therapy in early-stage Hodgkin's disease can significantly reduce long-term ovarian toxicity. Brusamolino and associates observed that after four courses of ABVD chemotherapy followed by local radiotherapy, fertility was preserved in young women. Transient amenorrhea was reported by 12 of 33 patients younger than 45 years, and no cases of permanent amenorrhea were observed in 17 patients younger than 25 years[84]. In 36 young patients (median age at diagnosis 14 years) treated by five cycles of COP (cyclophosphamide, vincristine and procarbazine) alternated with four cycles of ABVD and low-dose (20 Gy) regional radiotherapy, the majority had regular menstrual cycles following treatment. Six patients developed ovarian failure (17%), and ten had a total of 17 pregnancies[85] (Table 6).

In patients with high-grade non-Hodgkin's lymphoma who were younger than 45 years, gonadal dysfunction was documented in 10%[86]. A cohort of 37 women with aggressive non-Hodgkin's lymphoma was studied recently; the patients' mean age at diagnosis was 26 years and most were treated with the CHOP protocol. All but two women (40 years) resumed menses, which were regular in 65% of them, but the hormonal profile was not evaluated[87]. On the other hand, in a prospective study of 36 non-Hodgkin's lymphoma patients (mean age 34.8 ± 7.9 years), a significantly higher ovarian failure (sterilization) rate of 44% was found. The common protocols for

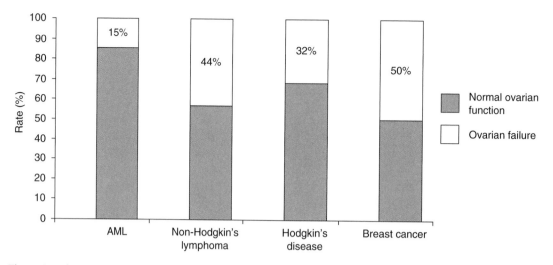

Figure 1 The rate of ovarian failure following chemotherapy to treat various conditions in 168 young cancer patients (mean age 29 years) with proven normal ovarian function prior to treatment. AML, acute myeloid leukemia

these patients were CHOP, MACOP-B (methotrexate, doxorubicin, cyclophosphamide, vincristine, prednisone and bleomycin) and VACOP-B[79]. This study also evaluated 47 patients with acute myeloid leukemia (mean age 38.4 ± 3.6 years), finding that 15% suffered from ovarian failure following treatment with different combinations of the following drugs: cytarabine, daunorubicin, mitoxantrone and vinblastine (Figure 1)[79].

Gershenson evaluated 40 patients treated for malignant ovarian germ cell tumors, their median age at diagnosis was 15 years and at the time of the study was 25.5 years. All patients had surgery and unilateral oophorectomy. Various regimens of chemotherapy were used, but the common protocol was VAC (vincristine, dactinomycin and cyclophosphamide). In this group 13% of patients had irregular menses, 15% oligomenorrhea or amenorrhea and 8% suffered from persistent amenorrhea[88].

Intensive high-dose multiagent chemotherapy has improved the prognosis of patients with osteosarcoma. Drugs commonly used are methotrexate, ifosfamide and cisplatin at high doses not routinely employed for other cancers. Very little information exists concerning ovarian function following chemotherapy for osteosarcoma. Wikstrom and co-workers reported on ten female osteosarcoma patients treated with chemotherapy. Median age at diagnosis was 13 years, five were postmenarchal. At discontinuation of therapy none of the girls experienced regular menstrual cycles. A few years later six had regular menses, three had irregular menstrual cycles and one was on hormone replacement therapy. Four patients, the ones who had been treated with high doses of ifosfamide, had hypergonadotropic hypogonadism[89]. Further studies with larger numbers are needed, especially among patients postpuberty and young adults.

Chemotherapy is a common treatment modality in some groups of patients with autoimmune diseases. Pulse cyclophosphamide therapy is frequently used for active lupus nephritis or neuropsychiatric lupus. The risk of secondary amenorrhea after pulse cyclophosphamide therapy was evaluated in 39 premenopausal women with systemic lupus erythematosus. Of the 16 women who received short cyclophosphamide pulses (0.5 to 1.0 g/m² body surface area) monthly for a total of seven doses, two (12%) developed

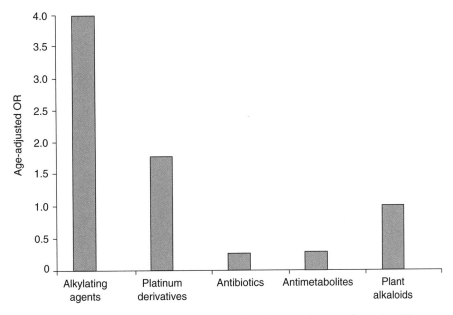

Figure 2 In 168 cancer patients treated by combination chemotherapy, the overall ovarian failure rate was 34%, representing an odds ratio (OR) of 1.0. Medications were in five drug categories (alkylating agents, platinum derivatives, plant alkaloids, antimetabolites and antibiotics) and analysis was performed on these groups. The fraction contributed by each of the chemotherapeutic classes was analyzed by the OR of exposed versus non-exposed patients. The results were adjusted for age

sustained amenorrhea, compared with nine of 23 women (39%) in the long cyclophosphamide pulse protocol (15 or more cycles). The increased risk of sustained amenorrhea with a long cyclophosphamide protocol was most evident in patients older than 25 years[90]. In another study of 70 patients suffering from systemic lupus erythematosus, 26% had premature ovarian failure after cyclophosphamide treatment. The major determinants for the development of ovarian failure in these patients were age at the start of therapy and cumulative cyclophosphamide dose[91].

Most cancer patients are treated with combination therapy that includes a few classes of chemotherapeutic agent. To evaluate ovarian failure rate according to the fraction contributed by each chemotherapeutic class (alkylating agents, platinum agents, plant alkaloids, antimetabolites and antibiotics), a group of 168 patients was analyzed by

examining the odds ratio (OR) of ovarian failure in exposed versus unexposed patients. Alkylating agents were found to impose the highest risk of ovarian failure (OR = 3.98), followed by cisplatin (OR = 1.77) (Figure 2)[79].

Partial ovarian injury

Chemotherapy and radiotherapy reduce the primordial follicle reserve, which can trigger ovarian failure. However, with many young patients, cyclic menses may proceed for a number of years after treatment but they are at risk of undergoing premature menopause. Several studies have observed that a significant proportion of younger patients who continued regular menstruation after chemotherapy had premature menopause[81,92,93]. The risk of premature menopause and infertility was evaluated in 719 female childhood cancer survivors; only females who were not

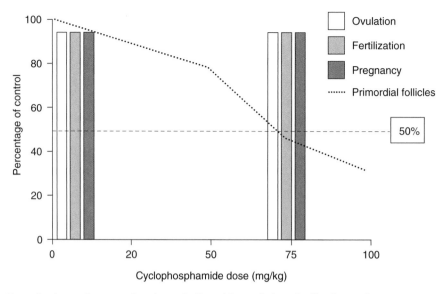

Figure 3 Reproductive performance in mice as indicated by ovulation, fertilization and pregnancy rates following exposure to 75 mg/kg cyclophosphamide, as a percentage of control values. Line graph represents the total number of primordial follicles counted in both ovaries of mice exposed to cyclophosphamide at doses of 0, 20, 50, 75 and 100 mg/kg. Reproductive performance was not altered despite the occult ovarian injury, even when more than 50% of follicles were destroyed[94]

menopausal at the end of treatment were analyzed. Survivors who had received both alkylating agents and abdominal–pelvic radiation were more likely to suffer from premature menopause than those who did not (relative risk = 2.58). The risk of premature menopause and infertility increased with increasing doses of abdominal–pelvic radiation and alkylating agent[73].

Clinical studies use indirect measurements such as menstrual history, endocrine profiles and pregnancy rates to examine the effects of chemotherapy on the ovary, necessarily defining the outcome in dichotomous terms – whether or not ovarian failure occurred. These studies do not demonstrate the effects of increasing doses of chemotherapy within a non-sterilizing range on the primordial follicle population and ovarian reserve.

In an animal study, primordial follicle loss following exposure to different doses of cyclophosphamide was measured directly and compared with reproductive outcome following treatment[94]. Young mice were treated with different doses of cyclophosphamide, and the total number of follicles remaining in both ovaries was counted. Results indicated that the effect of chemotherapy on the ovary is not an 'all or none' phenomenon; cyclophosphamide causes follicular destruction in proportion to dose. The study showed that exposure to doses of chemotherapy strong enough to destroy half of the ovarian primordial reserve did not affect reproductive performance (ovulation, mating and pregnancy rates) following treatment (Figure 3). These results strongly indicate that regular menses and normal reproductive outcome after chemotherapy are not reassuring parameters from which it is possible to conclude that the ovaries survived treatment unaffected. Reduced follicular reserve after treatment also explains the tendency of women subjected to chemotherapy to undergo premature menopause.

The clinical data and animal studies strongly support the recommendation that patients who regain ovarian function following high-dose chemotherapy or radiotherapy treatment should not delay childbearing.

These patients should try to conceive, if possible, after few disease-free years, although not less than 6–12 months after treatment due to possible toxicity of the treatment on growing oocytes[95].

Bone marrow transplantation

Patients treated with allogeneic/autologous stem cell transplantation suffer a very high sterilization rate[96]. Teinturier and co-workers[97] evaluated 21 girls who had received BMT without TBI for malignant tumors at the age 2–17 years. All ten girls who were treated with the alkylating agent busulfan (140 mg/m^2) with or without cyclophosphamide had persistent ovarian failure, even if treated before puberty. Of the 11 girls who were conditioned without alkylating agents, two had ovarian failure and three had gonadotropin levels above or at the upper normal limit. In another group of 31 girls aged 3.2–17.5 years who had BMT with or without irradiation, those who had menstruated before treatment suffered from permanent amenorrhea. Six years after BMT, 80% of this group had permanent ovarian failure[72].

We have studied a group of 63 female cancer patients (mean age 29.6 years) who were treated with ablative radiochemotherapy followed by BMT. All had previous chemotherapy treatment several months to years before BMT but all had cyclic menstrual activity with gonadotropin levels (FSH and LH) within normal limits. Continuous monitoring of these patients (menses cycles and gonadotropin levels) for more than 5 years following BMT has revealed persistent ovarian failure in all but five patients. There was no correlation with age, cytotoxic regimen given, or suppression of endogenous hormonal secretion during BMT by the administration of gonadotropin releasing hormone analogs (GnRH-a), oral contraceptives or progestins[98].

A common conditioning protocol for BMT that does not involve TBI is the busulfan–cyclophosphamide (Bu–Cy) regimen. Among adult females (mean age 38 years) who were treated with 'big Bu–Cy' (200 mg/kg

Table 7 Ovarian failure rates following bone marrow transplantation

Study	n	Age (years)	Ovarian failure rate (%)
Sanders et al., 1988[76]	73	38*	99
Teinturier et al., 1998[97]	21	2–17	72
Thibaud et al., 1998[72]	31	3.2–17	80
Meirow, 1999[79]	63	29*	79
Grigg et al., 2000[99]	19	30*	100

*Mean value

cyclophosphamide) only one out of 73 recovered ovarian function[66]. Moreover, even with decreased cyclophosphamide dose ('little Bu–Cy', 120 mg/kg) ovarian failure was the result in all 19 female patients aged 16–40 years (mean age 30) who were tested 2 or more years following BMT[99]. Use of a non-ablative approach for conditioning before BMT (high-dose melfalan) was shown to be as effective as more aggressive regimens in Hodgkin's disease and non-Hodgkin's lymphoma, but had the substantial advantage of preserving fertility in female patients. Of these 30 women, ten had successful pregnancies after BMT[100].

These studies indicate that there is an extremely high risk of persistent ovarian failure in female patients who undergo BMT. Growth and sexual development are impaired in children and sterility is common in adults (Table 7).

Final comments

The information provided herein is relevant for specialists in cancer and reproductive medicine. The data help to guide clinical judgement before and after cancer treatments, and emphasize when fertility preservation procedures, such as cryopreservation of gametes[101], are appropriate and can be offered. Also, these data aid in the critical evaluation of information regarding the protective effect of medications such as GnRH-a or hormones during chemotherapy administration[102]. During the last few years new chemotherapeutic agents such as taxol and its derivates, and new chemotherapeutic protocols such as AC-T for breast cancer (doxorubicin, cyclophosphamide and taxol), have emerged. However, there are currently insufficient data regarding the effect of these treatments on human reproduction. Future studies should focus on these medications and on patients treated by these protocols.

ACKNOWLEDGMENT

The authors deeply appreciate the assistance and information provided by Dr Liat Lerner Geva of the Women and Children Health Research Unit, Gertner Institute for Epidemiology and Health Policy Research, Sheba Medical Center, Israel.

References

1. Parking DM, Whelan SL, Ferlay J, et al., eds. *Cancer Incidence in Five Continents*, Vol. VIII. IARC Scientific Publications No. 155. Lyon: IARC, 2002
2. Boring CC, Squires TS, Tong J, Montgomery S. Cancer statistics 1994. *CA Cancer J Clin* 1994;44:7–26
3. McVie JG. Cancer treatment: the last 25 years. *Cancer Treat Rev* 1999;25:323–31
4. Chapman RM, Sutcliffe SB, Malpas JS. Male gonadal dysfunction in Hodgkin's disease. A prospective study. *J Am Med Assoc* 1981;245:1323–8
5. Vigersky RA, Chapman RM, Berenberg J, Glass AR. Testicular dysfunction in untreated Hodgkin's disease. *Am J Med* 1982;73:482–6
6. Viviani S, Ragni G, Santoro A, et al. Testicular dysfunction in Hodgkin's disease before and after treatment. *Eur J Cancer* 1991;27:1389–92
7. Barr RD, Clark DA, Booth JD. Dyspermia in men with localized Hodgkin's disease. A potentially reversible, immune-mediated disorder. *Med Hypotheses* 1993;40:165–8
8. Thachil JV, Jewett MA, Rider WD. The effects of cancer and cancer therapy on male fertility. *J Urol* 1981;126:141–5
9. Fossa SD, Klepp O, Molne K, Aakvaag A. Testicular function after unilateral orchiectomy for cancer and before further treatment. *Int J Androl* 1982;5:179–84
10. Hendry WF, Stedronska J, Jones CR, et al. Semen analysis in testicular cancer and Hodgkin's disease: pre- and post-treatment findings and implications for cryopreservation. *Br J Urol* 1983;55:769–73
11. Drasga RE, Einhorn LH, Williams SD, et al. Fertility after chemotherapy for testicular cancer. *J Clin Oncol* 1983;1:179–83
12. Jewett MA, Thachil JV, Harris JF. Exocrine function of testis with germinal testicular tumour. *Br Med J Clin Res Ed* 1983;286:1849–50
13. Fossa SD, Ous S, Abyholm T, Loeb M. Post-treatment fertility in patients with testicular cancer. I. Influence of retroperitoneal lymph node dissection on ejaculatory potency. *Br J Urol* 1985;57:204–9
14. Fritz K, Weissbach L. Sperm parameters and ejaculation before and after operative treatment of patients with germ-cell testicular cancer. *Fertil Steril* 1985;43:451–4
15. Horwich A, Nicholls EJ, Hendry WF. Seminal analysis after orchiectomy in stage I teratoma. *Br J Urol* 1988;62:79–81
16. Fossa SD, Aass N, Molne K. Is routine pretreatment cryopreservation of semen worthwhile in the management of patients with testicular cancer? *Br J Urol* 1989;64:524–9
17. Lampe H, Horwich A, Norman A, et al. Fertility after chemotherapy for testicular germ cell cancers. *J Clin Oncol* 1997;15:239–45
18. Hansen SW, Berthelsen JG, von der Maase H. Long-term fertility and Leydig cell function in patients treated for germ cell cancer with cisplatin, vinblastine, and bleomycin versus surveillance. *J Clin Oncol* 1990;8:1695–8
19. Witten FR, O'Brien DP 3rd, Sewell CW, Wheatley JK. Bilateral clear cell papillary cystadenoma of the epididymides presenting as infertility: an early manifestation of von Hippel-Lindau's syndrome. *J Urol* 1985;133:1062–4
20. Lehman D, Temminck B, Litmanen K, et al. Autoimmune phenomena and cytogenetic findings in a patient with carcinoma (seminoma) *in situ*. *Cancer* 1986;58:2013–7
21. Spermon JR, Kiemeney LA, Meuleman EJ, et al. Fertility in men with testicular germ cell tumors. *Fertil Steril* 2003;79(Suppl 3):1543–9
22. Pasqualotto FF, Pasqualotto EB, Agarwal A, Thomas AJ Jr. Detection of testicular cancer in men presenting with infertility. *Rev Hosp Clin Fac Med Sao Paulo* 2003;58:75–80

23. Berthelsen JG, Skakkebaek NE. Gonadal function in men with testis cancer. *Fertil Steril* 1983;39:68–72
24. Foster RS, Rubin LR, McNulty A, *et al.* Detection of antisperm antibodies in patients with primary testicular cancer. *Int J Androl* 1991;14:179–85
25. Guazzieri S, Lembo A, Ferro G, *et al.* Sperm antibodies and infertility in patients with testicular cancer. *Urology* 1985;26:139–42
26. Saint F, Leroy X, Graziana JP, Moukassa D, *et al.* Dendritic cell infiltration in a patient with seminomatous germ cell tumor of the testis: is there a relationship with infertility and tumor stage? *J Urol* 2002;167:1643–7
27. Narayan P, Lange PH, Fraley EF. Ejaculation and fertility after extended retroperitoneal lymph node dissection for testicular cancer. *J Urol* 1982;127:685–8
28. Pizzocaro G, Salvioni R, Zanoni F. Unilateral lymphadenectomy in intraoperative stage I nonseminomatous germinal testis cancer. *J Urol* 1985;134:485–9
29. Lass A, Akagbosu F, Brinsden P. Sperm banking and art treatment for couples following cancer treatment of the male partner. *Hum Reprod Update* 2001;7:370–7
30. Chung PH, Palermo G, Schlegel PN, *et al.* The use of intracytoplasmic sperm injection with electroejaculates from anejaculatory men. *Hum Reprod* 1998;13:1854–8
31. Ferreira U, Netto NR Jr, Esteves SC, *et al.* Comparative study of the fertility potential in men with only one testis. *Scand J Urol Nephrol* 1991;25:255–9
32. Howell SJ, Shalet SM. Testicular function following chemotherapy. *Hum Reprod Update* 2001;7:363–9
33. Jacobsen KD, Fossa SD, Bjoro TP, *et al.* Gonadal function and fertility in patients with bilateral testicular germ cell malignancy. *Eur Urol* 2002;42:229–38
34. Damewood MD, Growchow LB. Prospects for fertility after chemotherapy or radiation for neoplastic disease. *Fertil Steril* 1986;45:443–59
35. Howell S, Shalet S. Gonadal damage from chemotherapy and radiotherapy. *Endocrinol Metab Clin North Am* 1998;27:927–43
36. Littley MD, Shalet SM, Morgenstern GR, Deakin DP. Endocrine and reproductive dysfunction following fractionated total body irradiation in adults. *Q J Med* 1991;78:265–74
37. Petersen PM, Daugaard G, Rorth M, Skakkebaek NE. Endocrine function in patients treated for carcinoma *in situ* in the testis with irradiation. *APMIS* 2003;111:93–8
38. Howell SJ, Shalet SM. Effect of cancer therapy on pituitary–testicular axis. *Int J Androl* 2002; 25:269–76
39. Harris E, Mahendra P, McGarrigle HH, *et al.* Gynaecomastia with hypergonadotrophic hypogonadism and Leydig cell insufficiency in recipients of high-dose chemotherapy or chemo-radiotherapy. *Bone Marrow Transplant* 2001;28:1141–4
40. Martin RH, Hildebrand K, Yamamoto J, *et al.* An increased frequency of human sperm chromosomal abnormalities after radiotherapy. *Mutat Res* 1986;174:219–25
41. Martin RH. Detection of genetic damage in human sperm. *Reprod Toxicol* 1993;7(Suppl 1): 47–52
42. De Palma A, Vicari E, Palermo I, *et al.* Effects of cancer and anti-neoplastic treatment on the human testicular function. *J Endocrinol Invest* 2000;23:690–6
43. Brent RL. The effect of embryonic and fetal exposure to x-ray, microwaves, and ultrasound: counseling the pregnant and nonpregnant patient about these risks. *Semin Oncol* 1989;16:347–68
44. Fattibene P, Mazzei F, Nuccetelli C, Risica S. Prenatal exposure to ionizing radiation: sources, effects and regulatory aspects. *Acta Paediatr* 1999;88:693–702
45. Rautonen J, Koskimies AI, Siimes MA. Vincristine is associated with the risk of azoospermia in adult male survivors of childhood malignancies. *Eur J Cancer* 1992;28A: 1837–41
46. Byrne J, Mulvihill JJ, Myers MH, *et al.* Effects of treatment on fertility in long-term survivors of childhood or adolescent cancer. *N Engl J Med* 1987;317:1315–21
47. Spitz S. The histological effects of nitrogen mustard on human tumours and tissues. *Cancer* 1948;1:383–98
48. Kreuser ED, Harsch U, Hetzel D, Schreml W. Chronic gonadal toxicity in patients with testicular cancer after chemotherapy. *Eur J Cancer Clin Oncol* 1986;232:289–94
49. Nijman JM, Schraffordt Koops H, Kremer J, Sleijfer DT. Gonadal function after surgery and chemotherapy in men with stage II and III nonseminomatous testicular tumors. *J Clin Oncol* 1987;5:651–6
50. Naysmith TE, Blake DA, Harvey VJ, Johnson NP. Do men undergoing sterilizing cancer treatments have a fertile future? *Hum Reprod* 1998;13:3250–5
51. Hartmann JT, Albrecht C, Schmoll HJ, *et al.* Long-term effects on sexual function and fertility after treatment of testicular cancer. *Br J Cancer* 1999;80:801–7
52. Meirow D, Schenker JG. Cancer and male infertility. *Hum Reprod* 1995;10:2017–22
53. Pont J, Albrecht W. Fertility after chemotherapy for testicular cancer. *Fertil Steril* 1997;68:1–5

54. Rivkees SA, Crawford JD. The relationship of gonadal activity and chemotherapy-induced gonadal damage. *J Am Med Assoc* 1988;259: 2123–5

55. Whitehead E, Shalet SM, Blackledge G, *et al.* The effects of Hodgkin's disease and combination chemotherapy on gonadal function in the adult male. *Cancer* 1982;49:418–22

56. Chapman RM, Sutcliffe SB, Rees LH, *et al.* Cyclical combination chemotherapy and gonadal function. Retrospective study in males. *Lancet* 1979;1:285–9

57. Charak BS, Gupta R, Mandrekar P, *et al.* Testicular dysfunction after cyclophosphamide–vincristine–procarbazine–prednisolone chemotherapy for advanced Hodgkin's disease. A long-term follow-up study. *Cancer* 1990;65: 1903–6

58. Kreuser ED, Felsenberg D, Behles C, *et al.* Long-term gonadal dysfunction and its impact on bone mineralization in patients following COPP/ABVD chemotherapy for Hodgkin's disease. *Ann Oncol* 1992;3(Suppl 4):105–10

59. Viviani S, Santoro A, Ragni G, *et al.* Gonadal toxicity after combination chemotherapy for Hodgkin's disease. Comparative results of MOPP vs ABVD. *Eur J Cancer Clin Oncol* 1985; 21:601–5

60. Pryzant RM, Meistrich ML, Wilson G, *et al.* Long-term reduction in sperm count after chemotherapy with and without radiation therapy for non-Hodgkin's lymphomas. *J Clin Oncol* 1993;11:239–47

61. Muller U, Stahel RA. Gonadal function after MACOP-B or VACOP-B with or without dose intensification and ABMT in young patients with aggressive non-Hodgkin's lymphoma. *Ann Oncol* 1993;4:399–402

62. Longhi A, Macchiagodena M, Vitali G, Bacci G. Fertility in male patients treated with neoadjuvant chemotherapy for osteosarcoma. *J Pediatr Hematol Oncol* 2003;25:292–6

63. Meistrich ML, Wilson G, Brown BW, *et al.* Impact of cyclophosphamide on long-term reduction in sperm count in men treated with combination chemotherapy for Ewing and soft tissue sarcomas. *Cancer* 1992;1;70:2703–12

64. Palmieri G, Lotrecchiano G, Ricci G, *et al.* Gonadal function after multimodality treatment in men with testicular germ cell cancer. *Eur J Endocrinol* 1996;134:431–6

65. Wallace WH, Shalet SM, Lendon M, *et al.* Male fertility in long-term survivors of childhood acute lymphoblastic leukaemia. *Int J Androl* 1991;14:312–9

66. Sanders JE, Hawley J, Levy W, *et al.* Pregnancies following high-dose cyclophosphamide with or without high-dose busulfan or total-body irradiation and bone marrow transplantation. *Blood* 1996;87:3045–52

67. Jacob A, Barker H, Goodman A, *et al.* Recovery of spermatogenesis following bone marrow transplantation. *Bone Marrow Transplant* 1998; 22:277–9

68. Howell SJ, Radford JA, Smets EMA, Shalet SM. Fatigue, sexual function and mood following treatment for haematological malignancy – the impact of mild Leydig cell dysfunction. *Br J Cancer* 2000;82:789–93

69. Wallace WH, Shalet SM, Hendry JH, *et al.* Ovarian failure following ovarian irradiation in childhood: the radiosensitivity of the human oocyte. *Br J Radiol* 1989;62:995–8

70. Lushbaugh CC, Casarett GW. The effects of gonadal irradiation in clinical radiation therapy: a review. *Cancer* 1976;37:1111–25

71. Bath LE, Critchley HO, Chambers SE, *et al.* Ovarian and uterine characteristics after total body irradiation in childhood and adolescence: response to sex steroid replacement. *Br J Obstet Gynaecol* 1999;106:1265–72

72. Thibaud E, Rodriguez-Macias K, Trivin C, *et al.* Ovarian function after bone marrow transplantation during childhood. *Bone Marrow Transplant* 1998;21:287–90

73. Chiarelli AM, Marrett LD, Darlington G. Early menopause and infertility in females after treatment for childhood cancer diagnosed in 1964–1988 in Ontario, Canada. *Am J Epidemiol* 1999;150:245–54

74. Gosden RG, Wade JC, Fraser HM, *et al.* Impact of congenital hypogonadotropism on the radiation sensitivity of the mouse ovary. *Hum Reprod* 1997;12:2483–8

75. Moore HC. Fertility and the impact of systemic therapy on hormonal status following treatment for breast cancer. *Curr Oncol Rep* 2000; 2:587–93

76. Sanders JE, Buckner CD, Amos D, *et al.* Ovarian function following marrow transplantation for aplastic anemia or leukemia. *J Clin Oncol* 1988;6:813–8

77. Fisher B, Cheung AY. Delayed effect of radiation therapy with or without chemotherapy on ovarian function in women with Hodgkin's disease. *Acta Radiol Oncol* 1984;23:43–8

78. Lower EE, Blau R, Gazder P, Tummala R. The risk of premature menopause induced by chemotherapy for early breast cancer. *J Womens Health Gend Based Med* 1999;8: 949–54

79. Meirow D. Ovarian injury and modern options to preserve fertility in female cancer patients treated with high dose radio–chemotherapy for hemato-oncological neoplasias and other cancers. *Leuk Lymphoma* 1999;33:65–76

80. Bines J, Oleske DM, Cobleigh MA. Ovarian function in premenopausal women treated with adjuvant chemotherapy for breast cancer. *J Clin Oncol* 1996;14:1718–29

81. Jonat W. Amenorrhea with CMF. Presented at the *7th International Conference on Adjuvant Therapy of Primary Breast Cancer*, St Gallen, 2001

82. Goodwin PJ, Ennis M, Pritchard KI, *et al*. Risk of menopause during the first year after breast cancer diagnosis. *J Clin Oncol* 1999;17:2365–70

83. Burstein HJ, Winer EP. Primary care for survivors of breast cancer. *N Engl J Med* 2000; 343:1086–94

84. Brusamolino E, Lunghi F, Orlandi E, *et al*. Treatment of early-stage Hodgkin's disease with four cycles of ABVD followed by adjuvant radiotherapy: analysis of efficacy and long-term toxicity. *Haematologica* 2000;85:1032–9

85. Hudson MM, Greenwald C, Thompson E, *et al*. Efficacy and toxicity of multi-agent chemotherapy and low-dose involved-field radiotherapy in children and adolescents with Hodgkin's disease. *J Clin Oncol* 1993; 11:100–8

86. Bokemeyer C, Schmoll HJ, van Rhee J, *et al*. Long-term gonadal toxicity after therapy for Hodgkin's and non-Hodgkin's lymphoma. *Ann Hematol* 1994;68:105–10

87. Elis A, Tevet A, Yerushalmi R, *et al*. Infertility status among women treated for aggressive non Hodgkin's lymphoma. Presented at the *Annual Meeting of the Israeli Society of Hematology*, Tel Aviv, 2003

88. Gershenson DM. Menstrual and reproductive function after treatment with combination chemotherapy for malignant ovarian germ cell tumors. *J Clin Oncol* 1988;6:270–5

89. Wikstrom AM, Hovi L, Dunkel L, Saarian-Pikhala UM. Restoration of ovarian function after chemotherapy for osteosarcoma. *Arch Dis Child* 2003;88:428–31

90. Boumpas DT, Austin HA, Vaughan EM, *et al*. Risk for sustained amenorrhea in patients with systemic lupus erythematosus receiving intermittent pulse cyclophosphamide therapy. *Ann Intern Med* 1993;119:366–9

91. Mok CC, Lau CS, Wong RW. Risk factors for ovarian failure in patients with systemic lupus erythematosus receiving cyclophosphamide therapy. *Arthritis Rheum* 1998;41:831–7

92. Wallace WH, Shalet SM, Tetlow LJ, Morris-Jones PH. Ovarian function following the treatment of childhood acute lymphoblastic leukaemia. *Med Pediatr Oncol* 1993;21:333–9

93. Byrne J, Fears TR, Gail MH, *et al*. Early menopause in long-term survivors of cancer during adolescence. *Am J Obstet Gynecol* 1992; 166:788–93

94. Meirow D, Lewis H, Nugent D, Epstein M. Subclinical depletion of primordial follicular reserve in mice treated with cyclophosphamide: clinical importance and proposed accurate investigative tool. *Hum Reprod* 1999;14:1903–7

95. Meirow D, Nugent D. The effects of radiotherapy and chemotherapy on female reproduction. *Hum Reprod Update* 2001;7:535–43

96. Apperley JF, Reddy N. Mechanism and management of treatment related gonadal failure in recipients of high dose chemotherapy. *Blood Rev* 1995;9:93–116

97. Teinturier C, Hartmann O, Valteau-Couanet D, *et al*. Ovarian function after autologous bone marrow transplantation in childhood: high-dose busulfan is a major cause of ovarian failure. *Bone Marrow Transplant* 1998;22:989–94

98. Meirow D, Lewin A, Or R, *et al*. Ovarian failure post chemotherapy in young cancer patients – risk assessment indicate the need for intervention. Presented at the *53rd Annual Meeting of the American Society for Reproductive Medicine*, Cincinnati, OH, 1997

99. Grigg AP, McLachlan R, Zaja J, Szer J. Reproductive status in long-term bone marrow transplant survivors receiving busulfan–cyclophosphamide (120 mg/kg). *Bone Marrow Transplant* 2000;26:1089–95

100. Jackson GH, Wood A, Taylor PR, *et al*. Early high dose chemotherapy intensification with autologous bone marrow transplantation in lymphoma associated with retention of fertility and normal pregnancies in females. *Leuk Lymphoma* 1997;28:27–32

101. Nugent D, Meirow D, Brook PF, *et al*. Transplantation in reproductive medicine: previous experience, present knowledge and future prospects. *Hum Reprod Update* 1997;3: 267–80

102. Blumenfeld Z, Dann E, Avivi I, *et al*. Fertility after treatment for Hodgkin's disease. *Ann Oncol* 2002;13(Suppl 1):138–47

APPENDIX 1

The following table shows the influence of age, gender, geographical location and race on the incidence of different cancers, 1993–1997. Values are expressed as age standardized rate (ASR)/100 000 person-years. Adapted from the International Association of Cancer Registries (Parking DM, Whelan SL, Ferlay J, *et al.*, eds. *Cancer Incidence in Five Continents*, Vol. VIII. IARC Scientific Publications No. 155. Lyon: IARC, 2000).

Site	Children (< 14 years) Males	Females	Adults (< 50 years) Males	Females
USA, San Francisco, California (non-Hispanic, white)				
Hodgkin's disease	0.34	0.72	4.35	4.47
Non-Hodgkin's lymphoma	1.97	0.85	20.0	5.17
Leukemia				
AML	0.48	0.74	1.83	1.79
ALL	5.69	4.12	1.77	0.82
Soft tissue	0.83	0.86	1.24	1.62
Bone	0.45	0.47	1.2	0.7
Testes	0.23	—	11.7	—
Breast	0	0	0.21	56.07
Ovary	—	0	—	9.11
Endometrium	—	0	—	5.2
Cervix	—	0	—	7.58
USA, Connecticut				
Hodgkin's disease	0.97	0.59	5.49	5.15
Non-Hodgkin's lymphoma	1.5	0.78	9.45	5.5
Leukemia				
AML	1.04	0.97	2.24	1.84
ALL	2.88	3.33	1.79	0.98
Soft tissue	0.76	0.45	1.53	1.1
Bone	0.83	0.73	1.04	0.68
Testes	0.39	—	9.8	—
Breast	0	0.07	0.095	54.19
Ovary	0	0.33	—	8.37
Endometrium	—	0	—	5.93
Cervix	—	0	—	7.81
UK, England				
Hodgkin's disease	0.66	0.34	3.16	2.59
Non-Hodgkin's lymphoma	1.12	0.45	5.26	3.03
Leukemia				
AML	0.91	0.77	1.82	1.56
ALL	3.84	3.08	1.31	0.63
Soft tissue	0.4	0.44	1.1	0.85
Bone	0.53	0.56	0.82	0.56
Testes	0.32	—	9.13	—
Breast	0	0.02	0.13	46.15
Ovary	—	0.29	—	6.23
Endometrium	—	0	—	2.03
Cervix	—	0.02	—	10.41
Germany				
Hodgkin's disease	0.49	0.44	3.69	2.35
Non-Hodgkin's lymphoma	1.68	0.45	4.96	3.36
Leukemia				
AML	0.99	1.41	3.14	2.14
ALL	5.32	3.42	1.57	0.83
Soft tissue	1.06	0.99	2.05	1.12
Bone	0.41	0.7	1.28	1.0
Testes	0.2	—	13.25	—
Breast	0	0	0.11	43.35
Ovary	—	0.22	—	5.08
Endometrium	—	0	—	2.68
Cervix	—	0	—	13.39
Denmark				
Hodgkin's disease	0.63	0.26	3.23	2.45
Non-Hodgkin's lymphoma	1.56	0.57	5.86	3.74
Leukemia				
AML	0.82	0.74	1.78	1.65
ALL	4.07	3.22	1.32	0.69
Soft tissue	0.38	0.46	1.16	1.19
Bone	0.75	0.71	0.78	0.67
Testes	0.39	—	17.75	—
Breast	0	0	0.16	46.65
Ovary	—	0.13	—	6.29
Endometrium	—	0	—	2.47
Cervix	—	0.04	—	15.56
Singapore				
Hodgkin's disease	0.16	0.07	0.81	0.62
Non-Hodgkin's lymphoma	0.98	0.32	3.98	2.54
Leukemia				
AML	1.14	0.93	1.97	1.48
ALL	4.13	2.53	0.83	0.44
Soft tissue	0.37	0.13	1.04	0.78
Bone	0.21	0.28	0.65	0.33
Testes	0.69	—	1.27	—
Breast	0	0	0.17	36.06
Ovary	—	0.82	—	9.7
Endometrium	—	0	—	4.69
Cervix	—	0	—	9.61
Israel				
Hodgkin's disease	1.07	0.7	4.13	4.45
Non-Hodgkin's lymphoma	2.03	1.1	7.82	5.72
Leukemia				
AML	0.88	0.56	1.96	2.0
ALL	2.13	1.68	1.61	0.95
Soft tissue	0.17	0.15	0.54	0.48
Bone	0.92	0.55	1.70	1.19
Testes	0.3	—	5.1	—
Breast	0	0.02	0.48	50.86
Ovary	—	0.39	—	7.75
Endometrium	—	0	—	3.27
Cervix	—	0	—	5.41

AML, acute myeloid leukemia; ALL, acute lymphocytic leukemia

Vulnerability of the reproductive system to radiotherapy and chemotherapy
3

N. Salooja, N. Reddy and J. Apperley

INTRODUCTION

Advances in the treatment of cancer using radiotherapy and chemotherapy have improved the survival rate for many conditions. This is particularly evident in patients with childhood cancer or hematological and testicular malignancies. Radiotherapy and chemotherapeutic agents are toxic to healthy cells as well as to their target cancer cells, and successful treatment may be associated with long-term morbidity. Significant and in some cases permanent reproductive dysfunction creates a distressing long-term sequel to therapy in young people who make an otherwise good recovery.

Normal reproduction in both sexes requires a complex interplay between gonads and the hypothalamic–pituitary–endocrine axis. In addition, the uterus must be receptive to implantation and capable of effecting appropriate growth in pregnancy. Gonadotropin releasing hormone (GnRH) released from neurons of the hypothalamus regulates the synthesis and secretion of follicle stimulating hormone (FSH) and luteinizing hormone (LH) by the anterior pituitary. In males, these hormones stimulate spermatogenesis and the production of testosterone, which in turn is required for the development and maintenance of secondary sexual characteristics. The central functional unit of the mammalian ovary is the follicle, consisting of a germ cell (the oocyte) together with the surrounding somatic cells. Intrinsically linked to follicular development are the production of the hormones estrogen, progesterone and inhibin which are required for puberty, development of secondary sexual characteristics and normal functioning of the reproductive tract.

Tissues in the reproductive system which are vulnerable to damage from chemo/radiotherapy include the germ cells, the sex steroid-producing cells of the gonads, cells within the hypothalamus, pituitary, and, in women, the uterus and female reproductive tract. Destruction of germ cells can lead to failure to progress through puberty, or infertility in later life. In women, it can also result in a premature menopause with its associated endocrine, somatic and psychological changes. Damage to the reproductive tract and uterus can lead to sexual dysfunction, affect embryo implantation adversely and increase the risk of pregnancy complications.

THE FEMALE REPRODUCTIVE SYSTEM

Oogenesis

During fetal development the germ cells undergo a process of proliferation by a series of mitotic divisions to form oogonia. The oogonia differentiate into primary oocytes which progress to the diplotene stage of prophase of the first meiotic division where they remain arrested until after puberty. Condensation of mesenchymal cells (granulosa cells) around the diplotene oocyte gives rise to the primordial follicle. By mid-gestation the number of germ cells peak at 6–7 million.

Subsequently mitosis ceases and there is a massive depletion of germ cells by a process of programed cell death or apoptosis[1]. No similar rate of depletion is seen again. As a consequence of the termination of germ stem cell mitosis in fetal life, the loss of oocytes (either physiological or secondary to external insults) cannot be replaced. This is distinctly different from the male, where mitotic proliferation of spermatogonial stem cells continues throughout adult reproductive life (see below).

There are currently several paradigms for oocyte loss[2] and the specific pathway used by follicles to die may be determined by both the developmental status of the oocyte and the stimulus responsible for apoptosis[3]. Potential components of these pathways include p53[4,5] and members of bcl-2[6-9] and CASP gene families[3,8,10,11]. The protein Bax is a member of the bcl-2 family and its central role in some models of oocyte death has been highlighted by studies involving Bax-deficient female mice. The oocytes from these animals are resistant to developmental death during gametogenesis[12]. A role for the sphingolipid ceramide has been proposed upstream of Bax[13]. Mutant mice which lack the ceramide-generating enzyme, acid sphingomyelinase (ASMase), are also resistant to the normal apoptotic deletion of fetal oocytes and are born with a significantly larger reserve of primordial oocytes than their normal counterparts[14]. Conversely, a metabolite of ceramide, sphingosine-1-phosphate (S1P), has been shown to counterbalance apoptosis induced by ceramide analogs in some somatic cell types[15,16].

Because of the fixed initial endowment of germ cells the newborn female enters life still far from her reproductive potential yet having already lost 80% of her oocytes. Compartmentalization of the ovary into an outer cortex and inner medulla has occurred, with the cortex containing 1–2 million oocytes. These are contained in the primordial follicles, which are in varying states of maturation. By the onset of puberty the number of oocytes will have been reduced further to less than 500 000 and during the next 30–40 years of reproductive life, 400 to 500 will be selected to ovulate. The menopause occurs when the majority of functioning follicles have been lost.

Folliculogenesis

Prior to birth and throughout life, there is continual recruitment of small numbers of primordial follicles to differentiate and grow in a process called folliculogenesis. This process takes 6–9 months. As the primordial follicle grows it passes through three stages of development en route to ovulation: first, the primary or preantral follicle, then a secondary or antral follicle (which accounts for 95% of the estradiol production during the reproductive life of a woman) and finally a preovulatory follicle (Figure 1).

In childhood there are low levels of gonadotropin production, little response of the pituitary to GnRH and maximal suppression of the hypothalamus. Although follicles frequently reach the antral stage, the majority will undergo atresia because of inadequate gonadotropin stimulation. From about the age of 8 years, peripubertal increases in LH and FSH lead to increasing levels of follicular activity and estradiol production, culminating in menarche. Regular recruitment of primordial follicles into a pool of growing follicles first occurs at puberty (see legend to Figure 1). The number of follicles that enter the growth phase in each cycle appears to be a fixed proportion of the primordial follicles remaining in the ovary. This is a critical characteristic of the regulation of the ovarian follicular pool[18]. Only one follicle is selected to ovulate, however, while the rest undergo atresia. Immediately prior to ovulation meiosis resumes and the first meiotic division is completed giving rise to the secondary oocyte. The secondary oocyte is ovulated while proceeding to the second metaphase of meiosis. Completion of the second meiotic division occurs at fertilization.

The uterus

Pregnancy is possible without gonads, but not without the uterus. A uterus capable of normal function is essential for implantation,

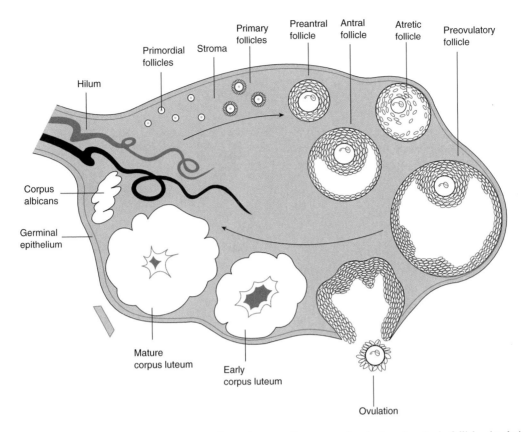

Figure 1 Folliculogenesis and the menstrual cycle. At the start of a menstrual cycle there is a rise in follicle stimulating hormone (FSH) levels followed by an increase in luteinizing hormone (LH). Under the influence of FSH, a cohort of follicles is recruited for development into secondary follicles. As the follicles grow the output of estradiol and the peptide inhibin increases. By about day 12 a threshold concentration of estradiol is exceeded and there is a surge in the release of gonadotropins triggering ovulation. The output of estrogen and inhibin decline and shortly after ovulation, under the influence of LH, the ruptured follicle develops into the corpus luteum which produces large amounts of progesterone, some estrogen and inhibin. In the absence of fertilization, the corpus luteum involutes forming the corpus albicans, estrogen and progesterone levels fall and a new cycle ensues. Reproduced with permission from reference 17

differentiation and growth of the fetus to term. The three major functional components of the uterus are the endometrium, the myometrium and cervix. The endometrium is further divided into two zones. A superficial functional layer, containing coiled 'spiral' blood vessels, undergoes characteristic changes in response to cyclic steroid hormones (estrogen and progesterone) to prepare the endometrium for pregnancy. The basal layer remains relatively unchanged during each menstrual cycle, but following menstruation provides stem cells for the renewal of the functional layer.

Both estrogen and progesterone act sequentially to regulate the cellular concentration of their individual receptors and to create an endometrium receptive to a developing embryo. Implantation involves a complex interaction between implanting embryo and the primed maternal endometrium. The endometrium is receptive to embryonic implantation during a defined window which is spatially and temporally restricted. Early studies have shown that in women this brief period of receptivity or 'implantation window' of 3–4 days occurs 7–8 days after ovulation. In the absence of implantation the corpus luteum regresses and the levels of estrogen and progesterone fall. The withdrawal of hormonal support leads to a breakdown of the endometrium and menstruation.

In the absence of sex steroids, the endometrium is completely inactive. If there is no functional damage it may still be capable of facilitating implantation and pregnancy if subsequently exposed to adequate doses of exogenous estrogen and progesterone.

THE MALE REPRODUCTIVE SYSTEM

The adult testis produces gametes (spermatogenesis) and synthesizes sex steroids (androgens and estrogen) and peptides (inhibin and activin). Androgens are required for the differentiation of male characteristics in the fetus, for pubertal development and for spermatogenesis. The bulk of the testis is made up of seminiferous tubules between which lie the Leydig cells, which synthesize testosterone. The seminiferous tubules contain two types of cells: the germ cells and the Sertoli cells. A physiological barrier in the form of tight gap junctions (blood–testis barrier) exists between adjacent Sertoli cells, producing two compartments. In the basal compartment spermatogonial stem cells reside and in the upper adluminal compartment cytodifferentiation or spermiogenesis occurs. This barrier enables the later stages of spermatogenesis to occur in a controlled chemical environment and, furthermore, it prevents sperm leaking into the systemic and lymphatic circulation. The barrier is absent prepubertally but develops prior to spermatogenesis. The seminiferous tubules lead to the epididymis where further maturation of the sperm occurs.

Spermatogenesis

In the prenatal period under the influence of human chorionic gonadotropin and subsequently pituitary gonadotropin, germ cells undergo rapid mitotic division. During childhood the levels of gonadotropin are

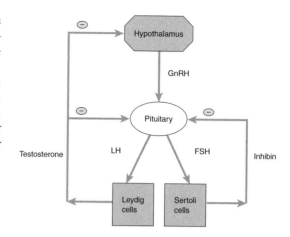

Figure 2 Hypothalamic–pituitary–endocrine axis in the male. GnRH, gonadotropin releasing hormone; LH, luteinizing hormone; FSH, follicle stimulating hormone

low, but cell proliferation continues albeit at a markedly reduced rate. Despite this low gonadotropic state, cell numbers increase significantly during the prepubertal period and infantile germ cells mature into spermatogonia. The number of Sertoli cells and spermatogonial stem cells produced during this time is important because, in large part, these cells will determine the maximum capacity of the testis to produce sperm during adulthood.

At puberty there is reactivation of hypothalamic GnRH secretion that stimulates pituitary FSH and LH. LH stimulates the synthesis of testosterone and it acts together with FSH on the Sertoli cells to initiate and maintain spermatogenesis. The secretion of hormones from the hypothalamic–pituitary unit is regulated by a negative feedback mechanism involving steroid hormones and the peptide inhibin, which is produced by the testes (Figure 2). Testosterone has a negative feedback effect on LH which is mediated by both inhibition of GnRH at the hypothalamic level and (more weakly) inhibition of LH secretion by the pituitary. Low levels of testosterone result in high levels of LH. When sperm production is impaired the level of FSH is elevated.

The germ cells in the basal compartment of the tubule are known as spermatogonia. Type A spermatogonia divide to both replenish

Table 1 Classes of chemotherapy and their action

Class of agent	Examples	Mechanism of action
Alkylating agents	cyclophosphamide mechlorethamine chlorambucil busulfan melphalan procarbazine*	crosslinks DNA strands, and inhibits RNA formation
Antimetabolites	methotrexate 5-fluorouracil cytarabine	inhibits pyrimidine or purine synthesis or incorporation into DNA
Vinca alkaloids	vincristine vinblastine	dissociation of microtubules leading to disruption of spindle
Antibiotics	daunorubicin bleomycin	various e.g. DNA intercalation, inhibition of transcription
Designer drugs	imatinib	tyrosine kinase inhibitor

*Mechanism of action not fully elucidated; probably alkylates DNA

the stem cell pool and to form type B spermatogonia. The latter move from the basal to the upper adluminal compartment of the seminiferous tubule, where they divide to form the primary spermatocytes. The type A spermatogonia are relatively resistant to external insults such as chemo/radiotherapy because of their low mitotic activity, while type B spermatogonia are highly radiosensitive. If damage to the testis occurs, type A spermatogonia undergo mitosis to replenish the affected spermatogonial population. Complete destruction of the type A spermatogonial stem cells, for example by radiotherapy or vascular compromise, will cause an irreversible loss of spermatogenic capacity.

The primary spermatocytes undergo meiosis, forming the secondary spermatocytes and then (following the second meiotic division) the spermatids. These undergo spermiogenesis to develop into spermatozoa. Although fully differentiated, further maturation occurs during passage through the epididymis. The fully motile sperm still remain incapable of fertilization until they undergo a further process of 'capacitation' in the female reproductive tract. The total duration of spermatogenesis up to the production of ejaculatory semen is approximately 65–75 days. This time period

has important implications for the duration of risk for the mutagenic effects of chemo/radiotherapy.

VULNERABILITY OF THE REPRODUCTIVE SYSTEM TO CANCER TREATMENT

Radiotherapy produces lethal cell damage, a large part of which is due to its production of double-strand DNA breaks that are not amenable to repair. Chemotherapy agents vary in their mode of action but all are capable of interrupting the normal cellular proliferation cycle (Table 1). The ongoing processes of cellular division and differentiation in male germ cell production renders them highly susceptible to damage by such agents. Within the ovarian follicle, both the germ cell and the somatic cells are vulnerable to damage from radiotherapy and chemotherapy. Postnatal oocytes are mitotically inactive, however, so the toxicity of radiotherapy and chemotherapy on this cell population is unlikely to occur via mechanisms which involve arrest of cell proliferation.

A second mechanism by which radiotherapy and chemotherapy cause cell death is the induction of apoptosis[19,20]. Data suggest that the toxicity of these agents to oocytes can be exerted via the same apoptotic pathways which account for the physiological oocyte losses described above. In support of this, genetically engineered Bax-deficient mice are resistant to apoptosis induced by chemicals such as doxorubicin[6], polycyclic aromatic hydrocarbons[21,22] and 4-vinylcyclohexene diepoxide[3]. Similarly, *ex vivo* oocytes lacking the gene for ASMase resist both developmental apoptosis and apoptosis induced by doxorubicin[14], and radiation-induced oocyte loss in female mice can be prevented by *in vivo* administration of S1P[23]. The enzyme Caspase-2 also has a role in oocyte death both during fetal ovarian development and after chemotherapy[2,24].

Changes to the uterus, cervix, vagina and vulva following chemo/radiotherapy are due to a combination of direct damage from treatment and secondary estrogen insufficiency. In patients who are treated with allogeneic peripheral blood or bone marrow transplants (stem cell transplants), a conditioning regimen is used to eradicate underlying malignant disease and suppress the host immune system. The subsequent infusion of donor-derived immune cells can lead to graft-versus-host disease (GVHD). This process can also contribute to vulvovaginal changes which occur following treatment. GVHD has been implicated in additional adverse reproductive sequelae of chemo/radiotherapy such as sexual dysfunction[25], reduced uterine and ovarian volumes[26] and decreased sperm counts[27].

Radiation to the hypothalamic–pituitary axis in both sexes can lead to irreversible deficiencies of the hormones of the anterior pituitary, which may be delayed by months or years following irradiation. Histological studies of the brain following external radiation indicate that the hypothalamus is particularly vulnerable to such damage compared to the pituitary, but the reasons for the relative resistance of the pituitary to damage are not fully understood[28].

Very recently, a new class of agents has been introduced into clinical practice in oncology – the so-called 'designer drugs'. These novel therapies are specifically designed to target parts of signal transduction pathways within malignant cells. By far the most successful of these drugs is imatinib (also known as Glivec®, Gleevec®, STI 571), which is used in the management of chronic myeloid leukemia[29,30]. Imatinib specifically inhibits a small number of tyrosine kinases, including abl, the platelet-derived growth factor receptors α and β, and c-kit. The clinical effects of their action on the human reproductive system are currently unknown but animal studies have indicated their potential to impair spermatogenesis and be teratogenic, at least in some species.

ASSESSMENT OF GONADAL DYSFUNCTION

In men, quantitative and qualitative semen analysis can provide useful information relating to preservation/restoration of fertility post-treatment, with the stipulation that abnormal parameters may improve with time. In women, direct end-stage assessment of the effects of chemo/radiotherapy is not routinely possible. Clinical studies therefore rely on indirect assessments of damage such as details of menstrual cycles, menopausal symptoms and pregnancy rates. While data on conception and successful pregnancy after treatment are a useful source of information for pretreatment counseling, rates of conception in patients with life-threatening illnesses may be low for reasons other than infertility, for example psychological or sexual factors and overall performance status. In addition, underlying disease can have a profound effect on the reproductive system even before treatment has been given.

Endocrine profiles in both sexes can provide additional information relating to gonadal function (Figures 2 and 3). Damage to the ovary is typically accompanied by a fall in estrogen levels and a compensatory increase in the gonadotropic hormones FSH and LH. Within the testis, sex steroid production occurs in a cellular compartment distinct from the germ cells which is less sensitive to the effects of chemo/radiotherapy. Damage to the germinal epithelium is therefore associated with

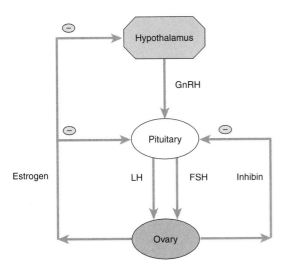

Figure 3 Hypothalamic–pituitary–endocrine axis in the female. GnRH, gonadotropin releasing hormone; LH, luteinizing hormone; FSH, follicle stimulating hormone

reduced sperm counts and an increased FSH level, but testosterone levels may be unaffected. Leydig cell dysfunction is typically accompanied by both a reduction in testosterone and raised LH levels.

Even in situations where these standard clinical and biochemical parameters fall within normal ranges, significant undetected gonadal damage may have occurred. Women with diminished ovarian reserve have a limited window of opportunity to conceive naturally because they are at risk of premature ovarian failure (POF). As such, it would be useful to be able to identify these patients so that they can be appropriately counseled regarding their prospects of fertility. Identifying this group of women is difficult. Recently, the use of three-dimensional ultrasound and power Doppler imaging to assess the number of antral follicles, ovarian volume and stromal blood flow has been introduced to assess ovarian reserve in patients with normal gonadotropin levels. Low antral follicle counts, reduced ovarian volume and decreased stromal blood flow are all considered to be a reflection of reduced ovarian follicular reserve[31–34].

Ultrasound and Doppler studies can also be used to assess uterine function. Additional information on endometrial function can be gained by histology and immunohistological techniques[35,36].

GONADAL DYSFUNCTION FOLLOWING RADIOTHERAPY

Adult men

Information on the effects of measured doses of radiation to the testes is available from several sources. First, there are experimental data relating to administration of graded doses of radiation to normal volunteers. Second, there are patients whose testes have been irradiated as treatment for malignant disease. Data from this source may be limited by the impact of the disease itself on gonadal function. Finally, there are data involving exposure of experimental animals to irradiation, although it is unlikely that information from this source could be fully extrapolated to man.

A study described by Rowley and colleagues[37] details the administration of 8–600 cGy radiation to 67 apparently healthy inmate volunteers from the Oregon State Penitentiary. Sperm counts and morphology were examined before the experiment together with testicular biopsy. Spermatogonia were the most radiosensitive cells, then spermatocytes and finally spermatids. The type B spermatogonia were the most radiosensitive cell type, showing quantitative and qualitative changes after only 8 cGy. From these data (Table 2) it is clear that damage to the testis by radiotherapy is dose-related. In addition, the speed of onset and chance of recovery depend on the dose received.

A considerable amount of data on the clinical effects of testicular irradiation have accrued from patients treated with radiotherapy for testicular cancer or Hodgkin's disease. In general these clinical studies support the data described by Rowley and co-workers, and highlight the greater sensitivity of the germinal epithelium to radiation damage compared to the testosterone-producing Leydig cells. Thus a transient fall in sperm count with

Table 2   The effects of irradiation on sperm counts of healthy volunteer males

Radiation dose* (cGy)	Cells damaged	Time for count to fall	Time for complete recovery of sperm count
8	spermatogonia (type B)		
100	spermatogonia	67 days	9–18 months
200–300	spermatocytes	46 days	30 months
400–600	spermatids	rapid	5 years or never

*Dose of radiation at which qualitative changes in sperm occur

full recovery within 24 months is frequently observed following doses of radiation below 1 Gy[38,39].

With higher doses of irradiation (20–30 Gy), falls in testosterone levels with concomitant increases in LH occur[40,41]. Raised LH and reduced testosterone levels have also been noted in adult men receiving radiotherapy in the range 14–20 Gy for testicular cancer. In a study including 44 patients receiving doses of 14 ($n = 13$), 16 or 18 ($n = 12$) and 20 Gy ($n = 19$), significant increases in LH levels together with a reduction in testosterone levels were seen at all doses. These persisted for more than 5 years without dose-dependency[42].

Animal data suggest that fractionation of radiotherapy can increase its gonadal toxicity at least in some species. In the mouse, a single dose of 16–30 Gy proves sterilizing compared to a cumulative fractionated dose of only 5–5.7 Gy. In the guinea pig a single dose of 45 Gy causes sterility compared to a fractionated total dose of 21 Gy[43]. There is some evidence to suggest fractionation is also deleterious for human testicular function. Of 10 men given inverted Y field inguinal irradiation for Hodgkin's disease, an estimated total testicular dose of 1.4–3 Gy was administered in 14–26 fractions. In the immediate postirradiation period, all patients were azoospermic[43]. Follow-up data were initially limited to a maximum of 15 months for four patients and 40 months for one, and azoospermia persisted throughout. Subsequent follow-up data have since been published and no recovery of spermatogenesis 17–43 months after irradiation was shown in patients who received

doses of 1.4–2.6 Gy. Recovery had occurred, however, in two patients who received radiation doses of 1.2 Gy[38].

Prepubertal males

As discussed above, the germinal epithelium of the testis is more sensitive to the effects of irradiation than the Leydig cells. As such, normal progression through puberty is common even where there is impairment of spermatogenesis. In two studies evaluating boys who had received total body irradiation (TBI) prior to bone marrow transplantation, all had normal testosterone levels following treatment and normal pubertal development[44,45]. Despite this, the chances of recovering fertility following TBI is low. In a study which evaluated eight boys who had progressed normally through puberty following 2–10 Gy for nephroblastoma, testicular volumes were reduced and sperm counts low[46].

Leydig cell function and testosterone production are at risk following higher doses of irradiation and the prepubertal Leydig cell may be more sensitive to damage than in the adult. In a study which encompassed patients of varying ages, children were more likely than adults to have elevated gonadotropin and reduced testosterone following testicular irradiation[47].

Adult women

The three major determinants of the clinical effects of irradiation on the ovary are the radiation field, the dose administered and the age of the patient at the time of treatment. Significant doses of irradiation may be received by the ovaries in the treatment of abdominal or pelvic malignancies, with the use of craniospinal irradiation for malignancies of the central nervous system (CNS) or acute lymphocytic leukemia (ALL), and with pelvic nodal irradiation in the treatment of Hodgkin's lymphoma. TBI used as conditioning for stem cell transplantation (SCT) also exposes the ovaries to significant doses of irradiation. In contrast, there is a low incidence of ovarian failure in women who receive irradiation above the pelvic brim[48,49].

Animal studies have indicated that increasing doses of radiation lead to loss of primordial follicles in a dose-dependent manner[50]. The dose at which 50% of human oocytes are lost (LD_{50}) has been quoted as close to 4 Gy[51] and more recently this estimation has been revised to < 2 Gy[52]. The clinical significance of losing 50% of the oocytes will depend on the number which remain following treatment. Reduction in oocyte numbers below a critical threshold will result in POF. Younger women with a high starting number of oocytes would be expected to tolerate higher doses of radiation before experiencing POF, and this is borne out in clinical practice. Chiarelli and colleagues evaluated the risk of POF and infertility in a group of young women who had received abdominal or pelvic irradiation in childhood, compared to women treated by surgery alone. The median age of the women evaluated was 28 years (range 18–49). The relative risk (RR) of POF was 1.02 (95% confidence interval (CI) 0.29–3.59) following radiation with doses < 20 Gy, 1.37 (95% CI 0.57–3.25) with 20–34.99 Gy and 3.27 (95% CI 1.57–6.81) with doses ≥ 35 Gy[53]. In the same study, a radiation dose-related reduction in age-adjusted fertility was also observed. In women receiving < 20 Gy of abdominopelvic irradiation the relative fertility was 1.42; following 20–34.99 Gy it was 0.78; and following 35 Gy or more the relative fertility was 0.68.

In women over the age of 40 years, considerably lower doses of irradiation cause ovarian failure. Doll and Smith[54] reported ovarian failure in 97% of 2068 patients who received between 5.0 and 10.5 Gy for dysfunctional uterine bleeding. Most (91%) of these women were over 40 years, with 20% older than 50 years.

Where TBI is used as conditioning for SCT, a dose of 8–15 Gy may be administered either as a single dose or in fractions. The Genoa transplant team followed up 79 women who had received TBI (8.4–12 Gy) containing conditioning protocols for leukemia with regular measurements of LH, FSH, estradiol levels and pelvic ultrasonography. Gonadal function was recovered in ten of 74 women who had been postmenarchal at the time of transplant, and there was one pregnancy. The actuarial chance of having a menstrual period at 10 years was 100% in women under the age of 18, compared to 15% in those over the age of 18 when transplanted[55]. Data from the Seattle transplant team[56] on 144 patients receiving TBI and cyclophosphamide revealed recovery of ovarian function in nine women between 3 and 7 years following transplant, all of whom were younger than 25 years of age at the time of transplant.

Prepubertal females

The prepubertal ovary is susceptible to damage from radiotherapy and this may manifest as failure to go through puberty or premature ovarian failure. Of 19 girls who received up to 30 Gy for abdominal malignancies, 12 required hormonal assistance through puberty and 18 developed primary ovarian failure[51]. Lower doses of irradiation are compatible with normal progression through puberty although these patients remain at risk of a premature menopause[57]. Girls treated with craniospinal irradiation for ALL are also at risk of arrested puberty and this risk is increased if abdominal irradiation is given concurrently. A follow-up study by Hamre and associates[58] included data on gonadal function in girls administered craniospinal irradiation alone or in combination with abdominal irradiation for ALL. Elevated gonadotropins and arrested or delayed puberty occurred in

93% of children receiving craniospinal plus abdominal irradiation and in 49% of children receiving craniospinal irradiation only.

HYPOTHALAMIC–PITUITARY DYSFUNCTION FOLLOWING RADIOTHERAPY

Patients at risk of pituitary hormone deficiencies following radiation include patients treated for pituitary or primary brain tumours, nasopharyngeal carcinomas, those receiving cranial irradiation for ALL and those who have received TBI. Cranial irradiation has dose-dependent effects on CNS function, some of which may be greater when radiation is administered at a younger age[41,59]. There is also some evidence that the brains of girls are affected more than boys; girls do less well than boys in cognitive tests following cranial irradiation[60] and they are more likely to experience weight gain and obesity[61]. Generally growth hormone (GH) is the first hormone to be affected, followed by gonadotropin, adrenocorticotropic hormone and finally thyroid stimulating hormone. In children, high doses of irradiation exceeding 50 Gy to the hypothalamic–pituitary axis may lead to gonadotropin deficiency[62]. Lower doses in the range 25–47.5 Gy, such as may be given for the treatment of brain tumours, may paradoxically be associated with precocious puberty in both sexes[63]. Following doses of 1.8–2.4 Gy, such as may be administered during the treatment of ALL, only girls are at risk of precocious puberty[64–66].

In adults with pituitary tumours, the risk of gonadotropin deficiency following doses in excess of 30 Gy is 60% at 4 years[67]. This high incidence of hormone deficit, however, may in part have been due to damage from the underlying pituitary malignancy.

Following the lower doses of cranial irradiation given to patients with ALL, central hypogonadism is rare. Birkebaek and colleagues[68] reported the long-term follow-up (10–21 years) of endocrine function in 30 patients (15 female) treated for ALL in childhood. All patients had been treated with

a combination chemotherapy, and 18 of 30 patients had also received cranial irradiation at a dose of 24 Gy in 15 fractions. FSH, LH and estradiol/testosterone measurements were used to evaluate gonadal function. Half (nine of 18) of the patient group receiving cranial irradiation had evidence of GH deficiency, compared to one of 12 patients treated with chemotherapy only. Although GH deficiency was common in the irradiated group, only one patient (male) had evidence of central hypogonadism. Another patient (male) had hypergonadotropic hypogonadism but all other patients had an apparently normal pituitary–gonadal axis.

A more detailed assessment of the hypothalamic–pituitary–ovarian axis in female survivors of childhood ALL indicates the presence of subtle ovulatory disturbances in some patients. Bath and associates[69] investigated the production of LH and the LH surge and estimated the length of the luteal phase in 12 women with regular menstrual cycles who had received 18–24 Gy cranial irradiation in childhood. The production of LH and the LH surge were reduced compared to a control group of healthy women, and the luteal phase was significantly shorter. These changes may be relevant to reproductive potential and further follow-up is required to evaluate this.

UTERINE AND UROGENITAL DYSFUNCTION FOLLOWING RADIOTHERAPY

In women who have been exposed to abdominal irradiation, uterine growth and function may also be compromised particularly when irradiation has occurred in childhood or adolescence when optimum growth of the uterus is normally achieved. The changes that occur not only adversely affect implantation but also increase the risk of miscarriage, premature labor and low-birth-weight infants. The physical characteristics of the uterus, such as length, endometrial thickness and blood flow (pulsatility index), were investigated in ten women aged 15–31 years with POF following 20–30 Gy abdominal radiotherapy. Data were compared with a control group of 22 women (median age 31 years, range 23–37) with POF who had not been exposed to abdominal radiotherapy. In the control group the uterine length was 7.3 ± 0.6 cm (mean ± 2 standard errors) versus 4.1 ± 0.8 cm in the radiotherapy group ($p < 0.01$). Bilateral Doppler signals were clearly seen from the uterine arteries in the control group, but were absent bilaterally in five out of ten and unilaterally in three of the remaining five patients who had received radiotherapy[70].

Even following TBI where the exposure to irradiation is considerably lower, significant impairment of uterine function has been described. Bath and co-workers[71] studied uterine characteristics of volume, endometrial thickness, uterine blood flow and endometrial histology in women who had received TBI in childhood in the context of SCT. They found that baseline uterine volume and vascularity were considerably decreased in these patients. Both of these parameters were improved, however, by a regimen of hormone replacement administered as transdermal estradiol patches and vaginal progesterone pessaries. Although uterine volumes were reduced to almost 40% of adult volume following three cycles of treatment, there was a significant increase from baseline readings of 6.5 ml (range 1.7–12.7) to 16.5 ml (range 8.3–27.4). Interestingly, the volume of the uterus after treatment correlated to the age at which exposure to irradiation occurred; those treated before puberty had a smaller increase in uterine volume than was noted in postpubertal women. It is possible that the basalis layer of the endometrium, which contains stem cells for development of the functional endometrium, is more easily affected in young girls where the uterus has not yet achieved complete growth.

The above study demonstrates that hormone replacement therapy is associated with re-establishment of uterine blood flow and increased uterine volume following radiotherapy. However, we do not know whether the currently recommended dose of estrogen replacement is adequate to achieve optimum uterine growth in the adolescent woman treated with radiotherapy in childhood. Prospective studies are required to assess the changes which can occur when the appropriate doses of hormone therapy are started at an early stage.

Urogenital problems following radiotherapy are frequent and include atrophic abnormalities, chronic cystitis-like symptoms and, in more severe cases, vaginal stenosis. In a study evaluating 44 female SCT recipients 261–4628 days following SCT, atrophic abnormalities were noted in 33/36 recipients of TBI compared to two out of eight women who had chemotherapy only as conditioning[72]. Changes included a reduction in size of the vagina, uterus and cervix, reduced vaginal elasticity, atrophic vulvovaginitis and introital stenosis. Marked vaginal stenosis requiring surgical intervention to correct menstrual obstruction has been described in a woman following SCT. In this case, chronic GVHD contributed to the severity of the clinical picture[73].

PREGNANCY OUTCOME FOLLOWING RADIOTHERAPY

From the discussion above it is clear that the effects of radiotherapy on the uterus would be expected to lead to an increased incidence of miscarriage, premature delivery and low-birth-weight babies. In clinical practice there is indeed an increased risk of adverse pregnancy outcome following abdominal or pelvic irradiation or TBI. Female survivors of Wilms' tumor who received abdominal radiation have been noted to have an increased risk of miscarriage and an increased incidence of low-birth-weight infants and perinatal morbidity[74–76].

The Childhood Cancer Survivor Study (CCSS) reported pregnancy outcome among 1915 female survivors of childhood cancer who had 4029 pregnancies between them[77]. Women who had received pelvic irradiation were at risk for low-birth-weight offspring. The relative risk of miscarriage was significantly increased in women who received craniospinal irradiation for ALL (RR = 3.63, 95% CI 1.7–7.78) compared to women who had no radiation. Women who received cranial irradiation only for ALL did not have a significantly increased risk of miscarriage (RR = 1.6, 95% CI 1.02–1.94).

An increased incidence of pregnancy complications has also been described in women who have received TBI together with chemotherapy as conditioning for SCT in the treatment of hematological malignancy. Data from the Seattle transplant team on 13 women conceiving after TBI indicated an increased incidence of miscarriage, premature labor and low-birth-weight babies[78]. Data from the European group for Blood and Marrow Transplantation (EBMT) on 12 women conceiving naturally after TBI also revealed an increased incidence of preterm delivery, reduced median gestation, and an increased risk of offspring who were small for their gestational age[79]. An increase in stillbirth has been noted in partners of male Sellafield workers exposed to irradiation prior to conception[80]. It is not clear whether this association represents a causal relation; nor is it clear what biological mechanism could explain such a link. Data from the CCSS on pregnancy outcome of partners of male survivors of childhood cancer did not identify adverse pregnancy outcomes following administration of radiotherapy. There were very few live births, however, among the partners of men whose testes were in the radiotherapy field[79].

ASSISTED CONCEPTION FOLLOWING RADIOTHERAPY

Women who are likely to be rendered infertile by their cancer treatment can undergo *in vitro* fertilization with cryopreservation of their embryos prior to chemo/radiotherapy. This, however, requires that the underlying disease can tolerate a minimum of 4 weeks delay in treatment for superovulation and egg collection. It also requires that the patient has a committed partner to provide sperm. For women who do not have a partner, cryopreservation of unfertilized oocytes may be considered. Unfertilized oocytes do not readily survive the freeze–thaw process[82], however, and subsequent fertilization and pregnancy rates are very low. In situations where a delay in treatment is unacceptable, the use of donor embryos offers hope of parenthood post-chemo/radiotherapy. In otherwise healthy women who are unable to conceive naturally, pregnancy rates using cryopreserved embryos are 15–20%[83]; following the use of donated oocytes with a normal uterus, pregnancy rates are 25–45%[84]. There is a lack of data on the success of assisted reproductive technologies (ART) following irradiation, however, and there are legitimate concerns about the ability of the irradiated uterus to facilitate implantation, growth and development of the fetus. A successful full-term pregnancy following the use of donor oocytes has been described in a woman with ovarian failure following 12 Gy TBI[85]. In our own unit there have been three pregnancies in five women treated with TBI undergoing ART using cryopreserved embryos (unpublished data). Two of these pregnancies ended in a miscarriage at 12–13 weeks' gestation. A third pregnancy was successful but premature (34 weeks)[86]. Data from the EBMT also highlight an increased incidence of preterm labor using ART following TBI[79]. Among nine women who had 12 pregnancies there were five live births, and incidences of premature labor and low-birth-weight infants were significantly higher than for a normal population.

GONADAL DYSFUNCTION FOLLOWING CHEMOTHERAPY

Adult men

Testicular damage due to chemotherapy was first reported in 1948, with a description of azoospermia in 27/30 men at autopsy following treatment with nitrogen mustard[87]. By the late 1960s there were also reports of testicular toxicity due to other alkylating agents (Table 1), namely busulfan, chlorambucil, cyclophosphamide and procarbazine[88]. Testicular biopsy

Table 3 Gonadal recovery in men following stem cell transplantation (SCT) conditioned with chemotherapy-only protocols

Type of SCT	Conditioning	n	Gonadal recovery (%)	Study
Allogeneic	CY	109	61	Sanders et al., 1996[78]
Allogeneic	BUCY	46	17	Sanders et al., 1996[78]
Allogeneic	BUCY*	26	42	Grigg et al., 2000[27]
Autologous	BEAM	11	0	Jacob et al., 1998[102]

CY, cyclophosphamide (200 mg/kg); CY*, cyclophosphamide (120 mg/kg); BU, busulfan; BEAM, BCNU, etoposide, cytarabine and melphalan

following such treatment shows aplasia of the germinal epithelium, atrophic tubules and peritubular fibrosis. These histological changes are associated with a reduction of testicular volume, reduced or absent sperm count and infertility. As with radiotherapy, chemotherapy is more toxic to the germinal epithelium than to the Leydig cells and animal studies indicate that the differentiating spermatogoonia are the most sensitive germ cells[89]. Although Leydig cells are more resistant to chemotherapy, significant rises in LH following chemotherapy indicative of Leydig cell dysfunction have been widely described[90–94].

In men the three most important factors in predicting gonadal dysfunction following chemotherapy-only protocols are the drug(s) used, the dose received and underlying disease. Most studies documenting reduced fertility prior to chemotherapy relate to patients with Hodgkin's disease or testicular cancer. A reduction in sperm count before treatment has been detected in 36–40% of patients with Hodgkin's disease[95–97] and in more than 50% of men with testicular cancer[98,99]. Studies which also take into account qualitative changes in sperm give higher overall estimates of sperm dysfunction. For example, in patients with Hodgkin's disease, up to 70% have abnormal sperm analysis (quantitative plus qualitative changes) prior to chemotherapy[96,98,100].

Cytotoxic agents within all chemotherapy classes may be associated with at least temporary impairment of spermatogenesis. Drugs regularly associated with permanent germ cell dysfunction include vinblastine, cytarabine, and the platinum analogs cisplatin and

carboplatin. The drugs most commonly implicated in causing infertility, however, are the alkylating agents.

Considerable data on gonadal dysfunction have accrued from studies using cyclophosphamide alone as an immunosuppressant for autoimmune disorders, as pre-SCT conditioning and from its use in multiagent chemotherapy protocols. An analysis of 30 published studies by Rivkees and Crawford[101] included data on 116 men who had received cyclophosphamide. Forty-five percent (52/116) had evidence of testicular dysfunction following treatment correlating with the total dose of cyclophosphamide. Of men receiving more than 300 mg/kg, more than 80% had gonadal dysfunction.

Recovery of gonadal function following administration of cyclophosphamide (CY), either alone or together with busulfan (BU), 16 mg/kg in the context of SCT, is summarized in Table 3. Of 109 men with aplastic anemia administered single-agent high-dose CY (200 mg/kg), 67 subsequently had normal LH, FSH and testosterone levels together with normal sperm counts, and the partners of 26/109 patients became pregnant[76]. Following the combination of BU and CY (200 mg/kg), recovery of spermatogenesis was less frequent, occurring in eight out of 46 patients; partners of only two became pregnant. The combination of BU with lower doses of CY (120 mg/kg) is more likely to be associated with recovery of gonadal function[26].

Gonadal function following treatment for testicular cancer and hematological malignancies (lymphoma and leukemia) have been widely investigated because these illnesses

Table 4 Gonadal toxicity in adult men receiving chemotherapy for lymphoma

Underlying illness	Regimen	Azoospermia	Recovery	Follow-up*	Study
HD	MVPP	27/27		1–14 months	Chapman et al., 1979[90]
			4/64	13–62 months	
HD	MVPP	13/14		30 months (4–83)	Clark et al., 1995[109]
HD	ChlVPP/EVA	20/21		30 months (4–83)	Clark et al., 1995[109]
HD	COPP	92/92		6 years (1–17)	Charak et al., 1990[92]
HD	ABVD	8/24		6 months (1–80)	Viviani et al., 1985[110]
			13[†]/13	10 months (1–18)[‡]	
HD	MOPP	28/29		8 months (2–37)	Viviani et al., 1985[110]
			3/21	24 months (4–67)[‡]	
NHL	CHOP based		67%	7 years	Pryzant et al., 1993[111]
NHL	VAPEC-B	2/14		13.5 months (5–30)	Radford et al., 1994[112]
NHL	VEEP		23/25	45 months (12–85)	Hill et al., 1995[113]

*Expressed as mean (range) where appropriate; [†]recovery occurred in eight azoospermic + five oligospermic patients; [‡]time from first assessment; HD, Hodgkin's disease; NHL, non-Hodgkin's lymphoma; MVPP, mechlorethamine, vinblastine, procarbazine and prednisone; ChlVPP/EVA, chlorambucil, vinblastine, procarbazine and prednisone/etoposide, vincristine and doxorubicin; COPP, cyclophosphamide, vincristine, procarbazine and prednisone; ABVD, doxorubicin, bleomycin, vinblastine and dacarbazine; CHOP, cyclophosphamide, doxorubicin, vincristine and prednisone; VEEP, vincristine, etoposide, epirubicin and prednisone

commonly affect adults of an age group in which fertility issues are relevant.

Compared to patients treated with orchiectomy alone, patients receiving chemotherapy for testicular cancer have a higher degree of testicular dysfunction[103–105]. In an analysis of 170 patients with testicular germ cell cancers treated with either cisplatin- or carboplatin-based drugs, Lampe and co-workers[105] revealed normal sperm counts in 89 (52%) patients before treatment. Of these[91], 57 (64%) retained normal sperm counts following chemotherapy. The probability of recovering a normal sperm count was increased if carboplatin- rather than cisplatin-based chemotherapy had been given and if fewer than five cycles of chemotherapy were administered. Cisplatin is frequently associated with poor semen quality and persistently low sperm counts. Although recovery may occur several years after treatment[106], permanent azoospermia is usual in patients who have received cumulative doses of 600 mg/m² or more[107].

The gonadotoxicity of treatment protocols for acute leukemia depend largely on the cumulative doses of alkylating agents. Several regimens which contain only anthracyclines and antimetabolites are associated with maintenance/recovery of gonadal function in the majority of patients. Wallace and associates[108] described germinal cell dysfunction in only six out of 36 (17%) patients treated for childhood ALL.

A variety of combination chemotherapy protocols have been employed in the management of lymphomas and these are summarized in Table 4. Recovery of spermatogenesis is low following treatment of Hodgkin's disease with combinations of drugs which include procarbazine and alkylating agents, for example MVPP (mechlorethamine, vinblastine, procarbazine and prednisone), ChlVPP/EVA (chlorambucil, vinblastine, procarbazine and prednisone/etoposide, vincristine and doxorubicin) and COPP (cyclophosphamide, vincristine, procarbazine and prednisone). Conversely, ABVD (doxorubicin, bleomycin, vinblastine and dacarbazine) is usually associated with only transient falls in sperm counts[110].

In general, regimens used in the treatment of non-Hodgkin's lymphoma (NHL) such as those based on CHOP (cyclophosphamide, doxorubicin, vincristine and prednisone) are less gonadotoxic than those used for Hodgkin's disease. In a study of 71 men treated with CHOP-based protocols, 47 (67%) had normal sperm counts at 5 years[111]. Other protocols for the treatment of NHL that are usually associated with normal post-treatment gonadal function include MACOP-B (methotrexate, doxorubicin, cyclophosphamide, vincristine, prednisone and bleomycin)[114], VAPEC-B (vincristine, doxorubicin, prednisone, etoposide, cyclophosphamide and bleomycin)[112] and VEEP (vincristine, etoposide, epirubicin and prednisone)[113].

Higher, myeloablative doses of chemotherapy with autologous stem cell rescue used in the treatment of patients with advanced NHL or Hodgkin's disease are more likely to cause permanent infertility. Gonadal function following the use of the protocol BEAM (BCNU, etoposide, cytarabine and melphalan) has been reported by two groups (Table 3). In a study which included 11 postpubertal males, all were azoospermic 2–3 months following BEAM and there was also evidence of reduced Leydig cell reserve[94]. A second study which included ten patients receiving BEAM evaluated sperm counts a median of 30 months (range 1–63) following treatment; again, all patients were azoospermic. Recovery of spermatogenesis following this regimen is possible, however, as inferred from pregnancies in the partners of male recipients of BEAM identified by the EBMT[79].

Prepubertal boys

Testicular damage from chemotherapy administered prior to puberty can lead to failure to progress through puberty. Even where puberty progresses normally, there may be subsequent evidence of testicular damage or even infertility. Gonadotoxic damage in younger boys may be less likely to prevent normal progression through puberty than damage close to the time of puberty itself. In a study involving 19 boys with Hodgkin's disease receiving combination chemotherapy, six prepubertal boys subsequently passed

through puberty normally. Of 13 boys who were pubertal at the time of chemotherapy, nine developed gynecomastia, eight had castrate levels of gonadotropic hormones and all six who underwent testicular biopsies had germinal aplasia[115]. A different pattern of damage was inferred from data from testicular biopsies on 44 boys with ALL. The number of seminiferous tubules containing viable sperm was lowest at 49% in boys treated before puberty, compared to 64% if treated during late puberty.

Adult women

In the late 1950s, three independent groups recorded premature menopause occurring in women receiving busulfan for chronic myeloid leukemia[116–118]. Following this, several other groups reported amenorrhea in association with the use of low-dose daily cyclophosphamide for rheumatoid arthritis, nephrotic syndrome and systemic lupus erythematosus[119–121]. As with men, alkylating agents have continued to be the drugs most commonly implicated in causing gonadal damage. Histological studies of ovarian tissue following chemotherapy demonstrate ovarian atrophy and a reduction in the number of follicles[121–124]. In vitro studies exposing human cortical ovarian slices to chemotherapy demonstrate apoptosis in pregranulosa cells together with disruption of the primordial follicle architecture[125]. The degree and frequency of ovarian failure depend on the drug used and dosage received, analogous to gonadal failure in men following chemotherapy. In women, age is of additional critical importance. Although chemotherapy destroys follicles in women of all ages, older women have a smaller follicular reserve and further losses resulting from chemotherapy are therefore more likely to cause complete and permanent ovarian failure.

Several studies have highlighted the adverse effect of age on ovarian function following chemotherapy in adult women. Data from 44 adult women treated for Hodgkin's disease using MOPP (mechlorethamine, vincristine, procarbazine and prednisone) highlighted the older median age of 17 women who

Table 5 Gonadal recovery in women following stem cell transplantation (SCT) conditioned with chemotherapy-only protocols

Type of SCT	Conditioning	n	Gonadal recovery (%)	Study
Allogeneic	CY	43	74 100 (< 26 years) 31 (> 26 years)	Sanders et al., 1988[56]
Allogeneic	CY	103	54	Sanders et al., 1996[78]
Allogeneic	BUCY	73	1	Sanders et al., 1996[78]
Allogeneic	BUCY*	19	0	Grigg et al., 2000[22]
Autologous	BEAM	10	60	Salooja et al., 1994[128]

BU, busulfan, 16 mg/kg; CY, cyclophosphamide, 200 mg/kg; CY*, cyclophosphamide, 120 mg/kg; BEAM, BCNU, etoposide, cytarabine and melphalan

became amenorrheic following treatment (median 30 years) compared to that of 17 women who continued regular menstrual cycles (median age 22 years). The remaining ten women (median age 23 years) developed oligomenorrhea[126]. In another study evaluating gonadal function in women with Hodgkin's, 21 of 25 women aged 30–51 years developed primary ovarian failure compared to only five of 16 aged less than 30 years[127].

Another source of data highlighting the importance of age comes from women receiving SCT with chemotherapy-only conditioning (Table 5). Of 43 women receiving conditioning with cyclophosphamide, ovarian function was normal following treatment in all 27 women under the age of 26 years, but in only five of 16 women over the age of 26[56]. Of ten women receiving the BEAM protocol for acute myeloid leukemia (AML), four women over the age of 32 years developed POF, while six women younger than this had normal gonadal function and five of the six became pregnant within 4–40 months of treatment[128]. The effect of age on ovarian failure has also been evaluated in 168 patients treated for hematological cancers (AML, NHL, Hodgkin's disease) or breast cancer[129]. All had normal ovarian function prior to treatment, but following combination chemotherapy 57 of 168 (34%) developed ovarian failure. The median age at the time of treatment was related to outcome, with a significantly higher median age in the group with ovarian failure (34.7 ± 8 years) compared to women who

retained normal ovarian function (27.4 ± 8.3 years).

The large number of chemotherapy protocols can make it difficult to acquire adequate longitudinal data on the toxicity of individual drugs. However, in an elegant analysis by Meirow[130], ovarian function was analyzed in 168 patients treated by combination chemotherapy and the effects of individual drugs were analyzed by the odds ratio of exposed against unexposed patients (see p. 31). The results were adjusted for age by logistic regression analysis. Ovarian failure was significantly related to the group of chemotherapeutic agent used, with alkylating agents and cisplatin giving the highest risks of ovarian failure with odds ratios of 3.98 and 1.77 respectively. No increased risk was identified with plant alkaloids and the odds ratios for other groups of chemotherapeutic agents, i.e. antimetabolites or antibiotics, were less than 1.0, indicating the possibility of safer options (if appropriate treatment for that cancer) for preservation of ovarian function.

The dose-dependent ovarian toxicity of alkylating agents has been demonstrated in both animal studies and clinical studies involving human subjects. In mice, increasing doses of cyclophosphamide lead to a dose-dependent destruction of primordial follicles[131]. A clinical study evaluating ovarian function in women with systemic lupus erythematosus treated with cyclophosphamide described sustained amenorrhea in nine of 23 (39%) women receiving more than

15 pulses of treatment, in contrast to only two of 16 women (12.5%) who received a total of seven doses[132]. Follow-up studies of female survivors of childhood cancer also indicate an increased risk of premature menopause and infertility with increasing doses of alkylating agents[53].

When cyclophosphamide is used together with other chemotherapeutic agents the incidence of ovarian failure may be increased. Of 109 premenopausal women receiving cyclophosphamide together with either methotrexate or an anthracycline for the treatment of breast cancer, persistent amenorrhea occurred in 45% and 46% respectively, 1 year following the completion of chemotherapy. Higher rates of amenorrhea (up to 68%) have been reported for regimens based on cyclophosphamide together with methotrexate and 5-fluorouracil[133]. The combination of cyclophosphamide and busulfan (BUCY) is particularly toxic to the ovary. BUCY is used as conditioning for allogeneic SCT (Table 5) with the CY component administered in one of two doses, 200 mg/kg or 120 mg/kg. The Seattle transplant team described recovery of ovarian function in only one of 73 women given BU (16 mg/kg) together with CY (200 mg/kg) conditioning[78] and the EBMT experience is similar in that there have been no pregnancies occurring in women following this regimen[79]. A single case report describing pregnancy following BUCY involved an 11-year-old girl who received SCT for thalassemia major. This patient received CY 200 mg/kg together with a lower dose of busulfan, 14 mg/kg, than is generally used in the treatment of leukemia[134].

The same multiagent protocols for Hodgkin's disease that are associated with gonadal dysfunction in male adults, such as MOPP[126], COPP[135,136] and ChlVPP[137], can lead to ovarian failure in women with an incidence of 38–57%[138]. The regimen ABVD is associated with preservation of fertility in younger women. Transient amenorrhea was reported by 12/33 women < 45 years old receiving four courses of ABVD and no cases

of permanent amenorrhea were observed in 17 patients aged < 25 years[139]. Of 36 young patients (median age at diagnosis 14 years) treated with five cycles of COP (cyclophosphamide, vincristine and procarbazine) alternating with four cycles of ABVD and low-dose (20 Gy) regional radiotherapy, the majority (30/36) had regular menstrual cycles following treatment[140].

Prepubertal females

It is difficult to detect gonadal damage in the prepubertal child and the first indication may be failure to progress through puberty. Other manifestations include primary amenorrhea or a premature menopause. In general, prepubertal females treated for childhood ALL progress normally through puberty. In a study evaluating 40 such patients, all had normal pubertal development and 37 had regular menstrual cycles[141]. Despite these apparently reassuring data, it is clear that these patients remain at risk of premature ovarian failure. An evaluation of more than 1000 women treated in childhood for malignancy revealed that, among women who were menstruating at the age of 21 years, 42% reached the menopause by the age of 31 years compared with only 5% of the control women[142].

More sophisticated assessment of ovarian function in adult survivors of childhood cancer may indicate dysfunction in patients who are menstruating normally and have normal baseline biochemistry. Larsen and colleagues[143] assessed ovarian reserve in 21 female survivors of childhood cancer using sonographic measurements of ovarian volume and antral follicle counts. These women had a significantly smaller ovarian volume compared to controls (4.9 vs. 6.8 cm^3) and a lower number of small antral follicles per ovary (4.5 vs. 8), indicative of reduced ovarian reserve. In addition, women in the study group had significantly shorter cycle lengths than the control group and this may also be indicative of ovarian follicular depletion[144,145]. The relevance of these data to subsequent reproductive potential requires further evaluation.

PREGNANCY OUTCOME FOLLOWING CHEMOTHERAPY

Most data suggest that chemotherapy administered prior to pregnancy is not associated with an adverse pregnancy outcome. A report from the CCSS, on the outcome of 4029 pregnancies among 1915 female childhood cancer survivors, evaluated the frequency of live birth, stillbirth, miscarriage and medical abortion according to patients' age, cancer diagnosis and cancer treatment. There were no significant differences in live birth rate and stillbirth rate according to treatment. The offspring were more likely to be of low birth weight, however, compared to the offspring of patients' female siblings. Significant variables affecting birth weight were pelvic irradiation, maternal education level and use of daunorubicin or doxorubicin. There was no evidence of a dose–response relationship with these latter drugs, however[77].

Women who have received high doses of chemotherapy as conditioning for SCT may have an increased incidence of pregnancy complications. Details of 56 pregnancies in 25 women who had received cyclophosphamide-only conditioning (200 mg/kg) were included in the report by Sanders and associates[78]. Of the 56 pregnancies, 12 did not go beyond 20 weeks because of either elective termination ($n = 5$), tubal pregnancy ($n = 3$) or spontaneous miscarriage ($n = 4$, 7%). There was an increased incidence of preterm and low-birth-weight babies compared to background populations, with eight of 44 (18%) live births occurring before 37 weeks and seven of these eight offspring being small for gestational age. The incidence of congenital anomalies was not increased (two of 44 infants). The EBMT describe 58 pregnancies in 46 women following non-TBI conditioning for aplastic anemia[79]. In agreement with the data from Sanders' group, the incidence of miscarriage was 7% and the incidence of

congenital anomalies was not increased. However, the EBMT study did not detect an increase in the incidence of preterm delivery.

The CCSS has also reported the pregnancy outcome of partners of male childhood cancer survivors, using offspring of the partners of siblings as the control group[81]. There were 2323 pregnancies among partners of 1227 male patients. A significantly lower proportion of pregnancies resulted in a live birth compared to the control group, and the use of the agent dactinomycin was specifically associated with a significantly lower rate of live birth. The use of procarbazine (> 5000 mg/m^2) was associated with a higher rate of miscarriage when compared to the control group. The M : F sex ratio of the offspring at 1.00 : 1.03 was significantly lower than in the control group (1.24 : 1.0). The altered sex ratio may have been a chance finding. However, other authors have also reported a reduction in the sex ratio of offspring to men who have been exposed to chemicals such as dibromochloropropane[146] or dioxin[147] prior to conception.

Patients using the designer drug imatinib are strongly advised to avoid conception. Despite this recommendation, 18 pregnancies have been reported in the partners of male patients taking this drug and 26 pregnancies have been reported in female recipients. Data are available for eight of the 18 pregnancies to partners of male patients: there were four normal infants, two therapeutic abortions for social reasons, one spontaneous abortion and one death *in utero* at 13 weeks. Data are also available for 19 of the 26 pregnancies in female patients following use of imatinib: there were 11 therapeutic abortions (one known to be because of congenital abnormalities), five spontaneous abortions, two normal infants and one infant born with hypospadias[148].

EFFECT OF CHEMOTHERAPY ON FUTURE GENERATIONS

Chemotherapy agents such as cyclophosphamide can cause gene mutations, chromosomal breaks and rearrangements. An increase in chromosomal abnormalities has been demonstrated several years after treatment for testicular cancer[149] and increased aneuploid frequency has been observed in human sperm following chemotherapy for Hodgkin's disease[150,151]. Animal studies have also demonstrated that cyclophosphamide causes injury to germ cells and can induce transmissible genetic damage[152–155]. These data raise concerns regarding transmitting genetic damage to the offspring of cancer survivors who retain fertility after treatment.

However, studies on pregnancy outcome in human survivors of cancer treatment indicate that such concerns may be unfounded. Patients exposed to cancer treatment do not appear to have a greater than normal risk of chromosomal or congenital abnormalities[78,79,156,157]. There are several explanations for this potential discrepancy. First, existing studies may not have sufficient power to detect a small difference. Alternatively, DNA repair mechanisms may be capable of correcting genomic damage during the time between exposure to mutagenic treatment and conception[158]. A third possibility is that there is a selection bias against genetically abnormal germ cells. It is, therefore, of some concern that techniques of assisted conception bypass the natural selection of healthy germ cells. Frozen semen banking is sometimes offered after the commencement of chemotherapy. If such a sample proves unsuitable for simple insemination, a single sperm may be selected artificially for use in the technique of intracytoplasmic sperm injection. Similarly, oocyte recovery for ART may be initiated in women who have already commenced chemotherapy programs. In animal studies where conception occurred soon after administration of chemotherapy there was a high incidence of malformation, implying damage to the oocytes[131]. Follicular growth takes several months in humans and it is likely that oocytes exposed to chemotherapy during this time will sustain significant damage. Currently there is no defined period of time after which it is safe to use such oocytes for ART. Long-term follow-up of offspring is required to evaluate this further.

SEXUAL DYSFUNCTION FOLLOWING CHEMO/RADIOTHERAPY

As survival rates for hematological, testicular and breast cancers improve, psychosocial and sexual sequelae assume greater importance to both the patient and clinician. Sexual function can be influenced by many factors in these patients, from the psychological impact of diagnosis to the consequences of gonadal failure, and studies indicate that there is a high rate of sexual dysfunction in treated cancer patients. The incidence of sexual problems following treatment for Hodgkin's disease was reported as 24% in a study by Kornblith and co-workers[159]. Following SCT, sexual dysfunction occurs in 20–50% of patients[25,160,161]. In a study that compared SCT with chemotherapy alone as treatment for AML[24], significantly more transplanted patients reported a decreasing interest in sex (48% vs. 24%), sexual activity (53% vs. 35%) and ability to have sexual intercourse (38% vs. 18%). In this latter study, patients with GVHD were significantly more likely to report a decreased ability to have sexual intercourse (64% vs. 39%) and women were more likely than men to report sexual dysfunction.

Sexual dysfunction in women following chemo/radiotherapy is multifactorial. The abrupt fall in estrogen levels which accompanies treatment in women can lead to marked menopausal symptoms and dyspareunia secondary to vaginal dryness. Dyspareunia may be further exacerbated by stenosis as a direct result of abdominal/pelvic irradiation or GVHD. Following chemotherapy an altered body image can contribute further to a reduction of libido. In a longitudinal study of sexual function and vaginal changes following radiotherapy for cervical or vaginal cancer, there was a high prevalence (55% of 118 patients) of dyspareunia throughout the 12 months following treatment. Reduced vaginal dimension was reported by 50% of patients and 45% were never or rarely able to complete sexual intercourse. Thirty-five percent described moderate to severe lack of lubrication and overall 30% were dissatisfied with their sexual life[162]. Following TBI the incidence of sexual dysfunction is also high. In a study evaluating 74 women during the first six months after TBI, 58 (78%) women had vasomotor symptoms, 45 (61%) reported genitourinary symptoms, and 49 of 52 sexually active women who gave information reported difficulties with intercourse[55].

SUMMARY

Patients treated with chemotherapy and/or radiotherapy are at significant risk of toxicity to the reproductive system. Females have no stem cell pool with which to replenish damaged oocytes, and in men the stem cell pool is particularly vulnerable to damage from agents designed to kill actively proliferating cell populations. The myriad of chemotherapy protocols, some of which include radiotherapy, can make it difficult to acquire sufficient longitudinal data on the toxicity of individual agents or protocols. As such, pretreatment counseling may prove difficult and is made harder by the paucity of data on the success of ART following chemo/ radiotherapy. Currently, these techniques require delays in treatment which may be unacceptable for patients with life-threatening diseases. There remains, therefore, a great need to develop effective treatments for patients with cancer that further reduce toxicity to the reproductive system.

References

1. Morita Y, Tilly JL. Oocyte apoptosis: like sand through an hourglass. *Dev Biol* 1999;213:1–17
2. Morita Y, Maravei DV, Bergeron L, *et al.* Caspase-2 deficiency rescues female germ cells from death due to cytokine insufficiency but not meiotic defects caused by ataxia telangiectasia-mutated (Atm) gene inactivation. *Cell Death Differ* 2001;8:614–20
3. Takai Y, Canning J, Perez GI, *et al.* Bax, Caspase 2 and Caspase 3 are required for ovarian follicle loss caused by 4-vinylcyclohexene diepoxide exposure of female mice *in vivo*. *Endocrinology* 2003;144:69–74
4. Tilly KI, Banerjee S, Banerjee PP, Tilly JL. Expression of the p53 and Wilms' tumour suppressor genes in the rat ovary: gonadotropin repression *in vivo* and immunohistochemical localization of nuclear p53 protein to apoptotic granulosa cells of atretic follicles. *Endocrinology* 1995;136:1394–402
5. Keren-Tal I, Suh BS, Dantes A, *et al.* Involvement of p53 expression in the cAMP-mediated apoptosis in immortalized granulosa cells. *Exp Cell Res* 1995;218:283–95
6. Perez GI, Knudson M, Leykin L, *et al.* Apoptosis-associated signalling pathways are required for chemotherapy-mediated female germ cell destruction. *Nat Med* 1997;3:1228–32
7. Perez GI, Robles R, Knudson CM, *et al.* Prolongation of ovarian lifespan into advanced chronological age by Bax-deficiency. *Nat Genet* 1999;21:200–3
8. Ratts VS, Flaws JA, Kolp R, *et al.* Ablation of bcl-2 gene expression decreases the number of oocytes and primordial follicles established in the post-natal female mouse gonad. *Endocrinology* 1995;136:3665–8
9. Morita Y, Perez GI, Maravei DV, *et al.* Targeted expression of bcl-2 in mouse oocytes inhibits ovarian follicle atresia and prevents spontaneous and chemotherapy-induced oocyte apoptosis *in vitro*. *Mol Endocrinol* 1999;13:841–50
10. Van Brocklyn JR, Tu Z, Esdall LC, *et al.* Sphingosine-1-phosphate-induced cell rounding and neural retraction are mediated by the G protein coupled receptor H218. *J Biol Chem* 1999;274:4626–32
11. Bergeron L, Perez GI, Macdonald G, *et al.* Defects in regulation of apoptosis in caspase-2-deficient mice. *Genes Dev* 1998;12:1304–14.
12. Rucker EB, Dierisseu P, Wagner KU, *et al.* Bcl-x and Bax regulate mouse primordial germ cell survival and apoptosis during embryogenesis. *Mol Endocrinol* 2000;14:1038–52
13. Kolesnick RN, Kronke M. Regulation of ceramide production and apoptosis. *Annu Rev Physiol* 1998;60:643–65
14. Morita Y, Perez GI, Paris F, *et al.* Oocyte apoptosis is suppressed by disruption of the acid

sphingomyelinase gene or by sphingosine-1-phosphate therapy. *Nat Med* 2000;6:1109–14

15. Olivera A, Kohama T, Esdall L, *et al.* Sphingosine kinase expression increases intracellular sphingosine-1-phosphate and promotes cell death and survival. *J Cell Biol* 1999; 147:545–58

16. Cuvillier O, Pirianov G, Kleuser B, *et al.* Suppression of ceramide-mediated programmed cell death by sphingosine-1-phosphate. *Nature* 1996;381:800–3

17. Speroff L, Glass RH, Kase NG. *Clinical Gynecological Endocrinology and Infertility,* 6th edn. Lippincott Williams & Wilkins, 1999

18. Scheffer GJ, Broekmans FJ, Dorland M, *et al.* Antral follicle counts by transvaginal ultrasonography are related to age in women with proven natural fertility. *Fertil Steril* 1999;72: 845–51

19. Solary E, Plenchette S, Sordet C, *et al.* Modulation of apoptotic pathways triggered by cytotoxic agents. *Therapie* 2001;56:511–18

20. Verheij MJ, Bartelink H. Radiation-induced apoptosis. *Cell Tissue Res* 2000;301:133–42

21. Matikainen T, Perez GI, Jurisicova A, *et al.* Aromatic hydrocarbon receptor-driven Bax gene expression is required for premature ovarian failure caused by biohazardous environmental chemicals. *Nat Genet* 2001;28:355–60

22. Matikainen TM, Moriyam T, Morita Y, *et al.* Ligand activation of the aromatic hydrocarbon receptor (AHR)-transcription factor drives Bax-dependent apoptosis in developing fetal ovarian germ cells. *Endocrinology* 2002;143: 615–20

23. Paris F, Perez G, Fils Z, *et al.* Sphingosine 1-phosphate preserves fertility in irradiated mice without propagating genomic damage in offspring. *Nat Med* 2002;8:901–2

24. Hahn ME. The aryl hydrocarbon receptor: a comparative perspective. *Comp Biochem Physiol C Pharmacol Toxicol Endocrinol* 1998;121:23–53

25. Watson M, Wheatley K, Harrison G, *et al.* Severe adverse impact on sexual functioning and fertility of bone marrow transplantation, either allogeneic or autologous, compared with consolidation chemotherapy alone. *Cancer* 1999;86:1231–9

26. Tauchmanova L, Sellieri C, De Rosa G, *et al.* Gonadal status in reproductive age women after haematopoietic stem cell transplantation for haematological malignancies. *Hum Reprod* 2003;18:1410–16

27. Grigg AP, McLachlan R, Zaja J, Szer J. Reproductive status in long-term bone marrow transplant survivors receiving busulfan–cyclophosphamide (120 mg/kg). *Bone Marrow Transplant* 2000;26:1089–95

28. Littley MD, Shalet SM, Beardwell CG. Radiation and hypothalamic–pituitary function. *Baillières Clin Endocrinol Metab* 1990;4:147–75

29. Druker BJ, Sawyers CL, Kantarjian H, *et al.* Activity of a specific inhibitor of the BCR-ABL tyrosine kinase in the blast crisis of chronic myeloid leukemia and acute lymphoblastic leukemia with the Philadelphia chromosome. *N Engl J Med* 2001;344:1038–42

30. O'Brien SG, Guilhot F, Larson RA, *et al.*, IRIS Investigators. Imatinib compared with interferon and low-dose cytarabine for newly diagnosed chronic-phase chronic myeloid leukemia. *N Engl J Med* 2003;348:994–1004

31. Faddy MJ, Gosden RG. A mathematical model of follicle dynamics in the human ovary. *Hum Reprod* 1995;10:770–5

32. Faddy MJ, Gosden RG. A model conforming the decline in follicle numbers to the age of menopause in women. *Hum Reprod* 1996;11: 1484–6

33. Pan HA, Cheng YC, Li CH, *et al.* Ovarian stroma flow intensity deceases by age: a three dimensional power Doppler ultrasonographic study. *Ultrasound Med Biol* 2002;28:425–30

34. Kupesic S, Kurjak A, Bjelos D, Vujisic S. Three dimensional ultrasonographic ovarian measurements and *in vitro* fertilisation outcome are related to age. *Fertil Steril* 2003;79:190–7

35. Noyes RW, Hertig AT, Rock J. Dating the endometrial biopsy. *Fertil Steril* 1950;1:3–25

36. Snidjers MPML, de Goeij AFPM, Debets-Te Baerts MJC, *et al.* Immunocytochemical analysis of estrogen receptors and progesterone receptors in the human uterus throughout the menstrual cycle and after the menopause. *J Reprod Fertil* 1992;94:363–71

37. Rowley MJ, Leach DR, Warner GA, Heller CG. Effect of graded doses of ionizing radiation on the human testis. *Radiat Res* 1974;59: 665–78

38. Centola GM, Keller JW, Henzler M, Rubin P. Effect of low-dose testicular irradiation on sperm count and fertility in patients with testicular seminoma. *J Androl* 1994;15:608–13

39. Kinsella TJ, Trivette G, Rowland J, *et al.* Long term follow up of testicular function following radiation therapy for early stage Hodgkin's disease. *J Clin Oncol* 1989;7:718–24

40. Giwercman A, von der Maase H, Berthelson JG, *et al.* Localized irradiation of testes with carcinoma *in situ*: effects of Leydig cell function and eradication of malignant germ cells in 20 patients. *J Clin Endocrinol Metab* 1991;73: 596–603

41. Shalet SM. Disorders of gonadal function due to radiation and cytotoxic chemotherapy in children. *Adv Int Med Ped* 1989;58:1–21

42. Peterson PM, Giwercman A, Daugaard G, *et al.* Effects of graded testicular doses of radiotherapy in patients treated for carcinoma *in situ* in the testis. *J Clin Oncol* 2002;20:1537–43

43. Speiser B, Rubin P, Casarett G. Aspermia following lower truncal irradiation in Hodgkin's disease. *Cancer* 1972;32:692–8

44. Leiper AD, Stanhope R, Lau T, *et al.* The effect of total body irradiation and bone marrow transplantation during childhood and adolescence on growth and endocrine function. *Br J Haematol* 1987;67:419–26

45. Ogilvy-Stuart AL, Clark DJ, Wallace WH, *et al.* Endocrine deficit after fractionated total body irradiation. *Arch Dis Child* 1992;67:1107–10

46. Shalet SM, Beardwell CG, Jacobs HS, Pearson D. Testicular function following irradiation of the human prepubertal testis. *Clin Endocrinol* 1978;9:483–90

47. Shalet SM, Tsatsoulis A, Whitehead E, Read G. Vulnerability of the human Leydig cell to radiation damage is dependent upon age. *J Endocrinol* 1989;120:161–5

48. Fisher B, Cheung AY. Delayed effect of radiation therapy with or without chemotherapy on ovarian function in women with Hodgkin's disease. *Acta Radiol Oncol* 1983;23:43–8

49. Madsen BL, Giudice L, Donaldson SS. Radiation-induced premature menopause: a misconception. *Int J Radiat Oncol Biol Phys* 1995;32:1461–4

50. Gosden RG, Wade JC, Fraser HM, *et al.* Impact of congenital hypogonadotropism on the radiation sensitivity of the mouse ovary. *Hum Reprod* 1997;12:2483–8

51. Wallace WHB, Shalet SM, Hendry JH, *et al.* Ovarian failure following ovarian irradiation in childhood. The radiosensitivity of human oocyte. *Br J Radiol* 1989;62:995–8

52. Wallace WHB, Thomson AB, Kelsey TW. The radiosensitivity of the human oocyte. *Hum Reprod* 2003;18:117–21

53. Chiarelli AM, Marrett LD, Darlington G. Early menopause and infertiliy in females after treatment for childhood cancer diagnosed in 1964–1988 in Ontario, Canada. *Am J Epidemiol* 1999;150:245–54

54. Doll R, Smith PG. The long-term effects of x irradiation in patients treated for metropathia haemorrhagica. *Br J Radiol* 1968;41:362–8

55. Spinelli S, Chiodi S, Bacigalupo A, *et al.* Ovarian recovery after total body irradiation and allogeneic bone marrow transplantation: long term follow up of 79 females. *Bone Marrow Transplant* 1994;14:373–80

56. Sanders JE, Buckner CD, Amos D, *et al.* Ovarian function following marrow transplantation for aplastic anemia or leukemia. *J Clin Oncol* 1988;6:813–8

57. Shalet SM, Beardwell CG, Jones PH, *et al.* Ovarian failure following abdominal irradiation in childhood. *Br J Cancer* 1976;33:655–8

58. Hamre MR, Robison LL, Nesbit ME, *et al.* Effects of radiation on ovarian function in long-term survivors of childhood acute lymphoblastic leukemia: a report from the Childrens Cancer Study Group. *J Clin Oncol* 1987;5:1759–65

59. Silber JH, Radcliffer J, Peckham V, *et al.* Whole brain irradiation and decline in intelligence: the influence of dose and age on IQ score. *J Clin Oncol* 1992;10:1390–6

60. Waber DP, Urion DK, Tarbell NJ, *et al.* Late effects of central nervous system treatment of acute lymphoblastic leukemia in childhood are sex-dependent. *Dev Med Child Neurol* 1990;32:238–48

61. Craig F, Leiper AD, Stanhope R, *et al.* Sexually dimorphic and radiation dose dependent effect of cranial irradiation on body mass index. *Arch Dis Child* 1999;81:500–4

62. Rappaport R, Brauner R, Czernichow P, *et al.* Effect of hypothalamic and pituitary irradiation on pubertal development in children with cranial tumors. *J Clin Endocrinol Metab* 1982;154:1164–8

63. Ogilvy-Stuart AL, Clayton PE, Shalet SM. Cranial irradiation and early puberty. *J Clin Endocrinol Metab* 1994;78:1282–6

64. Leiper AD, Stanhope R, Kitching P, Chessells JM. Precocious and premature puberty associated with treatment of acute lymphoblastic leukemia. *Arch Dis Child* 1987;62:1107–12

65. Quigley C, Cowell C, Jimenez M, *et al.* Normal or early development of puberty despite gonadal damage in children treated for acute lymphoblastic leukemia. *Arch Dis Child* 1989;62:1107–12

66. Didcock E, Davies HA, Didi M, *et al.* Pubertal growth in young adult survivors of childhood leukemia. *J Clin Oncol* 1995;13:2503–7

67. Littley MD, Shalet SM, Beardwell CG, *et al.* Hypopituitarism following external radiotherapy for pituitary tumours in adults. *Q J Med* 1989;70:145–60

68. Birkebaek NH, Fisker S, Clausen N, *et al.* Growth and endocrinological disorders up to 21 years after treatment for acute lymphoblastic leukemia in childhood. *Med Pediatr Oncol* 1998;30:351–6

69. Bath LE, Anderson RA, Critchley HO, *et al.* Hypothalamic–pituitary–ovarian dysfunction after prepubertal chemotherapy and cranial irradiation for acute leukaemia. *Hum Reprod* 2001;16:1838–44

70. Critchley HO, Wallace WH, Shalet SM, *et al.* Abdominal irradiation in childhood: the potential for pregnancy. *Br J Obstet Gynaecol* 1992;97:804–10

71. Bath LE, Critchley HO, Chambers SE, *et al.* Ovarian and uterine characteristics after total body irradiation in childhood and adolescence: response to sex steroid replacement. *Br J Obstet Gynaecol* 1999;106:1265–72

72. Schubert MA, Sullivan KM, Schubert MM, *et al.* Gynecological abnormalities following allogeneic bone marrow transplantation. *Bone Marrow Transplant* 1990;5:425–30

73. Corson SL, Sullivan KM, Batzer F, *et al.* Gynecologic manifestations of chronic graft-versus-host disease. *Obstet Gynecol* 1982;60: 488–92

74. Green DM, Fine WE, Li FP. Offspring of patients treated for unilateral Wilms' tumor in childhood. *Cancer* 1982;49:2285–8

75. Li FP, Gimbrere K, Gelber RD, *et al.* Outcome of pregnancy in survivors of Wilms' tumor. *J Am Med Assoc* 1987;257:216–19

76. Hawkins MM, Smith RA. Pregnancy outcomes in childhood cancer survivors: probable effects of abdominal irradiation. *Int J Cancer* 1989;43: 399–402

77. Green DM, Whitton JA, Stovall M, *et al.* Pregnancy outcome of female survivors of childhood cancer: a report from the Childhood Cancer Survivor Study. *Am J Obstet Gynecol* 2002;187:1070–80

78. Sanders JE, Hawley J, Levy W, *et al.* Pregnancies following high-dose cyclophosphamide with or without high-dose busulfan or total-body irradiation and bone marrow transplantation. *Blood* 1996;87:3045–52

79. Salooja N, Szydlo RM, Socie G, *et al.* Pregnancy outcomes after peripheral blood or bone marrow transplantation: a retrospective survey. *Lancet* 2001;358:271–6

80. Parker L, Pearce MS, Dickinson HO, *et al.* Stillbirths among offspring of male radiation workers at Sellafield nuclear reprocessing plant. *Lancet* 1999;354:1407–14

81. Green DM, Whitton JA, Stovall M, *et al.* Pregnancy outcome of partners of male survivors of childhood cancer: a report from the Childhood Cancer Survivor Study. *J Clin Oncol* 2003;21:716–21

82. Salha O, Picton H, Balen A, Rutherford A. Human oocyte cryopreservation. *Hosp Med* 2001;62:18–24

83. Salumets A, Tuuri T, Maliken S, *et al.* Effect of developmental stage of embryo at freezing on pregnancy outcome of frozen thawed embryo transfer. *Hum Reprod* 2003;18:1890–5

84. Soderstrom-Antila V, Vilska S, Makinen S, *et al.* Elective single embryo transfer yields good delivery rates in oocyte donation. *Hum Reprod* 2003;18:1858–63

85. Rio B, Letur-Konirsch H, Ajchenbaum-Cymbalista F, *et al.* Full-term pregnancy with embryos from donated oocytes in a 36-year-old woman allografted for chronic myeloid leukemia. *Bone Marrow Transplant* 1994;13: 487–8

86. Atkinson HG, Apperley JF, Dawson K, *et al.* Successful pregnancy after allogeneic bone marrow transplantation for chronic myeloid leukemia. *Lancet* 1994;344:199

87. Spitz S. The histological effects of the nitrogen mustards on human tumours and tissues. *Cancer* 1948;1:383–98

88. Chapman RM. Effect of cytotoxic therapy on sexuality and gonadal function. *Semin Oncol* 1982;9:84–94

89. Meistrich ML. Stage-specific sensitivity of spermatogonia to different chemotherapeutic drugs. *Biomed Pharmacother* 1984;38:137–42

90. Chapman RM, Sutcliffe SB, Rees LH, *et al.* Cyclical combination chemotherapy and gonadal function. Retrospective study in males. *Lancet* 1979;1:285–9

91. Whitehead E, Shalet SM, Blackledge G, *et al.* The effects of Hodgkin's disease and combination chemotherapy on gonadal function in the adult male. *Cancer* 1982;49:418–22

92. Charak BS, Gupta R, Mandrekar P, *et al.* Testicular dysfunction after cyclophosphamide–vincristine–procarbazine–prednisolone chemotherapy for advanced Hodgkin's disease. A long-term follow-up study. *Cancer* 1990;65: 1903–6

93. Bramswig J, Heimes U, Heiermann E, *et al.* The effects of different cumulative doses of chemotherapy on testicular function. Results in 75 patients treated for Hodgkin's disease during childhood or adolescence. *Cancer* 1990;65:1298–302

94. Chatterjee R, Mills W, Katz M, *et al.* Germ cell failure and Leydig cell insufficiency in post-pubertal male patients after autologous bone marrow transplantation with BEAM for lymphoma. *Bone Marrow Transplant* 1994;13: 519–22

95. Chapman RM, Sutcliffe SB, Malpas JS. Male gonadal dysfunction in Hodgkin's disease. A prospective study. *J Am Med Assoc* 1981;245: 1323–8

96. Vigersky R, Chapman R, Berenberg J, Glass A. Testicular dysfunction in untreated Hodgkin's disease. *Am J Med* 1982;73:482–6

97. Padron OF, Sharma RK, Thomas AJ, *et al.* Effects of cancer on spermatozoa quality after cryopreservation: a 12-year experience. *Fertil Steril* 1997;67:326–31

98. Hendry W, Stedronska J, Jones C, *et al.* Semen analysis in testicular cancer and Hodgkin's disease: pre- and post-treatment findings and implications for cryopreservation. *Br J Urol* 1983;55:769–73

99. Meirow D, Schenker JG. Cancer and male fertility. *Hum Reprod* 1995;10:2017–22

100. Viviani S, Ragni G, Santoro A, *et al.* Testicular dysfunction in Hodgkin's disease before and after treatment. *Eur J Cancer* 1991;27:1389–92

101. Rivkees SA, Crawford JD. The relationship of gonadal activity and chemotherapy-induced gonadal damage. *J Am Med Assoc* 1988;259:2123–5

102. Jacob A, Barker H, Goodman A, Holmes J. Recovery of spermatogenesis following bone marrow transplantation. *Bone Marrow Transplant* 1998;22:277–9

103. Hansen SW, Berthelsen JG, von der Maase H. Long term fertility and Leydig cell function in patients treated for germ cell cancer with cisplatin, vinblastine and bleomycin versus surveillance. *J Clin Oncol* 1990;8:1695–8

104. Palmieri G, Lotrecchiano G, Ricci G, *et al.* Gonadal function after multimodality treatment in men with testicular germ cell cancer. *Eur J Endocrinol* 1996;134:431–6

105. Lampe H, Horwich A, Norman A, *et al.* Fertility after chemotherapy for testicular germ cell cancers. *J Clin Oncol* 1997;15:239–45

106. Peterson PM, Giwercman A, Skakkebaek NE, Rorth M. Gonadal function in men with testicular cancer. *Semin Oncol* 1998;25:224–34

107. Peterson PM, Hansen SW, Giwercman A, *et al.* Dose-dependent impairment of testicular function in patients treated with cisplatin-based chemotherapy for germ cell cancer. *Ann Oncol* 1994;5:355–8

108. Wallace WH, Shalet SM, Lendon M, Morris-Jones PH. Male fertility in long-term survivors of childhood acute lymphoblastic leukemia. *Int J Androl* 1991;14:312–19

109. Clark ST, Radford JA, Crowther D, *et al.* Gonadal function following chemotherapy for Hodgkin's disease: a comparative study of MVPP and a seven-drug hybrid regimen. *J Clin Oncol* 1995;13:134–9

110. Viviani S, Santoro A, Ragni G, *et al.* Gonadal toxicity after combination chemotherapy for Hodgkin's disease. Comparative results of MOPP vs ABVD. *Eur J Cancer Clin Oncol* 1985;21:601–5

111. Pryzant RM, Meistrich ML, Wilson G, *et al.* Long term reduction in sperm count after chemotherapy with and without radiation therapy for non-Hodgkin's lymphomas. *J Clin Oncol* 1993;11:239–47

112. Radford JA, Clark S, Crowther D, Shalet SM. Male fertility after VAPEC-B chemotherapy for Hodgkin's disease and non-Hodgkin's lymphoma. *Br J Cancer* 1994;69:379–81

113. Hill M, Milan S, Cunningham D, *et al.* Evaluation of the efficacy of the VEEP regimen in adult Hodgkin's disease with assessment of gonadal and cardiac toxicity. *J Clin Oncol* 1995;13:387–95

114. Muller U, Stahel RA. Gonadal function after MACOP-B or VACOP-B with or without dose intensification and ABMT in young patients with aggressive non-Hodgkin's lymphoma. *Ann Oncol* 1993;4:399–402

115. Sherins RJ, Olweny CLM, Ziegler JL. Gynecomastia and gonadal dysfunction in adolescent boys treated with combination chemotherapy for Hodgkin's disease. *N Engl J Med* 1978;299:12–16

116. Louis J, Limarzi LR, Best WR. Treatment of chronic granulocytic leukemia with myleran. *Arch Intern Med* 1956;97:299–308

117. Galton DA, Till M, Wiltshaw E. Busulfan (1,4-dimethanesulfonyloxybutane, myleran); summary of clinical results. *Ann N Y Acad Sci* 1958;68:967–73

118. Belhorsky B, Siracky J, Sander L, *et al.* Comments on the development of amenorrhea caused by myleran in cases of chronic myelosis. *Neoplasma* 1960;7:397–402

119. Fosdick WM, Parsons JL, Hill DF. Long-term cyclophosphamide therapy in rheumatoid arthritis. *Arthritis Rheum* 1968;9:151–61

120. Uldall PR, Kerr DNS, Tacchi D. Sterility and cyclophosphamide. *Lancet* 1972;i:693–4

121. Warne GL, Fairly KF, Hobbs JB, Martin FIR. Cyclophosphamide induced ovarian failure. *N Engl J Med* 1973;289:1159–62

122. Himelstein-Braw R, Peters H, Faber M. Morphological study of the ovaries of leukaemic children. *Br J Cancer* 1978;38:82–7

123. Marcello MF, Nuciforo G, Romeo R, *et al.* Structural and ultrastructual study of the ovary in childhood leukemia after successful treatment. *Cancer* 1990;66:2099–104

124. Familiari G, Caggiati A, Nottoloa SA, *et al.* Ultrastructure of human ovarian primordial follicles after combination chemotherapy for Hodgkin's disease. *Hum Reprod* 1993;8:2080–7

125. Meirow D, Nugent D. The effects of radiotherapy and chemotherapy on female reproduction. *Hum Reprod* 2001;7:535–43

126. Whitehead E, Shalet SM, Blackledge G, *et al.* The effect of combination chemotherapy on ovarian function in women treated for Hodgkin's disease. *Cancer* 1983;52:988–93

127. Chapman RM, Sutcliffe SB, Malpas JS. Cytotoxic induced ovarian failure in women with Hodgkin's disease. I. Hormone function. *J Am Med Assoc* 1979;242:1877–81

128. Salooja N, Chatterjee R, McMillan AK, *et al.* Successful pregnancies in women following single autotransplant for acute myeloid leukemia with a chemotherapy ablation

protocol. *Bone Marrow Transplant* 1994;13: 431–5

129. Meirow D. Ovarian injury and modern options to preserve fertility in female cancer patients treated with high dose radio–chemotherapy for hemato-oncological neoplasias and other cancers. *Leuk Lymphoma* 1999;33:65–76

130. Meirow D. Reproduction post-chemotherapy in young cancer patients. *Mol Cell Endocrinol* 2000;169:123–31

131. Meirow D, Lewis H, Nugent D, Epstein M. Subclinical depletion of primordial follicular reserve in mice treated with cyclophosphamide: clinical importance and proposed accurate investigative tool. *Hum Reprod* 1999; 14:1903–78

132. Boumpas DT, Austin HA, Vaughan EM, *et al.* Risk for sustained amenorrhea in patients with systemic lupus erythematosus receiving intermittent pulse cyclophosphamide therapy. *Ann Intern Med* 1993;119:366–9

133. Bines J, Oleske DM, Cobleigh MA. Ovarian function in premenopausal women treated with adjuvant chemotherapy for breast cancer. *J Clin Oncol* 1996;14:1718–29

134. Borgna-Pignatti C, Marradi P, Rugolotto S, Marcolongo A. Successful pregnancy after bone marrow transplantation for thalassaemia. *Bone Marrow Transplant* 1996;18:235–6

135. Bokemeyer C, Schmoll HJ, van Rhee J, *et al.* Long-term gonadal toxicity after therapy for Hodgkin's and non-Hodgkin's lymphoma. *Ann Hematol* 1994;68:105–10

136. Kreuser ED, Xiros N, Hetzel WD, Heimpel H. Reproductive and endocrine gonadal capacity in patients treated with COPP chemotherapy for Hodgkin's disease. *J Cancer Res Clin Oncol* 1987;113:260–6

137. Mackie EJ, Radford M, Shalet SM. Gonadal function following chemotherapy for childhood Hodgkin's disease. *Med Pediatr Oncol* 1996;27:74–8

138. Howell S, Shalet S. Gonadal damage from chemotherapy and radiotherapy. *Endocrinol Metab Clin North Am* 1998;27:927–43

139. Brusamolino E, Lunghi F, Orlandi E, *et al.* Treatment of early stage Hodgkin's disease with four cycles of ABVD followed by adjuvant radiotherapy: analysis of efficacy and long term toxicity. *Haematologica* 2000;85:1032–9

140. Hudson MM, Greenwald C, Thompson E, *et al.* Efficacy and toxicity of multiagent chemotherapy and low dose involved field radiotherapy in children and adolescents with Hodgkin's disease. *J Clin Oncol* 1993;11: 100–8

141. Wallace WH, Shalet SM, Tetlow LJ, Morris-Jones PH. Ovarian function following the treatment of childhood acute lymphoblastic leukemia. *Med Pediatr Oncol* 1993;21:333–9

142. Byrne J, Fears TR, Gail MH, *et al.* Early menopause in long term survivors of cancer during adolescence. *Am J Obstet Gynecol* 1992;166:788–93

143. Larsen EC, Muller J, Rechnitzer C, *et al.* Diminished ovarian reserve in female childhood cancer survivors with regular menstrual cycles and basal FSH < 10 iu/l. *Hum Reprod* 2003;18:417–22

144. Treolar AE, Boynton RE, Behn BG, Brown BW. Variation of the human menstrual cycle through reproductive life. *Int J Fertil* 1967;12: 77–120

145. Munster K, Schmidt L, Helm P. Length and variation in the menstrual cycle – a cross-sectional study from a Danish county. *Br J Obstet Gynaecol* 1992;99:422–9

146. Potashnik G, Goldsmith J, Insler V. Dibro-mochloropropane-induced reduction of the sex-ratio in man. *Andrologia* 1984;16:213–18

147. Egeland GM, Sweeney MH, Fingerhut MA, *et al.* Total serum testosterone and gonadotropin in workers exposed to dioxin. *Am J Epidemiol* 1994;139:272–81

148. Hensley ML, Ford JM. Imatinib treatment: specific issues related to safety, fertility, and pregnancy. *Semin Hematol* 2003;40(Suppl 2): 21–5

149. Genesca A, Benet J, Caballin MR, *et al.* Significance of structural chromosome aberrations in human sperm: analysis of reduced aberrations. *Hum Genet* 1990;85:495–9

150. Monteil M, Rousseaux S, Chevret E, *et al.* Increased aneuploid frequency in spermatozoa from a Hodgkin's disease patient after chemotherapy and radiotherapy. *Cytogenet Cell Genet* 1997;76:134–8

151. Robbins WA, Meistrich ML, Moore D, *et al.* Chemotherapy induces transient sex chromosomal and autosomal aneuploidy in human sperm. *Nat Genet* 1997;16:74–8

152. Generoso WM, Stout SK, Huff SW. Effects of alkylating chemicals on reproductive capacity of adult female mice. *Mutat Res* 1971;13: 172–84

153. Becker K, Schoneich J. Expression of genetic damage induced by alkylating agents in germ cells of female mice. *Mutat Res* 1982;92: 447–64

154. Pydyn EF, Ataya KM. Effect of cyclophosphamide on mouse oocyte *in vitro* fertilization and cleavage: recovery. *Reprod Toxicol* 1991;5: 73–8

155. Meirow D, Epstien M, Lewis H, *et al.* Administration of cyclophosphamide at different stages of follicular maturation in mice: effects on reproductive performance

and fetal malformations. *Hum Reprod* 2001; 16:632–7

156. Hawkins MM. Pregnancy outcome and offspring after childhood cancer. *Br Med J* 1994; 309:1034

157. Robbins WA. Cytogenetic damage measured in human sperm following cancer chemotherapy. *Mutat Res* 1996;355:235–52

158. Ashwood-Smith MJ, Edwards RG. DNA repair by oocytes. *Mol Hum Reprod* 1996;2:46–51

159. Kornblith AB, Anderson J, Cella DF, *et al*. Comparison of psychological adaptation and sexual function of survivors of advanced Hodgkin's disease treated by MOPP, ABVD or MOPP alternating with ABVD. *Cancer* 1992; 70:2508–16

160. Hjermstad MJ, Kaasa S. Quality of life in adult cancer patients treated with bone marrow transplantation – a review of the literature. *Eur J Cancer* 1995;31A:163–73

161. Marks S, Friedman SH, Delli Carpini I, *et al*. A prospective study of the effects of high dose chemotherapy and bone marrow transplantation on sexual function in the first year after transplant. *Bone Marrow Transplant* 1997;19: 819–22

162. Jensen PT, Groenvold M, Klee MC, *et al*. Longitudinal study of sexual function and vaginal changes after radiotherapy for cervical cancer. *Int J Radiat Oncol Biol Phys* 2003; 56:937–49

Pharmacological protection
of female fertility

J. L. Tilly

4

INTRODUCTION

Female fertility can be compromised by a large number of factors, including advancing chronological age[1-3] and exposure to pathological insults of an environmental or clinical nature[4-7]. Some of these factors negatively affect the competency of oocytes to become fertilized and progress through the early stages of embryogenesis, while others disrupt key aspects of the ovarian cycle that are needed to successfully mature and release an egg for fertilization. However, an even more basic problem looms in many cases of female infertility, that being simply a loss of the ovarian follicle pool[7]. In many mammalian species, including mice, rats and humans, female germ cell numbers plateau at some point during the perinatal period and then steadily decline throughout juvenile and adult life to the point of exhaustion[8-18]. Further, a number of studies have shown that a variety of pathological insults cause premature ovarian failure by accelerating depletion of the ovarian follicle pool[6,7].

For example, a link between ovarian damage and conventional anticancer therapies has been recognized for decades. Indeed, the possibility of preserving ovarian function in women given radiotherapy was tested nearly 40 years ago using lead shields to surround each ovary[19], although unfortunately little progress has been made since then in meeting this essential aspect of care for female cancer patients. This point is more apparent now than ever as the efficacy of cancer treatments is improved and, hence, greater numbers of patients are provided with a much better prognosis for long-term survival. Given this, and the fact that one in 52 human females will be diagnosed with cancer at some point during their pre-reproductive or reproductive years[20], efforts must be made to ensure a high quality of life in female cancer survivors post-therapy – including the ability to become pregnant and conceive healthy offspring.

With knowledge of the problem and the need for a solution clearly evident for so long, it remains uncertain why so few strides have been made in developing strategies to preserve fertility in female cancer patients. One key issue has probably been the paucity of information available on mechanisms by which radiation and chemotherapy damage the ovaries. This is not to say that the basis of premature ovarian failure caused by these insults is not known – this was clearly established early on as excessive germ cell and follicle depletion[21,22], but rather that extremely little is known of *how* oocytes are lost in response to anticancer therapies. It is on this point that much of the following discussion focuses, under the supposition that a greater understanding of how cancer treatments damage the ovaries will lead to new ways of thinking about how to prevent it. Furthermore, the development of therapies aimed at preventing oocyte loss in female cancer patients will, in all likelihood, impact on the management of many other paradigms of ovarian failure, since similar intracellular events appear to be responsible for germ cell depletion under both physiological and pathological situations[7].

Accordingly, the first part of this chapter gives a brief overview of the progress made in elucidating the molecular biology and genetics of oocyte death – which, for all intents and purposes, resembles the programed cell death pathway of apoptosis[23] – and how manipulation of the oocyte death program with pharmacological agents has been used to successfully combat mouse models of premature ovarian failure and infertility. As a preface for these discussions, a brief review of the process of apoptosis is necessary and thus is also provided. These sections are followed by one of a more hypothetical nature, exploring the possibility that ovarian cellular targets other than oocytes should be considered in the future design of fertility-preserving strategies for female cancer patients. Although data are not yet available to support this latter contention, recent studies of other cell systems – with particular reference to vascular endothelial cell response to radiotherapy – suggest that anticancer treatments may inflict damage on the female germ cell population by both direct and indirect mechanisms.

THE CELL DEATH PROGRAM OF APOPTOSIS

In its truest sense, the term apoptosis is one most pertinent to histologists since the definition of apoptosis is based on morphological changes in dying cells visualized by light and electron microscopy[23,24]. However, the execution of apoptosis is now known to involve the actions and interactions of a wide spectrum of gene products and cellular organelles[25-41], and thus the use of the term apoptosis has taken on a much wider application reflective of the involvement of specific pathways and proteins needed to carry out cellular elimination in the absence of the inflammatory response classically associated with 'primary necrotic' cell death[42,43]. An important aspect of apoptosis, which is relevant to the discussion below, is that the body utilizes this program of cell death to delete cells under physiological *and* pathological situations. Hence, insight gained into how a particular cell lineage dies under normal conditions – whether it be associated with tissue remodeling or induced in the cell by growth factor insufficiency, irreparable damage or senescence – has considerable ramifications for designing therapeutic

strategies to control apoptosis in that cell in a much broader context.

Although a complete overview of the genes and pathways involved in the regulation of apoptosis is beyond the scope of this chapter (for further details in this regard, the reader is referred to recent reviews[25-43]), several salient features need to be addressed. At the outset, it is important to re-emphasize that both physiological and pathological cues are capable of activating apoptosis in cells. Regardless of the stimulus, however, in most cases some type of cellular stress response pathway becomes engaged, generating a number of pro-apoptotic amplification signaling cascades that eventually feed into one or more central integration steps required to commit the cell to apoptosis. As discussed in more detail below, the second messenger ceramide – a sphingolipid often produced either *de novo* or through the hydrolysis of membrane lipids under conditions of cellular stress[44,45] – is of particular relevance to the issue of fertility preservation in cancer patients. Once generated, ceramide can serve as a potent stimulator of apoptosis[44,45]; however, as a safeguard to prevent the unwanted activation of apoptosis, ceramide can be converted to sphingosine. This metabolic step serves to not only reduce ceramide levels but also to generate an additional second messenger, termed sphingosine-1-phosphate (S1P), through the phosphorylation of sphingosine[46]. In a number of cell types, S1P has been shown to antagonize intracellular signaling events activated by ceramide as well as to prevent apoptosis induced by cellular stresses known to trigger the production of ceramide[46-48].

After the initial stress response pathways are set in motion, integration of these signaling events is often accomplished by the actions of a group of proteins referred to as Bcl-2 family members[26-29]. These proteins, which interact to form hetero- and homodimers, can be separated into those that delay or inhibit apoptosis (e.g. Bcl-2, Bcl-x_L, Bcl-w, Mcl-1) and those that facilitate or induce apoptosis (e.g. Bax, Bak, Mtd/Bok, Bad, Bid, Bim). While many roles for Bcl-2 family members have been proposed, their principal function is probably to alter the integrity of mitochondria and the endoplasmic reticulum (ER) and/or regulate release of 'apoptogenic' factors from these organelles into the cytoplasm[26–32,35]. These latter proteins include both components and co-factors needed for initiating the final or execution phase of apoptosis, which is carried out by another functionally and structurally related group of proteins referred to as caspases[37–40]. Under normal conditions, caspases exist in cells either as inactive proforms or in functionally sequestered sites. However, following mitochondrial and ER destabilization induced by pro-apoptotic Bcl-2 family members, caspases are rapidly activated in a proteolytic cascade that leads to cleavage of key functional and structural proteins[37–40], followed by involution and fragmentation of the cell into small membrane-bound bodies that are cleared by phagocytosis[42,43].

It is important to emphasize from these discussions that apoptosis not only occurs in a stepwise fashion but that the process also possesses an inherent 'point of no return', after which therapeutic intervention may not be feasible or even desirable. For example, previous studies have shown that suppressing caspase activity in at least some cellular models of apoptosis eventually activates a default pathway of cell death resembling primary necrosis[49], probably due to the fact that mitochondria and other organelles are still 'damaged' by pro-apoptotic Bcl-2 family members in a caspase-independent manner. If such a situation were to occur *in vivo*, a severe inflammatory reaction would be expected due to non-specific cell rupture. Accordingly, to theoretically achieve the optimum therapeutic benefit of suppressing death of a given cell – such as of oocytes exposed to anticancer therapies – a pharmacological agent that acts at a 'pre-mitochondrial' step in the apoptosis program would be the most logical to develop[50].

THE ROLE AND REGULATION OF APOPTOSIS IN OOCYTE DEPLETION

Under normal physiological conditions, greater than 99% of the oocytes generated by the human female during gametogenesis degenerate at some point during fetal or postnatal life[10,11,13–15,17,18], a process that theoretically serves as a quality control mechanism to ensure survival of only the best germ cells for procreation[7]. Comparable levels of oocyte loss have been described in rats and mice[8,9,12,16,51,52], and studies of both fetal and postnatal ovaries of various species, including humans, have confirmed that apoptosis is the principal mechanism responsible for female germ cell loss[7,52–56]. Given, however, that this topic has recently been reviewed in detail elsewhere[7], the following discussion provides only a brief overview of the character of oocyte death via apoptosis and the regulation of this process from a genetic perspective.

Three principal directions have been taken in efforts to evaluate the role of apoptosis in female germ cell development. The first of these has been to define the involvement of apoptosis in germ cell loss in the developing fetal ovaries during the process of female gametogenesis. In addition to exploring the significance of fetal oocyte death in the context of genetic defects that cause gametogenic failure – such as monosomy X in Turner syndrome[57,58] or meiotic pairing abnormalities[59,60] – such studies are central to understanding what factors are responsible for setting size of the neonatal quota of oocytes and, as a consequence, ovarian longevity. As is the case with many of the studies to be discussed herein, genetically manipulated mice have proved invaluable for identifying functionally important signaling pathways that regulate prenatal germ cell apoptosis in the female[61]. For example, inactivation of the gene encoding the ceramide-generating enzyme, acid sphingomyelinase (ASMase), causes a germ cell-autonomous death defect in the fetal ovaries that leads to the birth of females with excess numbers of oocyte-containing follicles[62]. Similar results have been obtained in studies of mutant female mice lacking the pro-apoptotic enzyme, caspase-2[63], whereas compromised production of the anti-apoptotic Bcl-2 family member, Bcl-x, results in the opposite outcome: oocyte insufficiency in the neonatal ovaries[64]. Interestingly, the absence of certain pro-apoptotic genes, such as *caspase-2*, protects the developing female germline from death triggered by a lack of appropriate growth (survival) factor support but fails to sustain the survival of oocytes harboring extensive meiotic defects[65].

The second direction that has been explored in detail concerns the role of oocyte apoptosis as an initiating event in the elimination of immature follicles from the postnatal ovaries via atresia. Like prenatal germ cell death, several genes that comprise the basic machinery of apoptosis have been identified from studies of mutant mice as important modulators of oocyte degeneration during atresia, with the pro-apoptotic Bcl-2 family member, Bax, emerging as a central factor[52]. In fact, studies of *bax* mutant female mice have demonstrated that Bax deficiency not only slows the rate of immature follicle atresia but also dramatically extends ovarian function well into advanced chronological age[52]. Despite the persistence of follicles at all stages of development, however, aged *bax* mutant females fail to become pregnant when housed with wild-type males. Although the basis for this observation remains to be established, the phenotype most likely results from normal aging of the hypothalamic–pituitary axis in *bax*-null females, based on findings that exogenous gonadotropins could be used in aged Bax-deficient animals to induce ovulation of fertilization-competent eggs that develop to the blastocyst stage *in vitro*[52].

The third and final direction has investigated the role of apoptosis in oocyte loss and premature ovarian failure associated with exposure of females to toxic chemicals or other pathological insults such as radiation. Since the topic of anticancer therapies and oocyte depletion is addressed in detail in the following section, a few brief comments are made here with respect to recent studies of how chemicals in the environment may perturb female fertility via mechanisms involving germ cell apoptosis. Of particular interest due to their widespread presence in the environment are polycyclic aromatic hydrocarbons (PAH), which are produced during the incomplete combustion of fossil fuels such as wood and coal. Another primary route of human exposure to PAH is through tobacco smoking. In addition to being considered general human health hazards by the Agency for Toxic Substances and Disease Registry (www.atsdr.cdc.gov/tfacts69.html), the adverse effects of PAH on specifically female reproductive function have been well documented[6,66–68]. Interestingly, PAH can activate a transcription factor of the *Per-Arnt-Sim* gene family termed the aryl hydrocarbon receptor (AHR)[69,70]. Recent studies with mice have shown that PAH-driven activation of the AHR induces apoptosis in oocytes by increasing expression of the pro-apoptotic gene *bax*[71]. Oocytes within ovaries of *bax*-null mice were found to be resistant to the cytotoxic effects of PAH, as were oocytes of *ahr*-null mice, confirming the functional significance of the AHR and Bax to the ovotoxic response[71]. Similar data were derived from studies of mouse fetal ovarian germ cell death caused by *in utero* PAH exposure[72], suggesting that PAH–AHR-driven oocyte loss proceeds via a common genetic pathway irrespective of the developmental stage of the ovary. Importantly, using a human ovarian xenograft model, it was further shown that PAH induce *bax* expression and apoptosis in oocytes of human primordial and primary follicles *in vivo*[71], underscoring the evolutionary conservation of this pathway. Such findings may collectively explain the earlier menopause often observed in women smokers compared with non-smokers[73], as well as the reduced fecundity reported to occur in human female offspring exposed to cigarette smoke-derived chemicals *in utero*[74].

SPHINGOSINE-1-PHOSPHATE AND OOCYTE SURVIVAL

In addition to ovarian damage resulting from accidental exposure to toxicants in the environment or workplace, female fertility can, and frequently does, suffer irreparable harm from pathological insults of a clinical nature in the form of anticancer treatments[75–77].

In 1997, a study with mice was published establishing for the first time a direct causal link between chemotherapy and oocyte apoptosis[78]. This investigation was significant since it not only provided mechanistic insight into how oocytes are lost following exposure to cytotoxic drugs used to treat cancer, but also identified several specific steps in the apoptosis program that are needed for oocytes to die in response to this insult. One step in particular proved extremely important for later studies on the development of a pharmacological approach to preserve ovarian function and fertility following anticancer therapy: that step was generation of the stress sensor ceramide. Although the initial experiments were *in vitro* in nature, proof of the concept that S1P, a naturally occurring metabolite and potent antagonist of the pro-apoptotic messenger ceramide, could prevent oocyte death induced by chemotherapy was nonetheless set forth[78].

The crucial next step was application of the *in vitro* results with S1P to an *in vivo* model of premature ovarian failure and infertility resulting from anticancer treatment. The first of two such studies was published 3 years later[62], using ionizing radiation as the pathological insult. In this investigation, it was shown that the depletion of the immature follicle pool in young adult female mice exposed to radiation could be completely prevented *in vivo* by a single injection of S1P into the bursal sac surrounding each ovary 2 h prior to irradiation[62]. Moreover, oocytes retrieved from ovaries protected from radiation with S1P were found to fertilize normally and produce high-quality blastocysts *in vitro*, suggesting that the competency of the protected oocytes was fully retained. This latter point was explored in more detail in a subsequent publication[79], which evaluated the long-term reproductive performance of the protected females in natural mating trials, as well as the quality of the offspring conceived using oocytes protected from radiation with S1P. For both endpoints, no differences were noted between non-irradiated control female mice and female mice that had been irradiated after *in vivo* S1P

therapy, including an absence of any evidence for propagated genomic damage in the offspring of the S1P-treated mice[79]. These studies collectively demonstrated that long-term protection of ovarian function and fertility in female mice exposed to radiotherapy could be achieved *in vivo* using a small-molecule antagonist of apoptosis.

Several important questions arise from this conclusion. First, would S1P provide a comparable level of *in vivo* fertility protection in females treated with cytotoxic drugs? No published data yet exist that address this question; although it is of note that S1P does protect murine oocytes from apoptosis induced by the chemotherapeutic drug, doxorubicin, *in vitro*[78]. Moreover, the extent of damage to the gonads caused by radiotherapy is believed to be equivalent to, if not worse than, that caused by many chemotherapy drug regimens[80]. Indeed, it has been estimated that as little as 600 cGy of radiation is sufficient to destroy oocytes and cause sterility in human females[80]. As such, it is highly likely that S1P would function as a fertility-preserving agent under conditions of either radiotherapy or chemotherapy. Second, would the ability of S1P to protect the female gonads from anticancer treatments be evolutionarily conserved? Obviously, the underlying basis of this question is rooted in the prospects of eventual human application of such technology. Unfortunately, no published studies in this regard are currently available, and any consideration of human application should be dependent on the prior completion and outcomes of preclinical trials with non-human primates.

Finally, would S1P, or for that matter any other pharmacological agent capable of suppressing oocyte apoptosis, be amenable to development as a fertility-preserving compound in women other than cancer survivors? This represents an intriguing prospect for which there are at least circumstantial data available from rodent studies. Past work has shown that the pro-apoptotic Bcl-2 family member, Bax, is required for oocyte apoptosis induced by both developmental cues[52] and anticancer therapy[78]. If S1P functions in a similar capacity, it is possible that the fertility-preserving effects of S1P in the radiation experiments discussed earlier[62,79] could be extended to perpetuate normal ovarian function past the current time of menopause in a manner recently achieved, at least in mice, by *bax* gene knockout[52]. Indeed, S1P has been reported to reduce the incidence of developmental germ cell attrition in fetal mouse ovaries[62]; however, it remains to be determined if S1P could be used to slow the natural aging process of the female gonads in postnatal life.

ARE OOCYTES THE ONLY 'TARGETS' *IN VIVO*?

It is evident from a number of the studies discussed above that oocytes possess an intrinsic program of apoptosis that can be inappropriately activated by pathological insults in a cell-autonomous manner. In fact, the identification of specific gene products, such as ASMase and Bax, which are functionally required for radiation or chemotherapy to kill oocytes, has provided an important foundation for the testing of pharmacological agents like S1P as fertility-preserving therapies. However, an intriguing prospect worthy of investigation is the possibility that, at least *in vivo*, follicle depletion following anticancer therapy results not only from direct activation of apoptosis in oocytes by radiation or cytotoxic drugs but also from damage to non-germline cells within the ovary that are needed for oocyte or follicle survival. To this end, the following hypothesis is offered as a means to stimulate research interest in this question, and perhaps provide additional insight into how premature ovarian failure and infertility in female cancer patients can be overcome in the future with pharmacological agents.

In other cells and organ systems, such as the gastrointestinal (GI) tract[81] and, quite surprisingly, tumor masses[82], a prominent role for microvascular endothelial cell apoptosis in mediating tissue damage and degeneration following exposure to radiotherapy is emerging. Like the ovaries, the GI tract is

often damaged as a side-effect of anticancer treatments[83,84], producing a lethal syndrome involving death of the intestinal crypt stem cells that limits the efficacy of radiation or chemotherapy in the treatment of certain forms of cancer. Using mice as a model, recent studies demonstrated that apoptosis of intestinal microvascular endothelial cells occurs rapidly following radiation exposure[81]. More importantly, pharmacological or genetic approaches that suppress endothelial cell apoptosis were found to prevent GI tract damage and the lethality associated with high-dose radiotherapy, suggesting that a loss of vascular support rather than direct damage to the crypt is responsible for this side-effect of anticancer treatment[81]. A similar series of observations and conclusions was recently reported from a study in mice of the responses of fibrosarcomas and melanomas to radiotherapy[82]. In this investigation, it was shown that tumors generated in mutant mice lacking the ceramide-generating enzyme, ASMase, or the pro-apoptotic Bcl-2 family member, Bax, grew faster than comparable tumors generated in wild-type animals. Furthermore, these tumors failed to regress following radiotherapy due to defective apoptosis of the ASMase- or Bax-deficient endothelial cells that colonized the tumor tissue after transplantation into the mutant animals[82].

While these data are interesting and exciting for a number of reasons that are outside the scope of this chapter, one of the more striking aspects of this work is the finding that radiation-induced degeneration of either the GI tract[81] or tumors[82] *in vivo* was shown to be defective in mutant mice lacking the same apoptosis gene products required for oocyte apoptosis and premature ovarian failure following anticancer treatment[52,62]. Could, then, a case be made for microvascular collapse as being at least partly responsible for accelerated follicle depletion from the ovaries of female cancer patients post-therapy? Unfortunately, little information is available with respect to the role played by the microvascular system in regulating the growth and survival of *immature* follicles in the ovary of any species. Thus, the possibility that a direct cause–effect relationship exists between ovarian microvascular endothelial cell loss and follicle degeneration is a subject of pure speculation at the moment. But that may be changing. Preliminary work with mice has found that immunoneutralization of vascular endothelial growth factor-like activity in the ovaries *in vivo* causes a rapid and sharp decline in the number of primary and secondary follicles[85], providing a tantalizing link between the microvascular system and immature follicle survival in the ovary. Such findings, coupled with the clear genetic parallels drawn before with respect to the mechanisms involved in radiation-induced degeneration of the GI tract, tumor masses and ovaries *in vivo*, at least provide a strong impetus to further pursue this line of inquiry.

CONCLUSIONS AND FUTURE CONSIDERATIONS

Over the past decade, considerable progress has been made in elucidating the mechanisms responsible for normal and premature ovarian failure. In most cases, apoptosis has been identified as the mechanism underlying oocyte and follicle loss, and several discrete steps in the oocyte apoptosis pathway have been pinpointed as potential therapeutic targets to sustain female reproductive function[7]. One of these steps – signal transduction via the pro-apoptotic stress transducer ceramide – can be inactivated using a small lipid found naturally in the body (i.e. S1P), with an ensuing maintenance of normal ovarian function and fertility, at least in female mice, following radiation treatment[62,79]. Furthermore, this lipid is protective in human oocytes as well (A. Jurisicova and J. L. Tilly, unpublished data), suggesting that the mechanism responsible for ovarian failure caused by anticancer therapies is evolutionarily conserved.

It should be noted that alternative strategies to preserve fertility in female cancer patients are also being pursued by a number of other laboratories[77]. Most – but not all (see below) – of these efforts focus on auto-transplantation of frozen-banked ovarian tissue, a procedure first successfully documented in rodents, followed by work in sheep and most recently in humans[77,86]. However, it is critical to stress that ovarian tissue cryopreservation and grafting has two principal limitations. First, the procedure is designed to provide a short-term restoration of fertility, rather than long-term preservation of ovarian function. In other words, these patients will still suffer from a premature onset of menopause, and all of the health complications associated with ovarian failure. Second, in those patients with blood cell-borne cancers, the risk of re-introducing the cancer cells into the patient post-therapy by ovarian tissue auto-transplantation is of great concern.

In separate studies, the possibility that gonadotropin releasing hormone (GnRH) agonists could be used to inhibit chemotherapy (cyclophosphamide)-induced ovarian failure in humans has been pursued[76–78], spurred on in large part by the success of earlier studies conducted with rodents[87,88] and rhesus monkeys[89]. However, the extent of the fertility-sparing effects of GnRH agonists in human females treated for cancer remains to be established, due to the small size and the heterogeneous nature of the patients studied (e.g. wide age range, different chemotherapy protocols) in the limited published trials conducted to date[76,90–93]. While comprehensive clinical trials are still needed to determine the efficacy of GnRH agonist therapy in preserving fertility in female cancer patients, results from limited experiments in rhesus monkeys warrant brief discussion. It was reported that oocyte (follicle) destruction and ovarian failure caused by cyclophosphamide, but not that resulting from radiation, is attenuated in animals given GnRH agonists[89,94]. Although the reasons for this are unclear, one possibility is that GnRH agonists are believed to work indirectly by slowing the recruitment of follicles through alterations in endogenous gonadotropin secretion, thus minimizing the number of growing follicles that can be targeted for destruction by cyclophosphamide. Since, on the other hand, radiation preferentially destroys resting (primordial) and early growing (primary) follicles in primates and other species[62,95], the mechanism(s) by which GnRH agonists protect the ovary would become unimportant under these conditions. Whatever the case, it may be that combined therapies using a 'cocktail' of agents, such S1P and a GnRH agonist, will ultimately prove to be the most efficacious with respect to broad, long-term protection of the female gonads from the destructive side-effects of chemotherapeutic drugs and radiation.

Finally, what does the future hold in terms of developing other pharmacological agents for fertility preservation in females? Considering the promising results obtained with S1P thus far[62,79], other options should be, and are being, explored with respect to targeting additional steps in the oocyte apoptosis program to achieve some level of normal reproductive performance in the face of anticancer therapy. Although it is premature to discuss much of these new efforts in our own laboratory, ongoing studies from other groups have identified a number of small molecules, of either a manufactured or endogenous source, capable of interfering with one or more steps required for the initiation and execution of cell death in various model systems. For example, small peptide inhibitors of caspases are being preclinically evaluated in mouse models of a wide spectrum of human diseases ranging from neurodegeneration to sepsis[96–98]. Moreover, recent studies have shown that humanin, an anti-apoptotic peptide, exerts its effects in cells by directly binding to, and functionally inactivating, the pro-apoptotic Bax protein[99]. In light of the many reports implicating Bax as a required factor for oocyte depletion associated with normal and premature ovarian failure[52,64,71,72,100], the possibility that female fertility could be manipulated with humanin or structurally related analogs of the peptide capable of suppressing Bax function is certainly reasonable and well worth testing in the future.

ACKNOWLEDGMENTS

The author would like to thank the many past and current members of his laboratory, as well as a number of collaborators and colleagues, whose efforts were instrumental in seeing many of the studies discussed to completion. This work was supported by the National Institutes of Health (R01-AG12279, R01-ES08430), the Steven and Michele Kirsch Foundation, and Vincent Memorial Research Funds.

References

1. te Velde ER, Scheffer GJ, Dorland M, *et al*. Developmental and endocrine aspects of normal ovarian aging. *Mol Cell Endocrinol* 1998;145: 67–73
2. Fitzgerald C, Zimon AE, Jones EE. Aging and reproductive potential in women. *Yale J Biol Med* 1998;71:367–81
3. Te Velde ER, Pearson PL. The variability of female reproductive ageing. *Hum Reprod Update* 2002;8:41–54
4. Sharara FI, Seifer DB, Flaws JA. Environmental toxicants and female reproduction. *Fertil Steril* 1998;70:613–22
5. Hruska KS, Furth PA, Seifer DB, *et al*. Environmental factors in infertility. *Clin Obstet Gynecol* 2000;43:821–9
6. Tilly JL. Apoptosis in female reproductive toxicology. In Roberts R, ed. *Apoptosis in Toxicology*. London: Taylor and Francis, 2000:95–116
7. Tilly JL. Commuting the death sentence: how oocytes strive to survive. *Nat Rev Mol Cell Biol* 2001;2:838–48
8. Zuckerman S. The number of oocytes in the mature ovary. *Rec Prog Horm Res* 1951;6: 63–108
9. Beaumont HM, Mandl AM. A quantitative and cytological study of oogonia and oocytes in the foetal and neonatal rat. *Proc R Soc Lond B Biol Sci* 1961;155:557–79
10. Baker TG. A quantitative and cytological study of germ cells in human ovaries. *Proc R Soc Lond B Biol Sci* 1963;158:417–33

11. Baker TG, Franchi LL. The fine structure of oogonia and oocytes in human ovaries. *J Cell Sci* 1967;2:213–24

12. Gosden RG, Laing SC, Felicio LS, *et al.* Imminent oocyte exhaustion and reduced follicular recruitment mark the transition to acyclicity in aging C57BL/6J mice. *Biol Reprod* 1983;28:255–60

13. Gosden RG. Follicular status at menopause. *Hum Reprod* 1987;2:617–21

14. Richardson SJ, Senikas V, Nelson JF. Follicular depletion during the menopausal transition: evidence for accelerated loss and ultimate exhaustion. *J Clin Endocrinol Metab* 1987;65:1231–7

15. Forabosco A, Sforza C, De Pol A, *et al.* Morphometric study of the human neonatal ovary. *Anat Rec* 1991;231:201–8

16. Anderson LD, Hirshfield AN. An overview of follicular development in the ovary: from embryo to the fertilized ovum *in vitro*. *Md Med J* 1992;41:614–20

17. Faddy MJ, Gosden RG, Gougeon A, *et al.* Accelerated disappearance of ovarian follicles in mid-life: implications for forecasting menopause. *Hum Reprod* 1992;7:1342–6

18. Faddy MJ. Follicle dynamics during ovarian ageing. *Mol Cell Endocrinol* 2000;163:43–8

19. Fraser AC. Conservation of ovarian function during pelvic irradiation. *Proc R Soc Med* 1966;59:833

20. Greenlee RT, Murray T, Bolden S, *et al.* Cancer statistics, 2000. *CA Cancer J Clin* 2000;50:7–33

21. Peters H, Levy E. Radiation sensitivity of the mouse ovary: fertility and oocyte survival. *Fertil Steril* 1964;15:407–18

22. Miller JJ, Williams GF, Leissring JC. Multiple late complications of therapy with cyclophosphamide, including ovarian destruction. *Am J Med* 1971;50:530–5

23. Kerr JFR, Wyllie AH, Currie AR. Apoptosis: a basic biological phenomenon with wide-ranging implications in tissue kinetics. *Br J Cancer* 1972;26:239–57

24. Kerr JFR, Winterford CM, Harmon BV. Morphological criteria for identifying apoptosis. In Celis JE, ed. *Cell Biology: A Laboratory Handbook*. San Diego: Academic Press, 1994:319–29

25. Tittel JN, Steller H. A comparison of programmed cell death between species. *Genome Biol* 2000;1:3.1–3.6

26. Gross A, McDonnell JM, Korsmeyer SJ. BCL-2 family members and the mitochondria in apoptosis. *Genes Dev* 1999;13:1899–911

27. Antonsson B, Martinou JC. The Bcl-2 protein family. *Exp Cell Res* 2000;256:50–7

28. Huang D, Strasser A. BH-3-only proteins – essential initiators of apoptotic cell death. *Cell* 2000;103:839–42

29. Puthalakath H, Strasser A. Keeping killers on a tight leash: transcriptional and post-translational control of the pro-apoptotic activity of BH3-only proteins. *Cell Death Differ* 2002;9:505–12

30. Adrain C, Martin SJ. The mitochondrial apoptosome: a killer unleashed by the cytochrome seas. *Trends Biochem Sci* 2001;26:390–7

31. Kroemer G, Reed JC. Mitochondrial control of cell death. *Nat Med* 2000;6:513–19

32. Shi Y. A structural view of mitochondria-mediated apoptosis. *Nat Struct Biol* 2001;8:394–401

33. Nakagawa T, Zhu H, Morishima N, *et al.* Caspase-12 mediates endoplasmic-reticulum-specific apoptosis and cytotoxicity by amyloid-beta. *Nature* 2000;403:98–103

34. Rao RV, Castro-Obregon S, Frankowski H, *et al.* Coupling endoplasmic reticulum stress to the cell death program. An Apaf-1-independent intrinsic pathway. *J Biol Chem* 2002;277:21836–42

35. Scorrano L, Oakes SA, Opferman JT, *et al.* BAX and BAK regulation of endoplasmic reticulum Ca^{2+}: a control point for apoptosis. *Science* 2003;300:135–9

36. Cain K, Bratton SB, Cohen GM. The Apaf-1 apoptosome: a large caspase-activating complex. *Biochimie* 2002;84:203–14

37. Harvey NL, Kumar S. The role of caspases in apoptosis. *Adv Biochem Eng Biotechnol* 1998;62:107–28

38. Budihardjo I, Oliver H, Lutter M, *et al.* Biochemical pathways of caspase activation during apoptosis. *Annu Rev Cell Dev Biol* 1999;15:269–90

39. Salvesen GS, Dixit VM. Caspase activation: the induced-proximity model. *Proc Natl Acad Sci USA* 1999;96:10964–7

40. Leist M, Jäättela M. Four deaths and a funeral: from caspases to alternative mechanisms. *Nat Rev Mol Cell Biol* 2001;2:1–10

41. Shi Y. Mechanisms of caspase activation and inhibition during apoptosis. *Mol Cell* 2002;9:459–70

42. Conradt B. With a little help from your friends: cells don't die alone. *Nat Cell Biol* 2002;4:E139–43

43. Franc NC. Phagocytosis of apoptotic cells in mammals, *Caenorhabditis elegans* and *Drosophila melanogaster*: molecular mechanisms and physiological consequences. *Front Biosci* 2002;7:1298–313

44. Kolesnick RN, Kronke M. Regulation of ceramide production and apoptosis. *Annu Rev Physiol* 1998;60:643–65

45. Pettus BJ, Chalfant CE, Hannun YA. Ceramide in apoptosis: an overview and current perspectives. *Biochim Biophys Acta* 2002;1585:114–25

46. Maceyka M, Payne SG, Milstien S, *et al.* Sphingosine kinase, sphingosine-1-phosphate, and apoptosis. *Biochim Biophys Acta* 2002; 1585:193–201

47. Cuvillier O, Pirianov G, Kleuser B, *et al.* Suppression of ceramide-mediated programmed cell death by sphingosine-1-phosphate. *Nature* 1996;381:800–3

48. Spiegel S. Sphingosine 1-phosphate: a prototype of a new class of second messengers. *J Leukoc Biol* 1999;65:341–4

49. Xiang J, Chao DT, Korsmeyer SJ. BAX-induced cell death may not require interleukin-1beta-converting enzyme-like proteases. *Proc Natl Acad Sci USA* 1996;93:14559–63

50. Tilly JL, Kolesnick RN. Realizing the promise of apoptosis-based therapies: separating the living from the clinically undead. *Cell Death Differ* 2003;10:493–5

51. McClellan KA, Gosden RG, Taketo T. Continuous loss of oocytes throughout meiotic prophase in the normal mouse ovary. *Dev Biol* 2003;258:334–48

52. Perez GI, Robles R, Knudson CM, *et al.* Prolongation of ovarian lifespan into advanced chronological age by *Bax*-deficiency. *Nat Genet* 1999;21:200–3

53. Coucouvanis EC, Sherwood SW, Carswell-Crumpton C, *et al.* Evidence that the mechanism of prenatal germ cell death in the mouse is apoptosis. *Exp Cell Res* 1993;209:238–47

54. De Pol A, Vaccina F, Forabosco A, *et al.* Apoptosis of germ cells during human prenatal oogenesis. *Hum Reprod* 1997;12:2235–41

55. Morita Y, Manganaro TF, Tao X-J, *et al.* Requirement for phosphatidylinositol-3′-kinase in cytokine-mediated germ cell survival during fetal oogenesis in the mouse. *Endocrinology* 1999;140:941–9

56. Morita Y, Tilly JL. Oocyte apoptosis: like sand through an hourglass. *Dev Biol* 1999;213:1–17

57. Burgoyne PS, Baker TG. Perinatal oocyte loss in XO mice and its implications for the aetiology of gonadal dysgenesis in XO women. *J Reprod Fertil* 1985;75:633–45

58. Zinn AR, Ross JL. Turner syndrome and haploinsufficiency. *Curr Opin Genet Dev* 1998; 8:322–7

59. Speed RM. The possible role of meiotic pairing anomalies in the atresia of human fetal oocytes. *Hum Genet* 1988;78:260–6

60. Mittwoch U, Mahadevaiah SK. Unpaired chromosomes at meiosis: cause or effect of gametogenic insufficiency? *Cytogenet Cell Genet* 1992; 59:274–9

61. Pru JK, Tilly JL. Programmed cell death in the ovary: insights and future prospects using genetic technologies. *Mol Endocrinol* 2001;15: 845–53

62. Morita Y, Perez GI, Paris F, *et al.* Oocyte apoptosis is suppressed by disruption of the *acid sphingomyelinase* gene or by sphingosine-1-phosphate therapy. *Nat Med* 2000;6:1109–14

63. Bergeron L, Perez GI, Mcdonald G, *et al.* Defects in regulation of apoptosis in caspase-2-deficient mice. *Genes Dev* 1998;12:1304–14

64. Rucker EB, Dierisseau P, Wagner KU, *et al.* Bcl-x and Bax regulate mouse primordial germ cell survival and apoptosis during embryogenesis. *Mol Endocrinol* 2000;14:1038–52

65. Morita Y, Maravei DV, Bergeron L, *et al.* Caspase-2 deficiency rescues female germ cells from death due to cytokine insufficiency but not meiotic defects caused by *ataxia telangiectasia-mutated* (*Atm*) gene inactivation. *Cell Death Differ* 2001;8:614–20

66. Mattison DR, Thorgeirsson SS. Smoking and industrial pollution and their effects on menopause and ovarian cancer. *Lancet* 1978; 1:187–8

67. Mattison DR. Morphology of oocyte and follicle destruction by polycyclic aromatic hydrocarbons in mice. *Toxicol Appl Pharmacol* 1980; 53:249–59

68. Mattison DR, Plowchalk DR, Meadows MJ, *et al.* The effect of smoking on oogenesis, fertilization and implantation. *Semin Reprod Health* 1989;7:291–304

69. Hankinson O. The aryl hydrocarbon receptor complex. *Annu Rev Pharmacol Toxicol* 1995; 35:307–40

70. Wilson CL, Safe S. Mechanisms of ligand-induced aryl hydrocarbon receptor-mediated biochemical and toxic responses. *Toxicol Pathol* 1998;26:657–71

71. Matikainen T, Perez GI, Jurisicova A, *et al.* Aromatic hydrocarbon receptor-driven *Bax* gene expression is required for premature ovarian failure caused by biohazardous environmental chemicals. *Nat Genet* 2001;28:355–60

72. Matikainen TM, Moriyama T, Morita Y, *et al.* Ligand activation of the aromatic hydrocarbon receptor transcription factor drives Bax-dependent apoptosis in developing fetal ovarian germ cells. *Endocrinology* 2002;143: 615–20

73. Jick H, Porter J, Morrison AS. Relation between smoking and age of natural menopause. Report from the Boston Collaborative Drug Surveillance Program, Boston University Medical Center. *Lancet* 1977;1:1354–5

74. Weinberg CR, Wilcox AJ, Baird DD. Reduced fecundity in women with prenatal exposure to

cigarette smoking. *Am J Epidemiol* 1989;129: 1072–8

75. Blumenfeld Z, Avivi I, Ritter M, *et al*. Preservation of fertility and ovarian function and minimizing chemotherapy-induced gonadotoxicity in young women. *J Soc Gynecol Investig* 1999;6:229–39

76. Meirow D, Nugent D. The effects of radiotherapy and chemotherapy on female reproduction. *Hum Reprod Update* 2001;7:535–43

77. Revel A, Laufer N. Protecting female fertility from cancer therapy. *Mol Cell Endocrinol* 2002;187:83–91

78. Perez GI, Knudson CM, Leykin L, *et al*. Apoptosis-associated signaling pathways are required for chemotherapy-mediated female germ cell destruction. *Nat Med* 1997;3:1228–32

79. Paris F, Perez GI, Haimovitz-Friedman A, *et al*. Sphingosine-1-phosphate preserves fertility in irradiated female mice without propagating genomic damage in offspring. *Nat Med* 2002; 8:901–2

80. Garcia JE. Fertility after cancer treatment. In Trimble EL, Trimble CL, eds. *Cancer – Obstetrics and Gynecology*. Philadelphia: Lippincott Williams and Wilkins, 1999:53–86

81. Paris F, Fuks Z, Kang A, *et al*. Endothelial apoptosis as the primary lesion initiating intestinal radiation damage in mice. *Science* 2001;293: 293–7

82. Garcia-Barros M, Paris F, Cordon-Cardo C, *et al*. Tumor response to radiotherapy regulated by endothelial cell apoptosis. *Science* 2003;300: 1155–9

83. Potten CS. A comprehensive study of the radiobiological response of the murine (BDF1) small intestine. *Int J Radiat Biol* 1990;58: 925–73

84. Somosy Z, Horvath G, Telbisz *et al*. Morphological aspects of ionizing radiation response of small intestine. *Micron* 2002;33: 167–78

85. Danforth DR, Arbogast LK, Kaumaya PTP, *et al*. Endocrine gland vascular endothelial growth factor (EG-VEGF) regulates preantral follicle growth. *Biol Reprod* 2003;68(Suppl 1): 324–5

86. Gosden RG. Gonadal tissue cryopreservation and transplantation. *Reprod Biomed Online* 2002;4(Suppl 1):64–7

87. Montz FJ, Wolff AJ, Gambone JC. Gonadal protection and fecundity rates in cyclophosphamide-treated rats. *Cancer Res* 1991;51: 2124–6

88. Ataya K, Ramahi-Ataya A. Reproductive performance of female rats treated with

cyclophosphamide and/or LHRH agonist. *Reprod Toxicol* 1993;7:229–35

89. Ataya K, Rao LV, Lawrence E, *et al*. Luteinizing hormone-releasing hormone agonist inhibits cyclophosphamide-induced ovarian follicular depletion in rhesus monkeys. *Biol Reprod* 1995;52:365–72

90. Blumenfeld Z, Avivi I, Linn S, *et al*. Prevention of irreversible chemotherapy-induced ovarian damage in young women with lymphoma by a gonadotrophin-releasing hormone agonist in parallel to chemotherapy. *Hum Reprod* 1996; 11:1620–6

91. Blumenfeld Z, Shapiro D, Shteinberg M, *et al*. Preservation of fertility and ovarian function and minimizing gonadotoxicity in young women with systemic lupus erythematosus treated by chemotherapy. *Lupus* 2000;9:401–5

92. Recchia F, Sica G, De Filippis S, *et al*. Goserelin as ovarian protection in the adjuvant treatment of premenopausal breast cancer: a phase II pilot study. *Anticancer Drugs* 2002;13:417–24

93. Blumenfeld Z, Dann E, Avivi I, *et al*. Fertility after treatment for Hodgkin's disease. *Ann Oncol* 2002;13(Suppl 1):138–47

94. Ataya K, Pydyn E, Ramahi-Ataya A, *et al*. Is radiation-induced ovarian failure in rhesus monkeys preventable by luteinizing hormone-releasing hormone agonists? Preliminary observations. *J Clin Endocrinol Metab* 1995;80: 790–5

95. Baker TG. Radiosensitivity of mammalian oocytes with particular reference to the human females. *Am J Obstet Gynecol* 1971;110: 746–61

96. Robertson GS, Crocker SJ, Nicholson DW, *et al*. Neuroprotection by the inhibition of apoptosis. *Brain Pathol* 2000;10:283–92

97. Guttenplan N, Lee C, Frishman WH. Inhibition of myocardial apoptosis as a therapeutic target in cardiovascular disease prevention: focus on caspase inhibition. *Heart Dis* 2001;3:313–18

98. Hotchkiss RS, Chang KC, Swanson PE, *et al*. Caspase inhibitors improve survival in sepsis: a critical role of the lymphocyte. *Nat Immunol* 2000;1:495–501

99. Guo B, Zai D, Cabezas E, *et al*. Humanin peptide suppresses apoptosis by interfering with Bax activation. *Nature* 2003;423:456–61

100. Takai Y, Canning J, Perez GI, *et al*. Bax, caspase-2 and caspase-3 are required for ovarian follicle loss caused by 4-vinylcyclohexene diepoxide exposure of female mice *in vivo*. *Endocrinology* 2003;144:69–74

Pharmacological protection of male fertility

5

S. Howell and S. Shalet

INTRODUCTION

It has been recognized for many years that testicular dysfunction is relatively common following treatment with cytotoxic chemotherapy and radiotherapy. The number of malignancies which are potentially treatable has increased over the last few decades. This, coupled with the improving long-term survival rates following treatment for many cancers, has meant that the number of survivors who have received cytotoxic therapy or radiotherapy is growing rapidly, and cancer treatment is becoming an increasingly common cause of acquired testicular dysfunction.

Impairment of spermatogenesis has been demonstrated in patients with various malignancies prior to treatment. In addition, germinal epithelial damage resulting in oligo- or azoospermia is a recognized consequence of treatment with certain chemotherapeutic agents and radiotherapy. This has initiated a search for possible strategies to preserve fertility in men undergoing therapy.

Cryostorage of semen has become standard practice, and should be offered to all men who may be desirous of future fertility before undergoing potentially sterilizing therapy. Improvements in the techniques used to store semen[1] and advances in the field of assisted reproduction, such as intracytoplasmic sperm injection (ICSI), have increased the chance of successful pregnancies using cryopreserved sperm. However, there are some limitations to this method of preserving fertility. First, it is not a feasible option for prepubertal patients. Furthermore, testicular function in adult males with malignant disease is often impaired before treatment[2], resulting in poor sperm quality or difficulty providing semen for storage. Oligospermia is found in a third to a half of patients with Hodgkin's disease, non-Hodgkin's lymphoma and testicular cancer before treatment, and also occurs in men with leukemia and soft tissue cancer[3]. Sperm motility is also impaired in these patients, and the process of freezing and thawing semen further reduces the sperm quality. Whilst successful fertilization may be achieved with only a few viable sperm using ICSI, pregnancy rates using this method are lower with abnormal semen than with normal semen[4]. As a result, methods for protecting or enhancing the recovery of normal spermatogenesis following gonadotoxic therapy have been pursued.

ANIMAL STUDIES

The unsubstantiated belief that, compared with pubertal or postpubertal boys, prepubertal boys have a lower rate of permanent chemotherapy-induced testicular damage[5] has led many investigators to propose that suppression of testicular function in adult men (i.e. 'inducing a prepubertal state') will provide a degree of protection against cytotoxic-induced testicular damage. Irrespective of the validity of the hypothesis, data derived from animal models have been encouraging (see Table 1). Ward and colleagues[8] demonstrated enhanced recovery of spermatogenesis in procarbazine-treated rats by the administration of Zoladex®, a gonadotropin releasing hormone analog (GnRH-a), for 2 weeks before chemotherapy and during chemotherapy. Increased stem cell survival was evident by

Table 1 Animal studies which have demonstrated improved spermatogenesis with hormonal treatment in conjunction with cytotoxic therapy

Cytotoxic insult	Hormonal treatment	Timing of hormonal treatment	Study
Procarbazine	testosterone enanthate	6 weeks before chemotherapy	Delic et al., 1986[6]
Procarbazine	GnRH-a antagonist plus testosterone	3 weeks before chemotherapy	Pogach et al., 1988[7]
Procarbazine	GnRH-a agonist	2 weeks before chemotherapy	Ward et al., 1990[8]
Irradiation	testosterone plus estradiol	6 weeks before irradiation	Kurdoglu et al., 1994[9]
Procarbazine	GnRH-a agonist and flutamide	3 weeks before chemotherapy	Kangasniemi et al., 1995[10]
Irradiation, mesna and cyclophosphamide	GnRH-a antagonist and flutamide	after irradiation, before cyclophosphamide	Meistrich et al., 1995[11]
Irradiation	GnRH-a agonist or testosterone	immediately after irradiation	Meistrich and Kangasniemi, 1997[12]
Procarbazine	GnRH-a agonist	immediately after and 20 weeks after chemotherapy	Meistrich et al., 1999[13]
Busulfan	GnRH-a agonist	immediately after chemotherapy	Udagawa et al., 2001[14]

Mesna, sodium 2-mercaptoethanesulfonate; GnRH-a, gonadotropin releasing hormone analog

50 days, and at 90 days sperm count was close to normal values and significantly higher than in rats treated with procarbazine only.

Similar protective effects of hormonal treatment have been described following the use of testosterone[6], testosterone and estradiol[9], GnRH-a and testosterone[7], and GnRH-a and the antiandrogen flutamide[10,11], following testicular insult with procarbazine, cyclophosphamide or radiotherapy. Pogach and associates[7] suggested that testosterone administered after treatment with procarbazine enhanced the recovery of spermatogenesis. Meistrich and co-workers[12] have confirmed that treatment with either testosterone or Zoladex following testicular irradiation with 3.5 Gy markedly improves the recovery of spermatogenesis, even if treatment is delayed for 10–20 weeks after irradiation[13]. The same group had previously shown that spermatogenesis did not occur after a similar dose of radiation despite the presence of type A spermatogonia in the seminiferous tubules[15]; they postulated that the role of hormonal treatments in the 'protection' of germinal epithelial function may be to enhance the recovery of surviving type A spermatogonia and to facilitate their differentiation into more mature cells, rather than to protect them from damage during cytotoxic therapy or radiotherapy. More recent data[16] demonstrated a significant improvement in recovery of spermatogenesis in irradiated rats pretreated with testosterone and estradiol, despite no change in stem spermatogonial numbers following irradiation, compared with a control group given radiation only. This is further evidence for the concept that hormonal therapy does not protect stem cells from destruction by cytotoxic agents but enhances their ability to differentiate subsequently.

MECHANISMS OF STIMULATION OF SPERMATOGENIC RECOVERY

Further work by the same group has begun to elucidate the mechanisms by which hormonal therapy exerts its effects. They demonstrated that GnRH-a-stimulated spermatogonial differentiation was inhibited in a dose-dependent manner by testosterone[17]. Furthermore, this effect of testosterone was reversed by adding the androgen receptor blocker flutamide, suggesting that the suppression of spermatogonial differentiation by testosterone is mediated through the testosterone receptor rather than via a non-androgenic

Table 2 Human studies which have investigated the hypothetical protective impact on spermatogenesis of hormonal treatment in conjunction with cytotoxic therapy

Cytotoxic insult	Hormonal treatment	Timing of hormonal treatment	Outcome	Study
MOPP	GnRH-a agonist	during chemotherapy	no effect	Johnson et al., 1985[20]
MVPP	GnRH-a agonist	during chemotherapy	no effect	Waxman et al., 1987[21]
PVB	GnRH-a agonist	before, during and after chemotherapy	no effect	Kreuser et al., 1990[22]
Irradiation	GnRH-a agonist and cyproterone	before and during irradiation	no effect	Brennemann et al., 1994[23]
Cyclophosphamide	testosterone	during chemotherapy	improved spermatogenesis	Masala et al., 1997[24]
Procarbazine or irradiation	testosterone plus medroxyprogesterone	median 8.4 years after treatment	no effect	Thomson et al., 2002[25]

MOPP, mechlorethamine, vincristine, procarbazine and prednisone; MVPP, mechlorethamine, vinblastine, procarbazine and prednisone; PVB, cisplatin, vinblastine and bleomycin; GnRH-a, gonadotropin releasing hormone analog

metabolite. This was further supported by the observation that spermatogonial differentiation could be suppressed in GnRH antagonist-treated irradiated rats by the addition of other androgens[18]. Intratesticular testosterone levels within the normal range in these experiments were sufficient to produce significant inhibition of spermatogonial differentiation. Further work has also suggested a possible role of follicle stimulating hormone (FSH) in the inhibition of spermatogenesis. The addition of exogenous FSH to a regime of GnRH antagonist and flutamide partly abolished the improvements in spermatogonial differentiation but to a lesser extent than testosterone[19].

The data therefore suggest that changes to spermatogonial cells induced by cytotoxic agents affect their ability to differentiate subsequently. Intratesticular androgens appear to be responsible for the inhibition of spermatogonial differentiation, but whether this is due to a block in a step of differentiation or to apoptosis of the spermatogonia is not clear. Suppression of intratesticular testosterone in the rat model is effective in improving spermatogonial differentiation if induced both before and after cytotoxic insult, and this produces difficulty in formulating a unifying mechanism. Meistrich and colleagues[16] have hypothesized that failure of recovery of spermatogenesis may be a result of persistent

cytotoxic-induced alterations in gene expression by an androgen-responsive cell. These alterations may regulate production of paracrine factors important for spermatogonial differentiation or apoptosis. Hormonal pretreatment may protect the target cells from damage whilst treatment after cytotoxic insult may be able to reverse the phenomenon by temporarily suppressing testosterone and reinitiating appropriate gene expression.

HUMAN STUDIES

Despite the encouragement from animal experiments, results from studies in humans have so far been disappointing (see Table 2). Several groups have used GnRH-a, with and without testosterone, to suppress testicular function during MOPP (mechlorethamine, vincristine, procarbazine and prednisone)[20] or MVPP (mechlorethamine, vinblastine, procarbazine and prednisone)[21] chemotherapy for lymphoma, cisplatin-based chemotherapy for teratoma[22] and testicular irradiation for seminoma[23]. None of these studies has demonstrated any significant protective effect of these therapies in terms of maintenance of spermatogenesis or increasing the rate of recovery. Only one small study has demonstrated a beneficial effect of hormonal therapy. Masala and associates[24] studied five men who were given physiological testosterone therapy whilst receiving cyclophosphamide for treatment of nephrotic syndrome. All five had normal sperm counts 6 months following the completion of treatment, compared with only one of ten men treated with cyclophosphamide alone.

Part of the explanation for the lack of a consistent effect of gonadal-suppressive therapy on recovery of spermatogenesis is that none of the above studies involved the continuation of treatment for a significant period of time after the completion of chemotherapy or radiotherapy. There is only one study which has examined the effects of hormonal treatment given after cytotoxic insult. Thomson and co-workers[25] treated seven men who had previously received cytotoxic therapy for childhood cancer with testosterone implants and medroxyprogesterone acetate to suppress the hypothalamo–pituitary–testicular axis for at least 12 weeks. At 48 weeks they all remained azoospermic with no histological evidence of spermatogenesis on testicular biopsy. All of the patients, however, had been treated with relatively high dose cyclophosphamide or radiotherapy during childhood which is likely to have resulted in complete loss of stem cells; a situation that will result in irreversible azoospermia.

The selection of the appropriate patient group is likely to be important in determining the response to hormonal therapy. The animal data suggest that hormonal treatment administered after cytotoxic insult may enhance recovery of spermatogenesis from surviving stem cells rather than protect them from destruction during cytotoxic or radiation insult. A prerequisite for the success of this approach is therefore the survival of stem cells during the gonadotoxic therapy. There are, however, few testicular histology data after chemotherapy or radiotherapy. Following cis-platin-based chemotherapy and low-dose radiation, spontaneous recovery of spermatogenesis occurs in most patients, although there is often a latent period of azoospermia which may last several years. The eventual recovery of spermatogenesis, however, implies the survival of type A spermatogonia. Following

chemotherapy for Hodgkin's disease with procarbazine-containing regimens and high-dose radiotherapy, recovery to oligo- or nor-mospermia status is much less common. Testicular biopsies taken after standard chemotherapy (MVPP and COPP (cyclophosphamide, vincristine, procarbazine and prednisone)) for Hodgkin's disease have shown complete germinal aplasia with a Sertoli cell only pattern[2,26–29], and this is also the case in men treated with 20 Gy radiotherapy[30]. There have been some recent reports of the isolation of mature sperm in the testicular parenchyma of some men with biopsy evidence of Sertoli cell only pattern, suggesting that even in this situation there may be small foci of spermatogenesis[31]. In addition, recovery of spermatogenesis occurs in a minority of these patients indicating that some germ cells survive in some patients. However, the absence of histological evidence of any spermatogenesis at biopsy in many men suggests that all spermatogonia may be eradicated during chemotherapy.

Hormonal manipulation after treatment to enhance the recovery of spermatogenesis is therefore likely to be of most benefit to those patients in whom the testicular insult is less severe, as it is these patients in whom there is significant preservation of type A spermatogonia. This would include patients receiving cyclophosphamide alone, AVBD (doxorubicin, vinblastine, bleomycin and dacarbazine) for Hodgkin's disease or cisplatin-based chemotherapy for testicular cancer. The success of this approach in those patients who have undergone more intense gonadotoxic therapy will depend on whether any stem cells remain. Complete ablation of the germinal epithelium may occur in many men following treatment with procarbazine-based chemotherapy regimens for Hodgkin's disease and high-dose chemotherapy, and this will clearly be irreversible.

POTENTIAL FUTURE CLINICAL APPLICATION

Treatment protocols in appropriate patient groups should probably use GnRH-a agonists or the less widely available GnRH-a antagonists to produce suppression of the hypothalamo–pituitary–testicular axis. Use of these agents alone may result in symptoms associated with hypogonadism such as reduced libido and lethargy, and may also have deleterious effects on body composition (reduced muscle mass and increased fat mass) and bone density. These could be avoided by concurrent treatment with androgen replacement. Whilst animal studies have suggested a dose-dependent attenuation of the effects of GnRH-a on recovery of spermatogenesis with the addition of systemic testosterone, the combination of these treatments will still result in a much lower level of intratesticular testosterone compared with untreated men. As it is suppression of intratesticular testosterone levels which appears to be the most important factor in stimulating recovery of spermatogenesis, it is possible that treatment with both a GnRH-a agonist/antagonist and systemic testosterone may stimulate spermatogonial differentiation but avoid the adverse effects associated with androgen deficiency.

Given that the decline in testosterone and sperm production is slower in men than in mice, the duration of treatment in humans should probably be at least double that used in animal models. Animal data suggest a potential benefit of treatment given before, during and after cytotoxic insult. Starting hormonal treatment before chemotherapy is unlikely to be practical, so treatment during and for at least 20 weeks after chemotherapy is likely to be the optimum achievable protocol. Selection of the appropriate study population is one of the most important factors in determining the success of any hormonal treatment protocol in men. To adequately assess the impact of hormonal therapy, the patients must have received a cytotoxic insult which is sufficiently gonadotoxic to result in temporary or permanent azoospermia in a significant proportion of patients. This insult must also, however, be associated with spontaneous recovery of spermatogenesis in a significant proportion of men, which would imply preservation of spermatogonial stem cells in at least some patients. Proof of a positive effect of hormonal manipulation may be derived from an increase in the proportion of men recovering normal spermatogenesis or from an increase in the speed of recovery. In practice, it is likely that if benefit is derived from this approach it will be in men who already have a reasonable chance of a spontaneous return of spermatogenesis. Thus, paradoxically, the group who have the greatest need for a new method of preserving fertility during cancer treatment, i.e. those in whom recovery of spermatogenesis is very unlikely, are the least likely to benefit from this technique. Nonetheless, hormonal treatment may significantly improve the chances of retaining fertility following successful treatment for cancer in a proportion of men, and such research in humans would lead to a greater understanding of the basic process of spermatogenesis.

References

1. Royere D, Barthelemy C, Hamamah S, Lansac J. Cryopreservation of spermatozoa: a 1996 review. *Hum Reprod Update* 1996;2:553–9
2. Chapman RM, Sutcliffe SB, Malpas JS. Male gonadal dysfunction in Hodgkin's disease. A prospective study. *J Am Med Assoc* 1981;245:1323–8
3. Padron OF, Sharma RK, Thomas AJ Jr, Agarwal A. Effects of cancer on spermatozoa quality after cryopreservation: a 12-year experience. *Fertil Steril* 1997;67:326–31
4. Aboulghar MA, Mansour RT, Serour GI, *et al.* Fertilization and pregnancy rates after intracytoplasmic sperm injection using ejaculate semen and surgically retrieved sperm. *Fertil Steril* 1997;68:108–11
5. Rivkees SA, Crawford JD. The relationship of gonadal activity and chemotherapy-induced gonadal damage. *J Am Med Assoc* 1988;259:2123–5
6. Delic JI, Bush C, Peckham MJ. Protection from procarbazine-induced damage of spermatogenesis

in the rat by androgen. *Cancer Res* 1986;46:
1909–14
7. Pogach LM, Lee Y, Gould S, *et al.* Partial prevention of procarbazine induced germinal cell
aplasia in rats by sequential GnRH antagonist
and testosterone administration. *Cancer Res*
1988;48:4354–60
8. Ward JA, Robinson J, Furr BJ, *et al.* Protection
of spermatogenesis in rats from the cytotoxic
procarbazine by the depot formulation of
Zoladex, a gonadotropin-releasing hormone
agonist. *Cancer Res* 1990;50:568–74
9. Kurdoglu B, Wilson G, Parchuri N, *et al.*
Protection from radiation-induced damage
to spermatogenesis by hormone treatment.
Radiat Res 1994;139:97–102
10. Kangasniemi M, Wilson G, Huhtaniemi I,
Meistrich ML. Protection against procarbazine-
induced testicular damage by GnRH-agonist
and antiandrogen treatment in the rat.
Endocrinology 1995;136:3677–80
11. Meistrich ML, Parchuri N, Wilson G, *et al.* Hormonal protection from cyclophosphamide-
induced inactivation of rat stem spermatogonia.
J Androl 1995;16:334–41
12. Meistrich ML, Kangasniemi M. Hormone
treatment after irradiation stimulates recovery
of rat spermatogenesis from surviving spermatogonia. *J Androl* 1997;18:80–7
13. Meistrich ML, Wilson G, Huhtaniemi I.
Hormonal treatment after cytotoxic therapy
stimulates recovery of spermatogenesis. *Cancer
Res* 1999;59:3557–60
14. Udagawa K, Ogawa T, Watanabe T, *et al.* GnRH
analog, leuprorelin acetate, promotes regeneration of rat spermatogenesis after severe
chemical damage. *Int J Urol* 2001;8:615–22
15. Kangasniemi M, Huhtaniemi I, Meistrich ML.
Failure of spermatogenesis to recover despite
the presence of a spermatogonia in the irradiated LBNF1 rat. *Biol Reprod* 1996;54:1200–8
16. Meistrich ML, Wilson G, Kangasiemi M,
Huhtaniemi I. Mechanism of protection of rat
spermatogenesis by hormonal pretreatment:
stimulation of spermatogonial differentiation
after irradiation. *J Androl* 2000;21:464–9
17. Shetty G, Wilson G, Huhtaniemi I, *et al.*
Gonadotropin-releasing hormone analogs stimulate and testosterone inhibits the recovery of
spermatogenesis in irradiated rats. *Endocrinology* 2000;141:1735–45
18. Shetty G, Wilson G, Hardy MP, *et al.* Inhibition
of recovery of spermatogenesis in irradiated
rats by different androgens. *Endocrinology* 2002;
143:3385–96
19. Meistrich ML, Shetty G. Suppression of testosterone stimulates recovery of spermatogenesis
after cancer treatment. *Int J Androl* 2003;26:
141–6
20. Johnson DH, Linde R, Hainsworth JD, *et al.*
Effect of a luteinizing hormone releasing
hormone agonist given during combination
chemotherapy on posttherapy fertility in male
patients with lymphoma: preliminary observations. *Blood* 1985;65:832–6
21. Waxman JH, Ahmed R, Smith D, *et al.* Failure
to preserve fertility in patients with Hodgkin's
disease. *Cancer Chemother Pharmacol* 1987;19:
159–62
22. Kreuser ED, Hetzel WD, Hautmann R, Pfeiffer
EF. Reproductive toxicity with and without
LHRHA administration during adjuvant
chemotherapy in patients with germ cell
tumors. *Horm Metab Res* 1990;22:494–8
23. Brennemann W, Brensing KA, Leipner N, *et al.*
Attempted protection of spermatogenesis
from irradiation in patients with seminoma by
D-Tryptophan-6 luteinizing hormone releasing
hormone. *Clin Investig* 1994;72:838–42
24. Masala A, Faedda R, Alagna S, *et al.* Use of
testosterone to prevent cyclophosphamide-
induced azoospermia. *Ann Intern Med* 1997;
126:292–5
25. Thomson AB, Anderson RA, Irvine DS,
et al. Investigation of suppression of the
hypothalamic–pituitary–gonadal axis to restore
spermatogenesis in azoospermic men treated
for childhood cancer. *Hum Reprod* 2002;17:
1715–23
26. Charak BS, Gupta R, Mandrekar P, *et al.*
Testicular dysfunction after cyclophosphamide-
vincristine–procarbazine–prednisolone chemotherapy for advanced Hodgkin's disease. A
long-term follow-up study. *Cancer* 1990;65:
1903–6
27. Ortin TT, Shostak CA, Donaldson SS. Gonadal
status and reproductive function following
treatment for Hodgkin's disease in childhood:
the Stanford experience [see comments]. *Int J
Radiat Oncol Biol Phys* 1990;19:873–80
28. Chapman RM, Sutcliffe SB, Rees LH, *et al.*
Cyclical combination chemotherapy and gonadal function. Retrospective study in males.
Lancet 1979;1:285–9
29. Das PK, Das BK, Sahu DC, *et al.* Male gonadal
function in Hodgkin's disease before and after
treatment. *J Assoc Phys India* 1994;42:604–5
30. Giwercman A, von der Maase H, Berthelsen JG,
et al. Localized irradiation of testes with carcinoma *in situ*: effects on Leydig cell function
and eradication of malignant germ cells in
20 patients. *J Clin Endocrinol Metab* 1991;73:
596–603
31. Mulhall JP, Burgess CM, Cunningham D, *et al.*
Presence of mature sperm in testicular
parenchyma of men with nonobstructive
azoospermia: prevalence and predictive factors.
Urology 1997;49:91–5

Laparoscopy for preservation of fertility and ovarian cryopreservation

6

T. Tulandi

INTRODUCTION

Pelvic irradiation is often indicated in some women with Hodgkin's disease, genitourinary and low intestinal malignancies, and for preparation for bone marrow transplantation. Depending on the site and extent of the disease, radiation can be administered locally or to a larger area. It is highly effective but may result in the loss of ovarian function. The damage caused by radiotherapy depends on the type of radiation, the total dose of radiation and the dose per fraction.

The LD_{50} or lethal dose of radiation required to eliminate 50% of the human primordial follicles is estimated to be 2 Gy. In adolescent girls, an irradiation dose of > 30 Gy is likely to cause permanent ovarian damage[1].

To avoid radiation to the ovaries, ovarian transposition by either laparotomy or laparoscopy has been advocated. The ovaries can be transposed medially behind the uterus, laterally outside the radiation field or to distant sites[2-19]. The most simple and effective method is laparoscopic lateral ovarian transposition. Obviously, this technique will not work for women undergoing chemotherapy.

LAPAROSCOPIC OVARIAN SUSPENSION

Laparoscopy versus laparotomy

In the case of radiotherapy, there is a strategy that avoids danger to the ovary without removing it from the body. Ovarian transposition by laparotomy is associated with preservation of ovarian function in 83% of patients after pelvic radiation[9]. It can be done as a part of surgical staging or as a separate procedure[6,9,12,13]. Ovarian transposition by laparotomy is associated with a large abdominal incision, a long hospital stay, and an increased risk of adhesion formation and intestinal obstruction. Laparoscopic ovarian transposition is therefore a more favorable method.

Table 1 lists reported cases of laparoscopic ovarian transposition before irradiation[20]. Of the total 46 evaluable cases, only two patients were over 40 years of age and these patients became menopausal after irradiation. Laparoscopic ovarian transposition in women < 40 years was associated with preservation of ovarian function in 39 of the remaining 44 cases or 88.6%. This compares favorably to the similar procedure by laparotomy.

Surgical technique

Lateral ovarian transposition is more effective than transposing the ovaries behind the uterus and protecting them with a lead block[5], which may also shield affected nodes. Another method is exteriorization of the ovaries under the skin through an opening in the flank. This approach is not widely used and has been associated with ovarian cyst formation[12]. A more complicated technique is heterotopic ovarian transplantation[13]. In this procedure, vascular anastomosis is performed and the ovary is implanted on the inner face of the arm.

In 1998, we described a laparoscopic ovarian transposition in a 34-year-old

Table 1 Reported cases of laparoscopic ovarian transposition before radiation. Adapted with permission from reference 20

Study	n	Age (years)	Indication	Site of the ovaries after transposition	Outcome
Lee et al., 1995[17]	1	23	medulloblastoma	lower anterolateral abdomen (base of round ligaments)	normal menses
Covens et al., 1996[5]	3	24–29	cervical cancer	paracolic gutters	normal menses in two patients, one patient whose ovaries slipped back into the pelvis became menopausal
Clough et al., 1996[3]	20	22–44	cervical cancer (17 patients); Hodgkin's disease (two patients); ependymoma of the cauda equina (one patient)	right paracolic gutter (right ovary only)	normal ovarian function in all 12 patients aged < 40 years, two patients aged 43 and 44 years became menopausal
Treissman et al., 1996[15]	1	38	anal carcinoma	pelvic brim	transient ovarian failure
Howard, 1997[8]	1	21	Hodgkin's disease	paracolic gutters	transient ovarian failure
Tulandi and Al-Took, 1998[11]	1	34	rectal carcinoma	level of anterior–superior iliac spine	normal menses, spontaneous conception and delivery of a healthy baby (2 years later)
Hart et al., 1999[7]	1	18	medulloblastoma	pelvic brim	needed two operations, normal gonadotropins 12 weeks after radiotherapy
Classe et al., 1998[2]	4	22–37	Hodgkin's disease	paracolic gutters	regular menses
Morice et al., 1998[18]	19	15–40	carcinoma of cervix and/or upper vagina; sarcoma; ependymoma of the cauda equina; ovarian dysgerminoma	paracolic gutters	normal ovarian function in 15 of 19 of patients, three patients with intact uterus conceived
Schulz-Lobmeyr et al., 1999[19]	1	23	Non-Hodgkin's lymphoma	level of lower kidney pole; right ovary only	normal FSH 2 months after radiation

FSH, follicle stimulating hormone

woman with rectal carcinoma[11]. It is a simple procedure without dissection of the cecum. In this case, we transected the ovarian ligament and transposed the ovaries without cutting the fallopian tubes. The ovaries were positioned laterally and anteriorly to the level of the anterior–superior iliac spines. Despite receiving a large dose of pelvic radiation externally in combination with intrathecal brachytherapy, the patient's menstrual cycles were never interrupted. She conceived spontaneously 2 years following surgery and delivered a healthy baby[20].

Subsequently, we performed a similar procedure in a few other young women prior to pelvic irradiation. The patients' menstrual cycles were never interrupted and they continued to menstruate regularly. A similar technique in a 17-year-old female with non-Hodgkin's lymphoma was reported[14]. The patient continued to have regular menstruations.

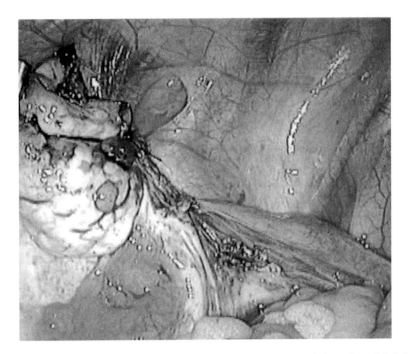

Figure 1 Laparoscopic ovarian transposition. The left ovary has been transposed above the pelvic brim

Sites of the transposed ovaries and the integrity of the fallopian tube

The ovaries have been transposed to a variety of sites and levels, from the base of round ligament to the level of the low kidney pole (Table 1). It seems that the ovaries should be transposed at least to a level above the pelvic brim (Figure 1). Transposition to this level can be achieved easily without separating the fallopian tubes from their uterine origin. This allows the possibility of spontaneous conception. To facilitate mobilization of the ovaries, the ovarian ligament should be divided. Unlike the fallopian tube, the ovarian ligament is not stretchable.

In a single reported case of ovarian transposition to the level of the pelvic brim, transient ovarian failure was encountered. Perhaps the final locations of the ovaries were lower than the authors had anticipated[15].

The transposed ovaries should be sutured securely to the peritoneum to prevent their return to the pelvic cavity. In a case where the ovaries were anchored with hemoclips only[5], the ovaries slipped back into the pelvic cavity

and the patient became menopausal after irradiation.

Radiation-induced cancer and cyst formation

One of the concerns of ovarian transposition is the possibility of radiation-induced cancer in the transposed ovaries. Anderson and colleagues[16] reported metastasis to the transposed ovary in a patient with cervical cancer. The ovarian cancer rate following radiation appears to be small. Another concern of ovarian transposition is ovarian cyst formation. However, it is usually a functional cyst. In women who have had an ovarian transposition, evaluation of the ovaries should be done by both abdominal and vaginal ultrasound.

LAPAROSCOPY FOR OVARIAN CRYOPRESERVATION

Another method to preserve ovarian function from the effects of radiation or chemotherapy is the retrieval of mature oocytes for *in vitro* fertilization. However, this is not applicable for prepubertal females and for those with no male partner. Furthermore, the time needed to achieve ovarian stimulation will delay cancer treatment. Retrieval of immature oocytes without hormonal stimulation, for *in vitro* maturation and fertilization followed by cryopreservation of the resulting embryos, can also be considered. However, in the absence of polycystic ovaries, only a few oocytes will be obtained.

Instead of cryopreserving oocytes, the ovarian tissue itself can be frozen[19,20]. Potentially, more oocytes will be obtained from thawed ovarian tissue. This technique is suitable for prepubertal women and is the most effective method for oocyte banking. It has been demonstrated that primordial follicles can be isolated from cryopreserved ovarian tissue and that they retain high viability rate. Also, in the case of ovarian failure, an autograft could be considered.

OVARIAN TRANSPLANTATION

In an animal model, cryopreservation and transplant of ovarian tissue have been followed by successful pregnancies and deliveries[21–23]. Follicular growth has also been observed with the use of human ovarian tissue as xenografts in immuno-deficient mice[24,25]. Recently, Bedaiwy and associates[21] reported that auto-transplantation of intact frozen–thawed sheep ovaries with microvascular anastomosis could restore the production of ovarian hormones. Vascular anastomosis is technically demanding and appears to be unnecessary.

Experience with allografts of ovarian tissue in humans is limited. The ovarian tissue can be placed in the ovarian fossa or in the subcutaneous tissue. Grischenko and co-workers[26] transplanted cryopreserved human ovarian tissue subcutaneously and demonstrated restoration of menstrual cycles. In another report, orthotopic transplantation of frozen–thawed ovarian cortical strips was associated with a return of ovarian hormone production[27]. A similar finding was reported with transplantation of ovarian tissue in the subcutaneous tissue of the inner arm and in a muscle pocket of the abdominal wall[28]. To date, however, there have been no live births reported with this technique.

One of the concerns with autotransplantation of ovarian tissue in cancer patients is the risk of transmission of microscopic disease. Therefore; it is important to examine the removed ovarian tissue histopathologically.

Ovarian resection or oophorectomy?

It would be logical to remove both ovaries if it was known that the treatment would make the patient menopausal. However, currently there is no method that can indisputably predict future ovarian function. Furthermore, surgical castration in young females might lead to psychological trauma. At present, we excise about a half of the ovary only (Figure 2). When the consulting oncologist feels strongly that the patient will become menopausal due to treatment, we remove an ovary.

Surgical technique

The technique depends on how much ovarian tissue will be excised. A few days prior to surgery, the embryologist should ascertain that the cryoprotective solution is available and not expired, and that he or she will be available to retrieve the specimen upon removal. The technique is done by laparoscopy. No special technique is required to remove the ovary[29].

Ovarian resection is performed by removing a portion of the ovary using laparoscopic scissors. Because it causes thermal damage to ovarian tissue, electrocoagulation should not be used. The excised specimen is left attached to the ovary until the embryologist is ready to receive it. The tissue is removed from the abdominal cavity through a 10 mm port. The ovarian opening is then sutured using a few interrupted sutures of 4-0 PDS. A small piece

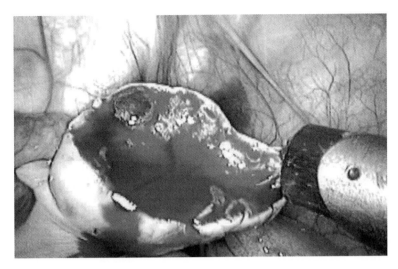

Figure 2 Laparoscopic ovarian resection for cryopreservation. Approximately a third to a half of the ovary has been excised

of ovarian tissue is sent for histopathological examination.

CONCLUSIONS

Laparoscopic ovarian transposition is simple and effective. In women aged < 40 years, it is associated with preservation of ovarian function in 88.6% of cases. This compares favorably to the similar procedure by laparotomy. Contrary to previous reports, ovarian transposition can be performed with preservation of the integrity of the fallopian tube, allowing future spontaneous conception. During laparoscopy, a portion of the ovary could be removed for ovarian cryopreservation. This allows the patient to maintain her options of fertility and of autografting her ovary if ovarian failure occurs. Ovarian cryopreservation is also indicated for women undergoing chemotherapy.

References

1. Janson PO. Possibilities of fertility preservation in children and young adults undergoing treatment for malignancy. *Acta Obstet Gynecol Scand* 2000;79:240–3
2. Classe J, Mahe M, Moreau P, *et al*. Ovarian transposition by laparoscopy before radiotherapy in the treatment of Hodgkin's disease. *Cancer* 1998;83:1420–4
3. Clough KB, Goffinet F, Labib A, *et al*. Laparoscopic unilateral ovarian transposition prior to irradiation: prospective study of 20 cases. *Cancer* 1996;77:2638–45
4. Ray GR, Trueblood HW, En Right L, *et al*. Oophoropexy: a means of preserving ovarian function following pelvic mega voltage radiotherapy for Hodgkin's disease. *Radiology* 1970; 96:175–80
5. Covens A, Putten H, Fyles A, *et al*. Laparoscopic ovarian transposition. *Eur J Gynaecol Oncol* 1996;3:177–82
6. Gabriel DA, Bernard SA, Lambert J, Croom RD III. Oophoropexy and the management of Hodgkin's diseases. *Arch Surg* 1986;121:1083–5
7. Hart R, Sawyer E, Magos A. Case report of ovarian transposition and review of literature. *Gynecol Endosc* 1999;8:51–4
8. Howard FM. Laparoscopic lateral ovarian transposition before radiation. Treatment of Hodgkin's disease. *J Am Assoc Gynecol Laparosc* 1997;5:601–4

9. Husseinzadeh N, Nahhas WA, Velkley DE, et al. The preservation of ovarian function in young women undergoing pelvic irradiation therapy. *Gynecol Oncol* 1984;18:373–9

10. Williams R, Mendenhall N. Laparoscopic oophoropexy for preservation of ovarian function before pelvic node irradiation. *Obstet Gynecol* 1992;80:541–3

11. Tulandi T, Al-Took S. Laparoscopic ovarian suspension before irradiation. *Fertil Steril* 1998;70:381–3

12. Kovacev M. Exterioration of ovaries under the skin of young women operated upon for cancer of the cervix. *Am J Obstet Gynecol* 1968; 101:756–9

13. Leporrier M, von Theobald P, Roffe JL, Mueller G. A new technique to protect ovarian function before pelvic irradiation. *Cancer* 1987;60:2201–4

14. Yarali H, Demirol A, Bukulmez O, et al. Laparoscopic high lateral transposition of both ovaries before pelvic irradiation. *J Am Assoc Gynecol Laparosc* 2000;7:237–9

15. Treissman MJ, Miller D, McComb PF. Laparoscopic lateral ovarian transposition. *Fertil Steril* 1996;65:1229–31

16. Anderson B, LaPolla J, Turner D, et al. Ovarian transposition in cervical cancer. *Gynecol Oncol* 1993;49:206–14

17. Lee C, Lai Y, Soong Y, et al. Laparoscopic ovariopexy before irradiation for medulloblastoma. *Hum Reprod* 1995;2:372–4

18. Morice P, Castaigne D, Haie-Meder C, et al. Laparoscopic ovarian transposition for pelvic malignancies: indications and functional outcomes. *Fertil Steril* 1998;70:956–60

19. Schulz-Lobmeyr I, Schratter-Sehn A, Huber J, Wenzl R. Laparoscopic lateral ovarian transposition before pelvic irradiation for a non-Hodgkin lymphoma. *Acta Obstet Gynecol Scand* 1999;78:350–2

20. Bisharah M, Tulandi T. Laparoscopic preservation of ovarian function: an underused procedure. *Am J Obstet Gynecol* 2003;188:367–70

21. Bedaiwy M, Jeremias E, Gurunluoglu R, et al. Restoration of function after auto transplantation of intact frozen–thawed sheep ovaries with microvascular anastomosis. *Fertil Steril* 2003; 79:594–602

22. Candy CJ, Wood MJ, Whittingham DG. Restoration of a normal reproductive life span after grafting of cryopreserved mouse ovaries. *Hum Reprod* 2000;15:1300–4

23. Salle B, Demirci B, Franck M, et al. Normal pregnancies and live births after autograft of frozen–thawed hemi-ovaries into ewes. *Fertil Steril* 2002;77:403–8

24. Oktay K, Newton H, Mullan J, Godsen RG. Development of human primordial follicles to antral stages in SCID/hpg mice stimulated with follicular stimulating hormones. *Hum Reprod* 1998;13:1133–8

25. Weissman A, Gotlieb L, Colgan T, et al. Preliminary experience with subcutaneous human ovarian cortex transplantation in the NOD-SCID mouse. *Biol Reprod* 1999;60:1462–7

26. Grischenko VI, Chub NN, Lobyntseva GS, et al. Creation of a bank of cryopreserved human ovarian tissue for allotransplantation in gynaecology. *Kriobiologia* 1987;3:7–11

27. Radford JA, Lieberman BA, Brison DR, et al. Orthotopic reimplantation of cryopreserved ovarian cortical strips after high-dose chemotherapy for Hodgkin's lymphoma. *Lancet* 2001;357:1172–5

28. Callejo J, Salvador C, Miralles A, et al. Long-term ovarian function evaluation after autografting by implantation with fresh and frozen–thawed human ovarian tissue. *J Clin Endocrinol Metab* 2001;86:4489–94

29. Tulandi T. Oophorectomy and laparoscopic orchiectomy. In Tulandi T, ed. *Atlas of Laparoscopy and Hysteroscopy Techniques.* London: WB Saunders, 1999:69–75

Strategies for gynecological cancers 7

G. Del Priore and G. S. Huang

INTRODUCTION

Less than a generation ago, women with cancer had little to hope for and even less to look forward to. Survival was low and expectations even lower. However, owing to significant therapeutic advances, a cancer diagnosis is no longer a death sentence. Greater treatment successes and the social phenomenon of later childbearing have presented us with an enviable problem. More and more women with cancer in their lives are now raising fertility preservation as a legitimate quality-of-life concern.

This chapter discusses the most common gynecological cancers as they relate to fertility. It includes basic information on traditional oncology treatments as well as promising alternative therapies to preserve or maximize fertility. Although conception after a cancer diagnosis is not new, it has not received the attention it deserves until now. The information below is limited but research and patient advocacy will undoubtedly change the current situation for the better.

BREAST CANCER

Breast cancer has been and will continue to be a leading cancer issue for women in the United States. Fortunately, breast cancer incidence and mortality have been declining in the USA since the late 1980s[1,2]. This is due at least in part to better screening and earlier detection, so that the majority of breast cancer detected in the USA today is by mammography[3,4]. Although the peak age of breast cancer diagnosis is later in life, approximately 10–20% of breast cancer patients are of childbearing age, when fertility is a major quality-of-life concern. The end result is that 5–10% of breast cancer patients become pregnant each year[5].

Fortunately, pregnancy is no longer considered contraindicated in breast cancer patients. In fact, survival for former breast cancer patients is higher among those who subsequently become pregnant[6,7]. Previous studies were limited by not controlling for confounders such as the time of diagnosis, failure to recognize the latency period between diagnosis and exposure to causative agents. The incident pregnancy cannot be easily implicated as a causative factor in a cancer diagnosed around delivery. Cancers diagnosed during pregnancy originated years before the incident pregnancy. They are obviously unrelated to the incident pregnancy as a causative factor. In acknowledging this relationship, 'therapeutic' abortions are no longer prescribed. Furthermore, recent data confirm there is no survival advantage to pregnancy termination or proscription. The uncertainty not withstanding, the recommendation against pregnancy has always hinted of patronism toward women and their ability to set their own priorities[8].

The optimal timing of conception after breast cancer treatment is still uncertain. This is not because of physiological concerns but rather a social and personal decision that balances the risk of recurrence, peak time to recurrence and the patient's reproductive priorities. The current arbitrary consensus is to wait some time between 6 and 24 months before attempting to conceive, although individual circumstances can justify any interval[9]. A specific example on the timing of conception is given in the section on ovarian cancer.

Timing of conception may lead to more anxiety for the patient and her physician if assisted reproductive technologies (ART) are contemplated. ART has been associated with ovarian cancers although the association is probably not causal[10,11]. Nevertheless, patients and physicians continue to be nervous when employing ART in cancer patients. It is not uncommon for an oncologist to be asked to 'clear' a cancer survivor for ART. Although institutions should be supportive of patients and the difficult decisions they face, promoting ART in cancer patients is not without risks. Therefore, a close collaboration between oncologists, perinatologists and reproductive endocrinologists is essential. Through this collaborative process, informed patients can be offered every possible option to achieve their family planning objectives while being cautioned about the largely unknown long-term consequences.

An illustrative but by no means unique case of fertility preservation in a cancer patient involved a woman and her attorney husband who had been treated unsuccessfully for infertility for 5 years with ART before finally delivering. Her father had died from breast cancer at age 48. During ART, she was diagnosed with stage IA, grade 1 ovarian cancer and treated with unilateral oophorectomy. Two years later, she successfully delivered twins. After a subsequent hysterectomy and oophorectomy, she remains free of disease on estrogen replacement therapy (ERT)[12].

Neither ART nor ERT is contraindicated in this clinical situation. In fact, successful ART is associated with a reduction in diagnoses of breast and ovarian cancer[13]. Physician and patient may be concerned about estrogen exposure from ART. However, it is reassuring that survival is actually improved in ovarian and breast cancer survivors subsequently treated with ERT[14-17]. Given the probable presence of an inherited mutation in this patient, her cancers were (i.e. ovarian) and are (i.e. breast) inevitable. ART allowed her to realize her reproductive objectives as determined by her and her partner. Certainly, in many patients with cancers that have a poor prognosis, quality of life is paramount when a cure may not be possible. Achieving her family planning objectives satisfied this patient's quality-of-life issues immensely, with no definitive increase in cancer risk.

Selective estrogen receptor modulators (SERMs) may delay the diagnosis of breast cancer in some risk groups. However, ERT is associated with a more important reduction in breast cancer death among at-risk groups[14-17]. A survival advantage for ERT is also consistent with the worsening survival seen after prolonged exposure to SERMs[18]. Based on the retrospective evidence of an ERT benefit on breast cancer survival, prospective, randomized clinical trials have accrued and continue to accrue breast cancer survivors to ERT versus placebo[19,20]. All of this may be reassuring to the patient and her physicians who are concerned about estrogen exposure during ART.

OVARIAN CANCER

As the previous example illustrates, women with a family history of breast cancer are often at increased risk for ovarian cancer. Ovarian cancer has long been perceived as a deadly disease; however, today's 5-year survival rate is double that of a generation ago[21]. The prognosis is actually very good for early-stage disease, with 90% of stage I cancer patients surviving 5 or more years. Often, those patients with the best prognosis are younger and have earlier stages of the disease. They usually do not present with the typical signs of ovarian cancer to a gynecological oncologist. Instead a general gynecologist may encounter them as a younger patient of reproductive age presenting with pelvic pain and an unexpected pelvic mass. Often in these situations fertility issues are unknown or at best known to be undecided.

Under these circumstances, aggressive surgical therapy, i.e. bilateral salpingo-oophorectomy, is best deferred until a definitive pathological diagnosis can be made. Frozen section should not be used as an indication for castration of a young person except in the clearest situation of advanced epithelial ovarian cancer. This delay in 'definitive' surgery will maximize the patient's chances of preserving fertility. Awaiting the final pathology result will also allow the patient to fully consider all her options with important members of her support network. After these discussions, referral to a specialist at a tertiary center may be a desirable option. For instance, tertiary referral centers may even consider fertility preservation in relatively advanced ovarian cancer under the right circumstances. Although successful pregnancies have been reported after the diagnosis and treatment of advanced ovarian cancer, it should be considered carefully[22].

However, the worse potential surgical outcome in a younger patient with unclear fertility objectives is to have a hysterectomy and bilateral oophorectomy, but no thorough dissection of the para-aortic lymph nodes. Too often this staging procedure is omitted because of the unavailability of a trained gynecological oncologist. This is the most important part of the surgical management of ovarian cancer, given that the high para-aortic nodes near the renal vessels are the most likely site of occult metastatic disease[23,24]. Clearly, if para-aortic nodes cannot be properly sampled, then removing an apparently normal uterus and normal contralateral ovary should not be done for the sake of 'staging'.

Once the diagnosis is confirmed by final pathological review, a repeat operation may be necessary to determine the need for additional chemotherapy treatment. The potential need for a repeat operation may be disappointing to the patient and the original treating physician. However, it may also be considered an essential risk needed to avoid unnecessary castration. Even if the diagnosis is clearly ovarian cancer at the initial surgery, should the patient desire future fertility, a unilateral salpingo-oophorectomy is acceptable as long as complete staging is performed including lymph node dissection.

Cystectomies have sometimes been performed for a presumed benign cyst in patients later found to have ovarian cancer. Cystectomies are often done in young patients

where the cancer diagnosis may not be suspected intra-operatively. Although these patients have done well with a good overall survival, the recurrence risk is greater than after unilateral salpingo-oophorectomy[25]. If the tumor was not completely resected at the time of cystectomy, a repeat operation for unilateral oophorectomy and staging may be indicated. Before any repeat operation, tumor surveillance should be initiated. This includes a computed tomography scan of the abdomen and pelvis plus serum tumor markers. Tumor markers should be drawn as soon as possible to determine if there are any circulating levels that can be used for surveillance. If the serum markers are negative after a long interval between surgery and the blood draw, immunostains on the pathology specimen may be useful to determine if the original tumor expressed any potential serum markers, e.g. CA125, CA19.9, CEA, etc.

The fertility-preserving management of ovarian cancer can also be looked at from the perspective of basic histological classifications, including epithelial, the most typical type of cancer, and germ cell, which is particularly relevant for younger patients and borderline tumors. In a large case series of epithelial ovarian cancers reported in 1997 among reproductive-aged women with stage I disease, 56 patients were managed with fertility-sparing surgery compared to 43 who underwent radical surgery[26]. Management was not randomized. Nulliparous women comprised 84% of the fertility-sparing group. Among conservatively managed patients, 19 were stage IC and 50% were grade 3, representing a high-risk group. Five patients (9%) in the fertility-sparing group recurred, while five patients (12%) in the radical surgery group recurred. Overall, 17 patients in the fertility-sparing group achieved pregnancy with a total of 25 conceptions. Among 36 patients with stage IA disease in the fertility-sparing group, three recurred, of which only one recurrence was in the retained ovary. A similar cohort was reported in 2002. In this multi-institutional observational study, patients with stage IA ($n = 42$) or stage IC ($n = 10$)

epithelial ovarian cancer were treated with fertility-sparing surgery[27]. The majority of tumors were well-differentiated. Five recurrences were observed (three in the contralateral ovary). At last follow-up, 50 patients were alive and two were dead from the disease, with an estimated 5-year survival rate of 98% and 10-year survival rate of 93%. Of 24 patients attempting pregnancy, 17 patients (71%) conceived, resulting in 26 term deliveries (no fetal anomalies) and five spontaneous abortions.

These data support the selective incorporation of fertility-sparing surgery for the management of stage IA or stage IC epithelial ovarian cancer in reproductive-aged patients who have been optimally staged and appropriately counseled. While the risk of recurrent ovarian cancer is significant, the overall cure rate does not appear to differ significantly between similar patients undergoing fertility-sparing versus radical surgery. The majority of conservatively managed patients who attempt pregnancy can be expected to conceive spontaneously and achieve successful term pregnancies.

The treatment of malignant ovarian germ cell tumors with fertility-sparing surgery has been accepted as the standard of care in these patients[21]. Ovarian germ cell tumors commonly present at an early stage and occur in children and young women. These tumors tend to be highly sensitive to chemotherapy, and even recurrent disease may be cured with second-line therapy. In a series of 31 patients with malignant germ cell tumors, only one of 21 patients treated with fertility-preserving surgery died from the disease, while three of ten patients treated with radical surgery died[28]. Patients with malignant germ cell tumors typically receive systemic adjuvant chemotherapy. The regimens in use do not appear to have an adverse effect on subsequent pregnancy outcome. In one report, a total of 38 children were born to women who had received systemic chemotherapy (either vincristine/actinomycin/cyclophosphamide or a multiagent cisplatin-containing regimen). No congenital anomalies were observed[29].

Borderline ovarian tumors often occur in reproductive-aged women, and the prognosis for all stages of disease is excellent. The literature contains well over 100 cases of conservative management of borderline ovarian tumors. They tend to be more often stage I. The risk of recurrence is less than that of frankly malignant epithelial ovarian cancer but not rare (8–36%). Ovarian cystectomy to preserve fertility rather than adnexectomy is associated with greater recurrences but the overall survival is unaffected[30,31].

In patients treated with fertility-preserving surgery to preserve fertility, it seems prudent to perform a completion hysterectomy and adnexectomy after childbearing objectives have been achieved. Theoretically, this may decrease risk of recurrence or of a second primary tumor in the retained residual ovary.

The timing of conception must be individualized for patients with cancer. As alluded to at the end of the preceding section on breast cancer, ovarian cancer illustrates the nuances of this counseling and decision making for the patient. For instance, the more common epithelial ovarian cancer has a poorer prognosis than borderline germ cell cancer. The traditional recommendation may have been to wait for 2 or more years to avoid conception before detection of an occult recurrence. However, these two years may actually represent a 'window of opportunity' for the patient who has a poor prognosis. Once ovarian cancer recurs for the first time, subsequent recurrences become more frequent and more difficult to treat. A patient with newly diagnosed ovarian cancer may not have another chance to conceive except immediately after her initial diagnosis.

Spontaneous pregnancy is certainly not contraindicated after an ovarian cancer diagnosis. However, ART may be more difficult to consider because of its previous association with ovarian cancer in the literature[11]. This association is probably not causal according to more recent research[10]. In fact, successful treatment with ART is now associated with a reduction of ovarian cancer.

Despite this reassurance, ART is perhaps most difficult to consider for the infertility patient with a genetic predisposition for ovarian cancer. This issue was raised earlier by the example above from the perspective of the patient herself. However, the potential expression of cancer after ART in the offspring of women ART patients with a genetic predisposition will undoubtedly complicate matters further[32].

Once childbearing is complete, these patients may experience early menopause. ERT may be considered in menopausal patients with ovarian cancer for quality-of-life benefits. In patients with a potentially fatal cancer and a shortened life expectancy, short-term symptomatic relief of menopausal symptoms and quality-of-life issues are perhaps more important than long-term theoretical concerns. Fortunately, for those hesitant to prescribe ERT to ovarian cancer patients, a well-conducted, prospective, randomized clinical trial has demonstrated that ERT has no negative impact on survival in these cases[33].

Ovarian transplant has been considered by patients and physicians for at least 100 years. There is an unconfirmed report of success that appears to have been based on good luck alone. The surgeon reportedly removed both ovaries but not the right fallopian tube. He then transplanted '... a small piece of the patient's diseased ovary ...' back into the retained tube. Menses and a subsequent pregnancy resulted. Further attempts around the same time to repeat the operation in other women were all failures. Animal models, however, have succeeded in all aspects of ovarian transplantation. These include fresh and frozen transplants with successful folliculogenesis, resumption of normal endocrine function, normal conception and even births[34–36]. Ovarian transplantation has the potential to become a 'natural' alternative to ART, with the advantage of avoiding embryo cryopreservation and the creation of excess embryos. Potential obstacles include the risk of reintroducing malignant cells (e.g. breast cancer patients harboring occult ovarian metastases) or potentially malignant germ cells (e.g. mutation carriers).

ENDOMETRIAL CANCER

Endometrial cancer would appear immediately to contraindicate future fertility. Fortunately, even these patients can hope to achieve their reproductive objectives. With nearly 15% of endometrial cancer patients being of reproductive age, any oncologist at a reasonably sized referral center will always have a patient with endometrial cancer in some stage of attempting conception. Many of these patients are diagnosed as part of their infertility evaluation and not because of the cancer symptoms. In other words, there may be a lead-time bias with endometrial cancer diagnosed as a result of an ART diagnostic test. This may also be true of all cancers diagnosed during ART. These cancers may therefore represent a very early 'preclinical' stage that may have an exceptionally good prognosis. After appropriate counseling which always includes recommendation for standard therapy, i.e. a hysterectomy, these patients often elect to be treated with prolonged high-dose progestins. While being supportive, it should be clear throughout the ART process that the standard oncological recommendation is hysterectomy and staging. The patient is reminded of this and given the option of surgery throughout the alternative therapy with progestins.

Before agreeing to prescribe the progestational agent, a thorough assessment of the tumor must be performed. This includes a magnetic resonance imaging (MRI) scan of the pelvis, which is the most accurate predictor of tumor size and depth of invasion. Other techniques may be less expensive, but MRI is more accurate than sonohysterogram or hysteroscopy in providing this information[37]. Both of the latter techniques have also been associated with the spread of cancer cells from the endometrium[38]. Peritoneal cytology is more likely to contain cancer cells after hysteroscopy. It is too early to tell if actual survival will also be worse for hysteroscopy patients.

If the tumor is small, well-differentiated and appears to not invade the uterus, a prescription for 12 weeks of high-dose oral megestrol may be acceptable. After the initial trial, a repeat office biopsy is performed. Any aspiration suction biopsy device along with an endometrial brush biopsy device (Tao Brush®, Cook Ob-Gyn) can be used to monitor accurately the effect of the hormonal therapy on the endometrial neoplasm. Using the two tests simultaneously in a single office visit yields a positive and negative predictive value of 100% for detecting or excluding endometrial carcinoma[39,40]. Rarely will it be necessary to repeat a dilatation and curettage (D&C) after the initial diagnosis of endometrial cancer is made if alternatives such as ultrasound, MRI, aspiration and brush biopsy are combined. Since the goal is fertility preservation, avoiding repeated D&Cs may reduce infertility secondary to endometrial scarring (i.e. Asherman's syndrome).

Hysteroscopy can be replaced by ultrasonography in the management of endometrial cancer since sonohistography has been reported to be more accurate and less invasive according to well-conducted randomized trials[40,41]. A recent study found that hysteroscopy did not contribute to the accurate diagnosis of endometrial cancer, as the sensitivity was only 27% with a negative predictive value of 25%[42]. Another concern regarding hysteroscopy is the theoretical potential of the procedure to worsen the prognosis for endometrial cancer patients[43].

Hormonal therapy has been utilized for the treatment of women with endometrial carcinoma who wish to preserve their uterus. This is based on a long history of successful progestin therapy for the prevention and treatment of endometrial hyperplasia, in anovulatory patients, or patients receiving estradiol replacement[44]. High-dose progestin therapy in carefully selected patients with early endometrial cancer results in moderate success, with complete response rates ranging from 50 to 75%. The median duration of treatment required to achieve remission is

estimated to be 6 to 9 months. Reported complications are uncommon. However, studies indicate that the number of patients lost to follow-up is up to 5–10%; a concerning finding given that disease persistence or progression may occur in this subgroup of patients years after initial treatment. Even among patients compliant with follow-up, disease recurrence has been documented in several cases. A portion of the documented recurrences may represent persistent disease that was not detected initially. Patients who continue to be anovulatory are at risk for disease recurrence, and long-term follow-up of patients with endometrial hyperplasia suggests that continuous progestational treatment for indefinite periods may be necessary to reduce the risk of recurrence. While some endometrial cancer recurrences are amenable to re-treatment with progestin therapy, some recurrences may require hysterectomy[45,46]. In addition, one patient who recurred was found to have extrauterine disease at laparotomy. In another report[47], a young woman successfully conceived by in vitro fertilization and delivered triplets following conservative management of endometrial cancer, but was incidentally found to have a mixed endometrioid/clear cell ovarian carcinoma at the time of completion hysterectomy and bilateral salpingo-oophorectomy. While the patient and her triplets ultimately did well, the case illustrates the important consideration of the increased risk these patients accept in trying to conceive.

Women diagnosed with endometrial cancer demonstrate an increased risk of malignancies including synchronous or metasynchronous ovarian carcinoma, intestinal malignancies, renal cell carcinoma, bladder carcinoma, squamous cell carcinoma, and others[48]. Genetic factors such as hereditary non-polyposis colorectal carcinoma may play a role. Nevertheless, treatment of early endometrial carcinoma with high-dose oral progestin therapy appears to be feasible and reasonably safe in carefully selected patients wishing to preserve their fertility.

Recently, intrauterine progesterone has been used for the treatment of early endometrial cancer[49]. A progesterone intrauterine device (IUD) was used to treat 13 patients with presumed stage IA, grade 1 endometrioid carcinoma, who were at high risk for perioperative complications. The majority of the patients had negative biopsies after 6 months, and there were no IUD-related complications, except for expulsion. Theoretical advantages of intrauterine progesterone include increased efficacy due to high local concentrations of progestin. In a series of 31 patients with endometrial hyperplasia treated with the levonorgestrel-releasing Nova T® IUD, all showed a complete histological regression[50]. In addition, symptoms related to high systemic progesterone levels are avoided by local administration.

Following successful non-surgical management of endometrial cancer, patients can be allowed to conceive using any means possible including ART. Achieving a successful pregnancy should further lower a patient's chance for recurrent endometrial cancer. At the time of delivery, a placental sample should be sent to pathology with the history of endometrial cancer noted for the examining pathologist. The endometrium is sampled postpartum with the same two office biopsy devices noted earlier (aspiration and brush). Once again hysterectomy should be recommended for definitive management, and considered either at the time of Cesarean delivery, i.e. a Cesarean hysterectomy, or postpartum. Until the patient is ready for that decision, the two office biopsy techniques should be performed at intervals no greater than every 6 months. Modern surveillance triages using complementary office biopsy devices and MRI have supplanted the need for repeated D&Cs. The D&C under general anesthesia may lead to impaired fertility and adds nothing to the combined sensitivity, specificity and positive and negative predictive value of the two office biopsy techniques.

CERVICAL CANCER

For the majority of the world's women, cervical cancer is by far more likely to impact on fertility than any of the other gynecological malignancies. Like endometrial cancer, cervical cancer has – until recent options – always resulted in the loss of fertility.

Surgical conservation of the uterine fundus is now routinely performed either abdominally or vaginally[51–53]. This procedure, known as a radical trachelectomy, has been reported for over 50 years but has lately become very popular because advances in laparoscopy have enabled surgeons to perform laparoscopic lymph node dissection. Although many prefer the vaginal route, an easier approach has been developed: abdominally. The abdominal radical trachelectomy approach is also an alternative if pelvic anatomy contraindicates the transvaginal approach or the operator is inexperienced in vaginal surgery[53–55]. Both approaches have reports indicating high survival and remarkable conception rates. A complete technical description of the procedures is available in most up-to-date surgical atlases[53].

Radiation with chemotherapy is increasingly utilized for advanced cervical cancers. Although effective therapy, radiation causes ovarian failure quickly in most patients. Oophoropexy to reposition the ovaries out of the pelvis before irradiation can reduce the incidence of ovarian failure but not eliminate it. Ovarian function is documented in as many as 75% of patients but as few as 0% following ovarian transposition[56]. Fertility after pelvic irradiation also depends on the type of cancer. In younger women, classically affected with germ cell tumors, conception rates of approximately 80% have been reported. However, because of the intense dose and location of the radiation treatment for cervical cancer, conceptions are exceedingly rare for this tumor site[57]. The best option to preserve fertility in advanced cervical cancer cases may be initial 'neoadjuvant' chemotherapy to convert a non-surgical case from primary radiation therapy to radical trachelectomy.

As a last resort, uterine transplantation may soon become an option. Already success of this operation has been reported in an actual patient[58,59]. The first successful uterine transplant was reported in 1966 using dogs[60] in which the vessels around the uterus and ovaries were isolated, divided and then reanastomosed, with subsequent uterine function. More recently, reports of successful orthotopic uteroovarian transplants in rats have appeared[61]. The success rate for this procedure was quite reasonable. However, there needs to be much more research before transplantation of reproductive organs becomes more than an investigational technique.

CONCLUSIONS

Fertility issues and options for cancer patients involve many controversial or experimental interventions. With additional studies some of the therapies and questions raised today will become irrelevant, and will be replaced by equally controversial therapies in the future. Throughout this evolution, it may be helpful to reflect on how different individuals and cultures view the importance of fertility. At the start of the third millennium, childbirth worldwide continues to cause the death of approximately 490 000 women each year from such preventable conditions as hemorrhage (123 000 deaths), sepsis (74 000 deaths), pregnancy-induced hypertension (62 000 deaths) and obstructed labor (38 000 deaths)[62]. These are very significant numbers but instead of the actual numbers of individuals affected, Western journal publications prefer to report the 'relative risk' (RR) or 'odds ratio'. Although

they are reported by the media with great drama, RR and p values can never fully communicate the risks and benefits of a medical intervention such as ART for a cancer survivor[63]. Certainly nothing discussed in this chapter comes anywhere near the risk of 'natural' childbearing as experienced by the majority of the world's population.

There are without question physical and emotional risks in pursuing a family under any circumstances. For the patient with a history of cancer or still with active disease, add an extra measure of anxiety to the process for all concerned. However, the actual magnitude of the excess or attributable risk is probably quite small. Most women are willing to accept some risk to achieve their reproductive goals. In truth it appears that there may actually be some advantages in conceiving for certain cancer patients (e.g. breast). Throughout all of these issues, physicians must focus on the patient's objectives. We have not even begun to grapple with the consequences of our actions on the subsequent generation. Do our responsibilities end with the cancer patient or her ART offspring?

Cancer patients do have options and time (although both are often limited). Physicians should urge family planning, not accidents, and bring up fertility issues with their cancer patients early to maximize the reproductive options.

References

1. Garfinkel L, Mushinski M. US cancer incidence, mortality and survival: 1973–1996. *Stat Bull Metrop Insur Co* 1999;80:23–32
2. Wingo PA, Ries LA, Rosenberg HM, *et al.* Cancer incidence and mortality, 1973–1995: a report card for the US. *Cancer* 1998;82: 1197–207
3. Evans WP 3rd, Starr AL, Bennos ES. Comparison of the relative incidence of impalpable invasive breast and ductal carcinoma *in situ* in cancers detected in patients older and younger than 50 years of age. *Radiology* 1997; 204:489–91
4. Wun LM, Feuer EJ, Miller BA. Are increases in mammographic screening still a valid explanation for trends in breast cancer incidence in the United States? *Cancer Causes Control* 1995;6: 135–44
5. Bernik SF, Bernik TR, Whooley BP, Wallack MK. Carcinoma of the breast during pregnancy: a review and update on treatment options. *Surg Oncol* 1998;7:45–9
6. Kroman N, Jensen MB, Melbye M, *et al.* Should women be advised against pregnancy after breast-cancer treatment? *Lancet* 1997;350: 319–22

7. Velentgas P, Daling JR, Malone KE, *et al*. Pregnancy after breast carcinoma: outcomes and influence on mortality. *Cancer* 1999;85: 2424–32

8. Michels KB, Willett WC. Does induced or spontaneous abortion affect the risk of breast cancer? *Epidemiology* 1996;7:521–8

9. Gemignani ML, Petrek JA, Borgen PI. Breast cancer and pregnancy. *Surg Clin North Am* 1999;79:1157–69

10. Del Priore G, Robischon K, Phipps W. Risk of ovarian cancer after treatment for infertility. *N Engl J Med* 1995;332:1300

11. Rossing MA, Daling JR, Weiss NS, *et al*. Ovarian tumors in a cohort of infertile women. *N Engl J Med* 1994;331:771–6

12. Challain R, Licciardi F, Rebarber A, Del Priore G. Ferility preservation in an ovarian cancer patient with a poor family history and infertility. *J Womens Health* 2004;in press

13. Venn A, Watson L, Bruinsma F, *et al*. Risk of cancer after use of fertility drugs with *in vitro* fertilization. *Lancet* 1999;354:1586–90

14. O'Meara E, Rossing MA, Daling JR, *et al*. Hormone replacement therapy after a diagnosis of breast cancer in relation to recurrence and mortality. *J Natl Cancer Inst* 2001;93: 754–62

15. Breast cancer and hormone replacement therapy: collaborative reanalysis of data from 51 epidemiological studies of 52 705 women with breast cancer and 108 411 women without breast cancer. Collaborative Group on Hormonal Factors in Breast Cancer. *Lancet* 1997;350: 1047–59

16. Jernstrom H, Frenander J, Ferno M, Olsson H. Hormone replacement therapy before breast cancer diagnosis significantly reduces the overall death rate compared with never-use among 984 breast cancer patients. *Br J Cancer* 1999; 80:1453–8

17. Fowble B, Hanlon A, Freedman G, *et al*. Postmenopausal hormone replacement therapy: effect on diagnosis and outcome in early-stage invasive breast cancer treated with conservative surgery and radiation. *J Clin Oncol* 1999;17:1680–8

18. Fisher B, Dignam J, Bryant J, *et al*. Five versus more than five years of tamoxifen therapy for breast cancer patients with negative lymph nodes and estrogen receptor-positive tumors. *J Natl Cancer Inst* 1996;88:1529–42

19. Cobau CD, Declercq K, Neuberg D, *et al*. A randomized trial of megestrol acetate with or without premarin in the treatment of potentially responsive metastatic breast cancer. A Study of the Eastern Cooperative Oncology Group (E2185). *Cancer* 1996;77:483–9

20. Vassilopoulou-Sellin R, Theriault RL. Randomized prospective trial of estrogen-replacement therapy in women with a history of breast cancer. *J Natl Cancer Inst Monogr* 1994;16:153–9

21. Gurski KJ, Del Priore G. Gynecologic malignancies. In Illig K, Cowles Husser W, eds. *The Rochester Manual: Practical Patient Care*. Cedar Grove, NJ: Laennec Publishing, 1997

22. Miller DM, Ehlen TG, Saleh EA. Successful term pregnancy following conservative debulking surgery for a stage IIIA serous low-malignant-potential tumor of the ovary: a case report. *Gynecol Oncol* 1997;66:535–8

23. Walter AJ, Magrina JF. Contralateral pelvic and aortic lymph node metastasis in clinical stage I epithelial ovarian cancer. *Gynecol Oncol* 1999;74:128–9

24. Sakai K, Kamura T, Hirakawa T, *et al*. Relationship between pelvic lymph node involvement and other disease sites in patients with ovarian cancer. *Gynecol Oncol* 1997;65: 164–8

25. Morris RT, Gershenson DM, Silva EG, *et al*. Outcome and reproductive function after conservative surgery for borderline ovarian tumors. *Obstet Gynecol* 2000;95:541–7

26. Zanetta G, Chiari S, Rota S, *et al*. Conservative surgery for stage I ovarian carcinoma in women of childbearing age. *Br J Obstet Gynaecol* 1997;104:1030–5

27. Schilder JM, Thompson AM, DePriest PD, *et al*. Outcome of reproductive age women with stage IA or IC invasive epithelial ovarian cancer treated with fertility-sparing therapy. *Gynecol Oncol* 2002;87:1–7

28. Kanazawa K, Suzuki T, Sakumoto K. Treatment of malignant ovarian germ cell tumors with preservation of fertility: reproductive performance after persistent remission. *Am J Clin Oncol* 2000;23:244–8

29. Tangir J, Zelterman D, Ma W, Schwartz PE. Reproductive function after conservative surgery and chemotherapy for malignant germ cell tumors of the ovary. *Obstet Gynecol* 2003;101:251–7

30. Donnez J, Munschke A, Berliere M, *et al*. Safety of conservative management and fertility outcome in women with borderline tumors of the ovary. *Fertil Steril* 2003;79:1216–21

31. Camatte S, Morice P, Pautier P, *et al*. Fertility results after conservative treatment of advanced stage serous borderline tumour of the ovary. *Br J Obstet Gynaecol* 2002;109:376–80

32. Lerner-Geva L, Toren A, Chetrit A, *et al*. The risk for cancer among children of women who underwent *in vitro* fertilization. *Cancer* 2000;88:2845–7

33. Guidozzi F, Daponte A. Estrogen replacement therapy for ovarian carcinoma survivors: a randomized controlled trial. *Cancer* 1999;86: 1013–18

34. Meirow D. Ovarian injury and modern options to preserve fertility in female cancer patients treated with high dose radio–chemotherapy for hemato-oncological neoplasias and other cancers. *Leuk Lymphoma* 1999;33:65–76

35. Shaw JM, Cox SL, Trounson AO, Jenkin G. Evaluation of the long-term function of cryopreserved ovarian grafts in the mouse, implications for human applications. *Mol Cell Endocrinol* 2000;161:103–10

36. Del Priore G, Zhang JJ, Grifo J. Ovary transplant and oocyte cryopreservation. *Contemp Ob Gyn* 2003;48:85–91

37. Frei KA, Kinkel K, Bonel HM, *et al.* Prediction of deep myometrial invasion in patients with endometrial cancer: clinical utility of contrast-enhanced MR imaging – a meta-analysis and Bayesian analysis. *Radiology* 2000;216: 444–9

38. Yang GC, Wan LS. Endometrial biopsy using the Tao Brush method. A study of 50 women in a general gynecologic practice. *J Reprod Med* 2000;45:109–14

39. Del Priore G, Williams R, Harbatkin CB, *et al.* Endometrial brush biopsy for the diagnosis of endometrial cancer. *J Reprod Med* 2001;46: 439–43

40. Cicinelli E, Romano F, Anastasio PS, *et al.* Transabdominal sonohysterography, transvaginal sonography, and hysteroscopy in the evaluation of submucous myomas. *Obstet Gynecol* 1995;85:42–7

41. Karlsson B, Granberg S, Hellberg P, Wikland M. Comparative study of transvaginal sonography and hysteroscopy for the detection of pathologic endometrial lesions in women with postmenopausal bleeding. *J Ultrasound Med* 1994; 13:757–62

42. Del Priore G, Feinstein S, Williams FS, Liu A. Accuracy of hysteroscopic visual impression for diagnosing endometrial complex atypical hyperplasia or cancer. *Int J Gynaecol Obstet* 2000;70(Suppl 1):57

43. Zerbe MJ, Zhang J, Bristow RE, *et al.* Retrograde seeding of malignant cells during hysteroscopy in presumed early endometrial cancer. *Gynecol Oncol* 2000;79:55–8

44. Janicek MF, Rosenshein NB. Invasive endometrial cancer in uteri resected for atypical endometrial hyperplasia. *Gynecol Oncol* 1994; 52:373–8

45. Wang CB, Wang CJ, Huang HJ, *et al.* Fertility-preserving treatment in young patients with endometrial adenocarcinoma. *Cancer* 2002; 94:2192–8

46. Kim YB, Holschneider CH, Ghosh K, *et al.* Progestin alone as primary treatment of endometrial carcinoma in premenopausal women. Report of seven cases and review of the literature. *Cancer* 1997;79:320–7

47. Pinto AB, Gopal M, Herzog TJ, *et al.* Successful *in vitro* fertilization pregnancy after conservative management of endometrial cancer. *Fertil Steril* 2001;76:826–9

48. Hemminki K, Aaltonen L, Li X. Subsequent primary malignancies after endometrial carcinoma and ovarian carcinoma. *Cancer* 2003;97:2432–9

49. Montz FJ, Bristow RE, Bovicelli A, *et al.* Intrauterine progesterone treatment of early endometrial cancer. *Am J Obstet Gynecol* 2002; 186:651–7

50. Scarselli G, Tantini C, Colafranceschi M, *et al.* Levo-norgestrel-nova-T and precancerous lesions of the endometrium. *Eur J Gynaecol Oncol* 1988;9:284–6

51. Smith JR, Boyle DC, Corless DJ, *et al.* Abdominal radical trachelectomy: a new surgical technique for the conservative management of cervical carcinoma. *Br J Obstet Gynaecol* 1997; 104:1196–200

52. Roy M, Plante M. Pregnancies after radical vaginal trachelectomy for early-stage cervical cancer. *Am J Obstet Gynecol* 1998;179:1491–6

53. Boyle DM, Ungars L, Del Priore G, Smith JR. Radical abdominal trachelectomy. In Smith JR, Del Priore G, Curtin JP, Monaghan J, eds. *Gynaecological Oncology: An Atlas of Investigation and Surgery.* London: Martin Dunitz, 2001

54. Del Priore G, Ungar L, Boyle DM, Smith JR. Abdominal radical trachelectomy for fertility preservation in cervical cancer patients. *Obstet Gynecol* 2003;101:2

55. Palfavi L, Ungar L, Boyle DCM, *et al.* Announcement of a healthy baby boy born following abdominal radical trachelectomy (ART). *Int J Gynecol Cancer* 2003;13:249

56. Chambers SK, Chambers JT, Kier R, Peschel RE. Sequelae of lateral ovarian transposition in irradiated cervical cancer patients. *Int J Radiat Oncol Biol Phys* 1991;20:1305–8

57. Martin XJ, Golfier F, Romestaing P, Raudrant D. First case of pregnancy after radical trachelectomy and pelvic irradiation. *Gynecol Oncol* 1999;74:286–7

58. Fageeh W, Raffa H, Jabbad H, Marzouki A. Transplantation of human uterus. *Int J Gynaecol Obstet* 2002;76:245–51

59. Keith L, Del Priore G. First human uterine transplantation. *Int J Gynaecol Obstet* 2002;76: 243–4

60. Eraslan S, Hamernik RJ, Hardy JD. Replantation of uterus and ovaries in dogs, with successful pregnancy. *Arch Surg* 1966;92:9–12

61. Lee S, Mao L, Wang Y, *et al*. Transplantation of reproductive organs. *Microsurgery* 1995;16: 191–8

62. Sciarra JJ. Reproductive health: a global perspective. *Am J Obstet Gynecol* 1993;168: 1649–54

63. Del Priore G, Zandieh P, Lee MJ. Treatment of continuous data as categorical variables in obstetrics and gynecology. *Obstet Gynecol* 1997;89:351–4

In vitro fertilization and embryo banking

8

S. M. Kelly, D. Rao, N. L. Dean and S. L. Tan

INTRODUCTION

The cryopreservation of surplus embryos is an integral component of modern assisted reproductive technologies (ART). Current ovarian stimulation protocols for most couples undergoing *in vitro* fertilization (IVF) treatment result in the production, on average, of between ten and 12 oocytes. The ability to cryopreserve surplus embryos has meant that it is possible to avoid wastage of embryos as well as maximize the fertility potential of any one cycle of treatment. The first human pregnancy as a result of a frozen–thawed embryo was reported in 1983[1], with the first successful live birth in 1985[2]. In the year 2000 there were more than 13 000 cycles of assisted reproduction using frozen–thawed embryos in the United States alone. This represents approximately 13% of all ART treatments performed in that year[3].

Theoretically, embryos may be cryopreserved indefinitely and although pregnancy rates using frozen–thawed embryos are lower than with fresh embryos, there is no significant evidence of any increased prevalence of congenital or developmental problems in the offspring[4]. In addition, there have been a number of advances in cryobiology since the widespread introduction of assisted reproduction, and these have led to improvements in the survival rates of frozen embryos and higher concomitant pregnancy rates.

More recently, cryopreservation of embryos obtained from IVF treatment has been advocated as a potential method of fertility preservation. It has been estimated that in the USA alone there are in excess of 50 000 women under the age of 40 who are diagnosed with a malignancy each year. Additionally, over 4000 preadolescent females receive chemo- or radiotherapy annually for a variety of childhood cancers[5]. Over the past two decades the survival rates for many of the cancers that affect young adults have improved dramatically. Indeed, for many of the common cancers that affect young adults and children, survival rates well in excess of 60% have been reported. The mortality rate for childhood leukemia has fallen by over 70% in the developed world from 1960 until the mid-1990s[6].

However, these improvements in survival have not come without cost. The late effects of cancer treatment are an issue that has received a good deal of recent interest[7]. In both males and females one of the unfortunate potential consequences of cancer therapy is premature gonadal failure. This is particularly so with the use of radiotherapy or aklylating chemotherapeutic agents, which are often harmful to the gonads. The issue of fertility preservation is one that should be discussed with these patients prior to the commencement of any therapy. An awareness of the recent developments in this field among health professionals is essential so that these patients (and, in many situations, their parents or guardians) are given every opportunity to make an informed decision. For females faced with potentially fertility-damaging treatment, it is now possible to cryopreserve not only embryos but also oocytes and ovarian tissue. The optimum approach will vary from patient to patient, and the remainder of this chapter focuses primarily on the current status of embryo cryopreservation and its application to fertility preservation.

EMBRYO CRYOPRESERVATION – CURRENT TECHNOLOGY

Cryobiology is not a new concept but most of its current success owes its origins to the somewhat fortuitous discovery of cryoprotectants in the late 1940s[8]. The results of further research over the following 50 or so years have given us a greater understanding of the critical biological effects of cryopreservation[9,10]. Among the critical factors important for successful cryopreservation include the extent of intra- and extracellular ice crystal formation, the toxicity of the cryoprotectant solution and the cellular changes that may result from the osmotic alterations in cell volume.

Most cryopreservation protocols for embryo freezing utilize a traditional slow-cooling technique, which involves the following basic steps:

(1) Addition of cryoprotective agent prior to cooling;

(2) Cooling the embryos to a temperature at which they can be stored but at a rate that minimizes intracellular ice formation;

(3) Embryo thawing, generally done rapidly to room temperature;

(4) Removal of the cryoprotectant.

Damage to the embryo may occur at any of these stages. The addition and removal of the cryoprotectant may lead to osmotic changes across the cell membrane, causing intracellular damage or even lysis. The rate of cooling is also extremely important since the cells are unable to exchange water at a rate fast enough to maintain equilibrium if the decline in temperature is too rapid. Intracellular ice crystal formation may result, leading to further cytoplasmic damage. If the cooling process is too slow, cell shrinkage may occur and expose the embryos to potentially toxic cytoplasmic solute concentrations.

The optimal rate of cooling is generally obtained using commercially available programable freezers. In fact, most units use a slow freeze and a relatively rapid thaw protocol adhering to the basic principles outlined above. Propanediol is the most commonly used cryoprotectant and is generally used in conjunction with a sucrose solution, which aids transport of water from the cells. Glycerol and dimethyl sulfoxide are alternative cryoprotectants that have also been used widely. After using the programable freezer in a stepwise fashion down to $-30°C$, the embryos are then placed and stored in liquid nitrogen at $-196°C$. When thawing the embryos for replacement, this is done relatively rapidly using a water bath initially, then at room temperature with progressively decreasing solute concentrations to aid removal of the cryoprotectant and sucrose. Finally, the embryos are placed in a culture medium and returned to the incubator. Depending on the initial embryo quality, survival rates of the order of 70 to 80% can be expected.

Embryos may be cryopreserved at the pronucleate, cleaved or blastocyst stage of development[11]. Although the criteria for embryo cryopreservation may vary between units, in general it will be determined by the total number of embryos available, the number of embryos required for fresh transfer and the quality of the remaining embryos after transfer. Where there are large numbers of embryos available for freezing, it is generally preferable to freeze the embryos at the pronucleate stage. Embryos cryopreserved at this stage of development are more resistant to cryoinjury than cleavage-stage embryos[12]. This relates particularly to the risk of damage involving the mitotic spindle, which is more vulnerable in dividing cells. For cleavage-stage embryos the decision to freeze will largely be dependent on the embryo quality. The embryos should preferably have an even number of blastomeres with less than 10% cytoplasmic fragmentation. Successful freezing of blastocyst-stage embryos has also been achieved and one potential advantage of this approach lies in the fact that blastocyst formation is a selection process where poorer-quality embryos arrest or degenerate prior to this stage. Although fewer numbers of embryos develop to the blastocyst stage, their individual competency – as far as implantation potential is concerned – is significantly higher[13].

There are a number of important factors that will influence both the survival and the potential for implantation of frozen–thawed embryos. The quality of the embryo prior to freezing is uppermost in terms of importance; it is recognized that pronucleate embryos have a higher implantation potential upon thawing, compared with cleaved embryos, most likely as a consequence of their resilience to cryoinjury[14].

When patients elect for replacement of frozen–thawed embryos, they may be transferred in either a natural menstrual cycle or in a controlled hormone replacement cycle. In women who have undergone premature ovarian failure as the result of sterilizing medical treatment, the latter method would obviously be required. Success rates are not significantly different between the two methods[15].

Patients who elect to cryopreserve embryos for reasons of fertility preservation should also be made aware that pregnancy rates using frozen–thawed embryos remain lower than for fresh embryos. In general, the studies that have assessed pregnancy rates for cryopreserved embryos have involved infertile patients who have previously replaced the best-quality fresh embryos from the IVF cycle, leaving the remaining possibly lower-quality embryos to be cryopreserved. Notwithstanding the impact of cryopreservation itself on implantation rates, patients utilizing this method of fertility preservation may well be very fertile (prior to medical treatment for their specific condition) and since all embryos are cryopreserved, there would not be the negative impact of having the best-quality embryos used prior to their subsequent freeze–thaw cycle.

With strict control over freezing protocols, pregnancy rates of the order of 20–25% per

cycle can be achieved. In addition, there is a mounting body of evidence that implantation rates with frozen–thawed embryos can be augmented with assisted hatching to overcome the hardening of the zona pellucida, which is a consequence of embryo cryopreservation[16].

Most recent interest in cryopreservation technology has been focused on rapid freezing techniques or, more specifically, vitrification. Vitrification essentially means the solidification of a solution. In the context of intracellular water, this can be formed into a solid 'glass-like' state by rapid cooling which leads to an extreme increase in viscosity without intracellular ice formation[17]. This process of vitrification is achieved by increasing both the rate of cooling and the concentration of cryoprotectant solution, both of which help to minimize intracellular ice formation. Vitrification is not a new concept but it has only been with the recent developments of less toxic cryoprotectant solutions that there has been renewed interest in this technology as an alternative to traditional slow-cooling techniques. In fact, in nature, vitrification is seen as a natural form of protection for some varieties of plants that survive in subzero environments[18]. The key to successful vitrification of any cell type is to maintain a balance between maximal cooling rate and the reduction in potential cryoprotectant toxicity that may occur. It has been determined that most cryoinjury to cells occurs between 15°C and −5°C, and most vitrification techniques aim to cool very rapidly through this danger zone. Ethylene glycol is the most widely used cryoprotectant for vitrification purposes. It has a relatively low toxicity as demonstrated by a number of murine studies, and in addition its rapid diffusion and equilibration properties make it ideal for this purpose[19,20].

Successful vitrification of both pronucleate and cleaved human embryos has been reported, with very good survival and cleavage rates[20,21]. Pregnancies have also been reported following vitrification and thawing of human cleavage-stage embryos[23,24]. Blastocyst vitrification has also been successfully achieved, and there are several reports of live births as a result[25-27]. However, the blastocoele, which is a large fluid-filled cavity within the blastocyst, is prone to ice crystal formation; the larger the cavity, the lower the survival rate and the poorer the outcome following vitrification. Recent reports suggest that aspiration of blastocoele fluid prior to vitrification may improve survival rates on thawing[28].

As a technique, vitrification also has the advantage of being technically easier and less expensive as it does not require a programable freezer that is essential for the slow-cooling method.

Vitrification has also shown considerable promise for oocyte cryopreservation, with significant improvements in the survival and development of subsequent embryos compared to traditional slow-cooling techniques[29,30].

EMBRYO BANKING FOR FERTILITY PRESERVATION

For females, the options for fertility preservation are to cryopreserve embryos, immature or mature oocytes, or ovarian tissue itself. Embryo cryopreservation is of course a well-established process and for a number of couples this would be the first choice based on its proven success. There have been a number of reported cases of successful pregnancies using embryo cryopreservation as a method of maintaining fertility prior to a variety of cancer treatments[31,32].

However, cryopreservation of embryos for fertility preservation is suitable only for women with a partner and ideally in a stable relationship. It is not suitable for young adolescent females (or children), for whom either oocyte or ovarian tissue cryopreservation may be more applicable. In addition, in order to obtain mature oocytes that can be fertilized to form embryos, patients may need to undergo ovarian stimulation.

There is a variety of ovarian stimulation protocols that can be utilized to obtain mature oocytes; however, the use of gonadotropin releasing hormone agonists (GnRH-a) in a long protocol with gonadotropin stimulation is the most commonly used. Early IVF studies had shown this protocol to be superior to either agonist-free cycles or the short GnRH-a flare protocol. Both the number of oocytes collected and the clinical pregnancy rates were better with the long protocol[33,34]. However, for many cancers it is desirable to commence therapy as soon as possible after diagnosis and this may not allow sufficient time for a cycle of IVF to be performed, especially using the long GnRH-a protocol. More recently, the introduction of GnRH antagonists has afforded an alternative ovarian stimulation protocol that is much shorter than the traditional long protocol, as there is no requirement for pituitary suppression prior to the commencement of gonadotropin stimulation. Initial results from antagonist treatment cycles demonstrated somewhat lower pregnancy rates than with standard long protocol cycles[35,36]. With improvement in the understanding of the mechanism of GnRH antagonists and their optimal protocol of usage, comparable pregnancy rates have been reported along with improved patient satisfaction[37]. In addition, it has also been demonstrated that whether the long GnRH-a protocol or the antagonist protocol is used, there appears to be minimal difference in the ability of resultant cryopreserved embryos to implant subsequently[38,39]. This means that shorter protocols using gonadotropin-releasing antagonists may be more suitable where time is an important consideration. Ovarian stimulation with tamoxifen has also been reported in patients with breast cancer undergoing embryo cryopreservation[40]. This raises an important issue, since there is concern about the potential deleterious effect of ovarian stimulation on the malignancy itself, especially if it is hormone-sensitive, such as estrogen receptor-positive breast cancer. In these patients the use of ovarian stimulation needs to be considered with caution.

As a means of obtaining oocytes without ovarian stimulation, the collection and *in vitro* maturation of immature oocytes (IVM) has gained a lot of interest. Essentially developed as an alternative fertility treatment to traditional IVF, it has also been advocated as a method of obtaining oocytes for cryopreservation, or for fertilization to form embryos for cryopreservation. Clinical pregnancy rates in excess of 25% per cycle have been reported in women with polycystic ovaries undergoing IVM treatment for infertility[41–43]. For women faced with potentially gonadotoxic treatment, this can be performed at relatively short notice and obviates the potential harmful effect of gonadotropin treatment.

Patients undergoing an IVM cycle have immature oocytes collected from the small antral follicles of the ovary without ovarian stimulation. They begin with a baseline ultrasound scan performed between days 2 and 4 of their cycle. At this point the total number of antral follicles > 2–4 mm is assessed. It has been demonstrated that the success of IVM in the context of fertility treatment is heavily dependent upon the number of immature oocytes obtained, which in turn can be predicted by the antral follicle count[44]. Pregnancy rates comparable with conventional IVF may be obtained when ten or more immature oocytes are collected. Oocytes can be retrieved from about 50% of visible follicles. This implies that patients who have an antral follicle count > 20 could be offered IVM treatment as an alternative to IVF[45]. The patient is normally scanned again on day 8 and oocyte retrieval is planned for between days 10 and 14. Thirty-six hours prior to oocyte collection, a subcutaneous injection of human chorionic gonadotropin is given. This has been shown to improve the rate of maturation of the immature oocytes and the final number of mature oocytes obtained[46].

The collection of immature oocytes is performed under ultrasound guidance with a reduced aspiration pressure. Although similar to IVF it is a more technically challenging procedure.

Following collection of the immature oocytes, they can either be cryopreserved at this stage or matured in a specialized culture media to the metaphase II stage, and then either cryopreserved or fertilized to form embryos. Although IVM has proved most successful as a fertility treatment for women with polycystic ovaries, it is still an option for fertility preservation in women with normal numbers of antral follicles. For women with a low antral follicle count, or where the risk of premature ovarian failure is very high, then combining IVM with ovarian tissue cryopreservation may offer the best solution (see below).

The cryopreservation of oocytes has gained a lot of recent interest in terms of fertility preservation, as it is an option for women who are not in a stable relationship where embryo cryopreservation would be inappropriate. Initial results with cryopreserving mature oocytes were rather poor, with an expected live-birth rate of less than 1%[47]. This appears to be due to the fact that mature oocytes are particularly susceptible to cryoinjury as the chromosomes at the metaphase II oocyte are arranged on a delicate spindle, which is very sensitive to low temperatures and cryoprotectant toxicity. This leads to a significant risk for aneuploidy as a result of damage to the spindle[48]. Immature oocytes, on the other hand, appear to be less susceptible to cryoinjury as the chromosomes are within the nuclear membrane and not arranged on a spindle (prophase I). Initial results for survival, maturation and fertilization were somewhat variable[49], but the recent revival of interest in vitrification has proven to be particularly effective with both immature and mature oocytes. High post-thaw survival rates as well as improved rates of maturation have been reported, and indeed there are live births recorded from the use of vitrified oocytes[50,51].

A further potential option for women wanting to preserve their fertility is to cryopreserve ovarian tissue itself. As a technique, this option is in its infancy in terms of development, and there remain some doubts concerning both its efficacy and its safety[52]. To date there have been no reported cases of human pregnancy, although it has been successful in the animal model. What is known is that the primordial follicles within the ovarian cortex can be successfully cryopreserved, and they are significantly less susceptible to cryoinjury than either mature or immature oocytes[53]. A sample of ovarian cortex can be removed laparoscopically during a planned surgical procedure or performed during unrelated surgery, and is feasible in both pre- and postpubescent patients. One of the major concerns regarding ovarian tissue cryopreservation in cancer patients is the possibility of transmission of cancer cells at the time of transplantation. Cancers such as leukemia and breast cancer carry a not insignificant risk of ovarian metastasis, and caution concerning cryopreservation and transplantation should be exercised in these patients. There are more reliable methods becoming available to detect the presence of neoplastic cells in ovarian tissue samples, and hence this option may become more applicable as the safety improves[54,55].

In humans, transplantation of ovarian tissue has resulted in the return of ovarian function for a limited duration. However, as mentioned, the animal studies have shown more success with return of ovarian function and indeed pregnancies and live births in a number of species[56–60].

Nevertheless, the progress in this field means that cryopreservation and banking of ovarian tissue for preserving fertility should be discussed with all women facing potentially sterilizing treatment. It may also be a consideration for prepubescent females who may particularly gain future benefit from such a procedure. It should be discussed in an informative and sensitive manner with the parents or guardians, so they can be fully informed of any decision.

It is also worth noting that while most of the discussion concerning fertility preservation is focused on women being treated for a variety of malignancies, there are a number of other conditions where some form of fertility preservation may be appropriate. Women with severe endometriosis may require oophorectomy where conservative medical or surgical therapy has failed. Women of reproductive age are more commonly affected by autoimmune conditions such as systemic lupus and, in severe cases, cyclophosphamide therapy

may be advocated, which is often gonadotoxic. These patients should have the various options of fertility preservation discussed with them prior to their specific treatment[61]. It has even been suggested that women who carry the BRCA-1 or BRCA-2 gene mutations, who are often advised to have prophylactic oophorectomy because they are at high risk of developing ovarian cancer, may benefit from some form of fertility preservation[62].

In summary, whilst embryo banking may not be appropriate for every patient, it has a number of advantages over oocyte or ovarian tissue cryopreservation. These are its proven success with regard to the likelihood of subsequent pregnancy and a potentially more reassuring safety profile.

EMBRYO BANKING: SAFETY AND ETHICAL ISSUES

Following the first successful IVF birth in 1978, there was a delay of several years before embryo cryopreservation became a routine method of preserving excess embryos. Whilst the technology existed, there were obvious concerns about the safety of human embryo cryopreservation, including worries over the susceptibility of frozen embryos to background radiation levels or other potentially harmful environmental toxins. In addition, the outcome of any subsequent pregnancies and the development of the offspring were unknown.

There were several key studies that helped to allay these fears and enable embryo cryopreservation gradually to become commonplace. The effect of radiation on mouse embryos was studied, whereby the level of background ionizing radiation was enhanced to the equivalent of 2000 years' duration[63]. There appeared to be no effect on morphology, developmental potential, implantation rates or indeed the ratio of live births to the number of embryos transferred. Moreover, there are a number of studies that have demonstrated no detrimental effect of long-term storage of cryopreserved human embryos[64,65]. Pregnancies resulting from the transfer of cryopreserved embryos were shown to have similar characteristics – in terms of mean gestational age, birth weight, perinatal mortality and the incidence of congenital malformations – to pregnancies resulting from transfer of fresh embryos or indeed natural conceptions when adjusted for age and parity[66–68]. Thus, reassuringly, the general health and development of offspring at least into early childhood does not appear to be adversely affected by cryopreservation[69,70].

Contamination of the storage tanks with viruses or bacteria is a potential concern. There has been a case report of hepatitis B contamination involving a liquid nitrogen tank[71]. The risk appears to be higher when open freezer containers are used and can be minimized by hermetically sealing storage containers to prevent direct contact of the freezing media with the liquid nitrogen[72]. Embryos from patients known to be carriers of viruses such as hepatitis and HIV should be stored in separate tanks to avoid cross-contamination.

One of the consequences of having an effective embryo cryopreservation program is that it leads to large numbers of stored embryos that will not necessarily be utilized. In the USA alone the results of a recent survey of assisted reproduction clinics estimated that there are approximately 400 000 cryopreserved embryos in storage[73]. In fact, many more embryos are cryopreserved annually than are used in frozen–thawed embryo replacement cycles. The storing of embryos as a means of fertility preservation may contribute to this pool of 'unwanted' embryos, especially as the mortality rate for some patients is not inconsiderable. The heart of the issue is what should become of these embryos in the event that the original couple no longer requires them or is able to use them. In many countries there is a maximum storage period of usually between 5 and 10 years, although there may be some provision for extension beyond this period. In the case of young women utilizing this method of fertility preservation, these restrictions may obviously be unreasonable. It has been advocated that

many of these unwanted embryos should be either donated to other infertile couples or to approved research programs. In terms of research, there has been a lot of interest in this pool of cryopreserved embryos as a source of embryonic stem cells that may be useful to develop cell or tissue lines to treat a variety of illnesses. Interestingly, however, the recent survey in the USA revealed that only 2.8% of the stored embryos were targeted for research.

The issue of excess embryo storage is an emotive one, which is complicated by the complexity of the moral and legal status of the embryo itself. In terms of the moral status, the most widely accepted definition is that the embryo is a potential human being and as such should be handled with dignity, with its rights respected as long as they do not interfere with major maternal or social interests[74]. The legal status is even less clear and in some situations appears to be at odds with the moral status. In criminal law, the destruction of an embryo is not a criminal act, thereby implying it does not have the status of a human being. Many clinics now insist on disposition agreements prior to cryopreservation of embryos, but even these have been subject to differences in legal interpretation[75]. Opinions regarding the status of the embryo vary widely and are influenced by a variety of social, legal and religious factors.

These problems surrounding the storage of embryos is certainly an important factor to consider when counseling young women regarding their options in terms of fertility preservation. In general, where there is any doubt about the stability of the relationship then oocyte or ovarian tissue cryopreservation is preferable, as many of these ethical problems can be avoided.

CONCLUSION

The possibility of requiring a potentially harmful treatment for a malignancy or serious medical condition during the reproductive or pre-reproductive years is a frightening situation for anyone. To compound this with the knowledge that the individual's future capacity to have children may be significantly impaired exacerbates this stressful situation.

However, with the advances in both assisted reproduction and cryobiology over recent years, the ability to preserve future fertility is becoming more realistic.

Embryo cryopreservation has a long and established history and is the most successful option at present in terms of achieving a desired pregnancy at a later date. However, it is applicable only to couples in a stable relationship and there are ethical concerns about long-term storage of embryos. More recent options of cryopreservation of oocytes or ovarian tissue are promising alternatives, particularly for

single women. It must be emphasized, however, that the success rates are currently significantly below that for embryo cryopreservation, and there have been no recorded pregnancies as a result of transplantation of cryopreserved ovarian tissue to date.

The rapid pace of development in this area of fertility preservation means that it is essential that health professionals dealing with these patients be fully informed of the options. These options should be discussed with patients in a timely and sensitive manner, so that they are able to come to an informed decision that suits their individual situation.

References

1. Trounson A, Mohr L. Human pregnancy following cryopreservation, thawing and transfer of an eight-cell human embryo. *Nature* 1983;305:707–9
2. Cohen J, Simons RS, Fehilly CB, *et al.* Birth after replacement of a hatching blastocyst cryopreserved at the expanded blastocyst stage. *Lancet* 1985;8249:647
3. www.cdc.gov/nccdphp/drh/ART00 (accessed July 2003)
4. FIVNAT. Bilan des transfert d'embryons congelés de 1987 à 1994. *Contracept Fertil Sex* 1996;24:700–5
5. Ries LAG, Eisner MP, Kosary CL, *et al.*, eds. *SEER Cancer Statisitics Review 1973–1999*. Bethesda, MD: National Cancer Institute, 2002
6. Garattini S, LaVecchia C. Perspectives in cancer chemotherapy. *Eur J Cancer* 2001;Suppl 8: S128–47
7. Schwartz CL. Long-term survivors of childhood cancer: the late effects of therapy. *Oncologist* 1999;4:45–54
8. Polge C, Smith AU, Parkes AS. Revival of spermatozoa after vitrification and dehydration at low temperatures. *Nature* 1949;164:666
9. Lovelock JE. The haemolysis of human red blood cells by freezing and thawing. *Biochim Biophys Acta* 1953;10:414–26
10. Mazur P, Rall WF, Rigopoulos N. The relative contributions of the fraction of unfrozen water and of salt concentration to the survival of slowly frozen human erythrocytes. *Biophys J* 1981;36:653–75
11. Troup SA, Matson PL, Critchlow JD, *et al.* Cryopreservation of human embryos at the pronucleate, early cleavage or expanded blastocyst stage. *Eur J Obstet Gynecol Reprod Biol* 1991;38:133–9
12. Veeck LL, Amundson CH, Brothman LJ. Significantly enhanced pregnancy rates per cycle through cryopreservation and thaw of pronuclear stage oocytes. *Fertil Steril* 1993;59: 1202–7
13. Nakayama T, Goto Y, Kanzaki H. Developmental potential of frozen thawed human blastocysts. *J Assist Reprod Genet* 1995;12:239–43
14. Senn A, Vozzi C, Chanson A, *et al.* Prospective randomized study of two cryopreservation policies avoiding embryo selection: the pronucleate stage leads to higher cumulative delivery rate than the early cleavage stage. *Fertil Steril* 2000;74:946–52
15. Sathanandan M, Macnamee MC, Rainsbury P, *et al.* Replacement of frozen–thawed embryos in artificial and natural cycles: a prospective semi-randomized study. *Hum Reprod* 1991;6: 685–7
16. Check JH, Hoover L, Nazari A, *et al.* The effect of assisted hatching on pregnancy rates after frozen embryo transfer. *Fertil Steril* 1996;65:254–7
17. Fahy GM, MacFarlane DR, Angell CA, *et al.* Vitrification as an approach to cryopreservation. *Cryobiology* 1984;21:407–26
18. Hirsch AG. Vitrification in plants as a natural form of cryoprotection. *Cryobiology* 1987;24: 214–28

19. Zhu S, Kasai M, Otoge H, *et al.* Cryopreservation of expanded mouse blastocysts by vitrification in ethylene glycol. *J Reprod Fertil* 1993;98:139–45

20. Emiliani S, Van den Bergh M, Vannin A, *et al.* Comparison of ethylene glycol, 1,2-propanediol and glycerol for cryopreservation of slow-cooled mouse zygotes, 4-cell embryos and blastocysts. *Hum Reprod* 2000;15:905–10

21. Liebermann J, Tucker M, Graham J, *et al.* Blastocyst development after vitrification of multipronucleate zygotes using the Flexipet denuding pipette. *Reprod Biomed Online* 2002; 4:148–52

22. Park SP, Kim EY, Oh JH, *et al.* Ultrarapid freezing of human multipronuclear zygotes using electron microscope grids. *Hum Reprod* 2000; 15:1787–90

23. Jelinkova L, Selman HA, Arav A, *et al.* Twin pregnancy after vitrification of 2-pronuclei human embryos. *Fertil Steril* 2002;77:412–14

24. Selman HA, El-Danasouri I. Pregnancies derived from vitrified human zygotes. *Fertil Steril* 2002;77:422–3

25. Yokota Y, Sato S, Yokota M, *et al.* Successful pregnancy following blastocyst vitrification. *Hum Reprod* 2000;15:1802–3

26. Choi D, Chung H, Lim J, *et al.* Pregnancy and delivery of healthy infants developed from vitrified blastocysts in an IVF–ET program. *Fertil Steril* 2000;74:838–9

27. Mukaida T, Nakamura S, Tomiyama T, *et al.* Vitrification of human blastocysts using cryoloops: clinical outcome of 223 cycles. *Hum Reprod* 2003;18:384–6

28. Vanderzwalmen P, Bertin G, Debauche C, *et al.* Births after vitrification at morula and blastocyst stages: effect of artificial reduction of the blastocoelic cavity before vitrification. *Hum Reprod* 2002;17:744–51

29. Kuleshova L, Lopata A. Vitrification can be more favorable than slow cooling. *Fertil Steril* 2002;78:449–54

30. Kuwayama M, Kato O. All-round vitrification method for human oocytes and embryos. *J Assist Reprod Genet* 2000;17:477

31. Atkinson HG, Apperley JF, Dawson K, *et al.* Successful pregnancy after embryo cryopreservation after BMT for CML. *Lancet* 1994; 344:199

32. Gallot D, Pouly JL, Janny L, *et al.* Successful transfer of frozen–thawed embryos obtained immediately before radical surgery for stage IIIa serous borderline ovarian tumour. *Hum Reprod* 2000;15:2347–50

33. Tan S, Maconochie N, Doyle P, *et al.* Cumulative conception and live-birth rates after *in vitro* fertilization with and without the use of long, short, and ultrashort regimens of the gonadotropin-releasing hormone agonist buserelin. *Am J Obstet Gynecol* 1994;171:513–20

34. Tan SL, Kingsland C, Campbell S, *et al.* The long protocol of administration of gonadotropin-releasing hormone agonist is superior to the short protocol for ovarian stimulation for *in vitro* fertilization. *Fertil Steril* 1992;57:810–14

35. Ludwig M, Katalinic A, Diedrich K. Use of GnRH antagonists in ovarian stimulation for assisted reproductive technologies compared to the long protocol. *Arch Gynecol Obstet* 2001;265:175–82

36. Al-Inany H, Aboulghar M. GnRH antagonist in assisted reproduction: a Cochrane review. *Hum Reprod* 2002;17:874–85

37. Shapiro DB. GnRH antagonists in normal responder patients. *Fertil Steril* 2003;80(Suppl 1): S8–15

38. Nikolettos N, Al-Hasani S, Felderbaum R, *et al.* Comparison of cryopreservation outcome with human pronuclei stage oocytes obtained by the GnRH antagonist, cetrorelix, and GnRH agonists. *Eur J Obstet Gynecol Reprod Biol* 2000; 93:91–5

39. Seelig AS, Al-Hasani S, Katalinic A, *et al.* Comparison of cryopreservation outcome with gonadotropin-releasing hormone agonists or antagonists in the collecting cycle. *Fertil Steril* 2002;77:472–5

40. Oktay K, Buyuk E, Davis O, *et al.* Fertility preservation in breast cancer patients: IVF and embryo cryopreservation after ovarian stimulation with tamoxifen. *Hum Reprod* 2003; 18:90–5

41. Cha K, Koo J, Ko J, *et al.* Pregnancy after *in vitro* fertilization of human follicular oocytes collected from nonstimulated cycles, their culture *in vitro* and their transfer in a donor oocyte program. *Fertil Steril* 1991;55:109–13

42. Tan SL, Child TJ. *In vitro* maturation of oocytes from unstimulated polycystic ovaries. *Reprod Biomed Online* 2001;4(Suppl 1):18–23

43. Child TJ, Abdul-Jalil AK, Gulekli B, Tan SL. *In vitro* maturation and fertilization of oocytes from unstimulated normal ovaries, polycystic ovaries, and women with polycystic ovary syndrome. *Fertil Steril* 2001;76:936–42

44. Tan SL, Child TJ, Gulekli B. *In vitro* maturation and fertilization of oocytes from unstimulated ovaries: predicting the number of immature oocytes retrieved by early follicular phase ultrasonography. *Am J Obstet Gynecol* 2002; 186:684–9

45. Child TJ, Abdul-Jalil AK, Gulekli B, Tan SL. *In vitro* maturation and fertilization of oocytes from unstimulated normal ovaries, polycystic ovaries, and women with polycystic ovary syndrome. *Fertil Steril* 2001;76:936–42

46. Chian R, Gulecki B, Buckett W, Tan SL. Priming with human chorionic gonadotrophin before retrieval of immature oocytes in women with infertility due to polycystic ovarian syndrome. *N Engl J Med* 1999;341:1624–6

47. Porcu E, Fabbri R, Ciotti PM, *et al.* Cycles of human oocyte cryopreservation and intracytoplasmic sperm injection: results of 112 cycles. *Fertil Steril* 1999;72:2

48. Pickering S, Braude P, Johnson M. Transient cooling to room temperature can cause irreversible disruption of the meiotic spindle in the human oocyte. *Fertil Steril* 1990;54:102–8

49. Toth TL, Baka SG, Veeck LL. Fertilization and *in vitro* development of cryopreserved human prophase I oocytes. *Fertil Steril* 1994;61:891–4

50. Chian RC, Kuwayama M, Tan LHL, *et al.* High survival rates of bovine and human oocytes matured *in vitro* following vitrification. Submitted for publication

51. Yoon TK, Kim TJ, Park SE, *et al.* Live births after vitrification of oocytes in a stimulated *in vitro* fertilization–embryo transfer program. *Fertil Steril* 2003;79:1323–6

52. Kim SS. Ovarian tissue banking for cancer patients: to do or not to do? *Hum Reprod* 2003; 18:1759–61

53. Abir R, Franks S, Mobberley MA, *et al.* Mechanical isolation and *in vitro* growth of preantral and small follicles. *Fertil Steril* 1997; 68:682–8

54. Poirot C, Vacher-Lavenu MC, Helardot P, *et al.* Human ovarian tissue cryopreservation: indications and feasibility. *Hum Reprod* 2002; 17:1447–52

55. Newton H, Aubard Y, Rutherford A, *et al.* Low temperature storage and grafting of human ovarian tissue. *Hum Reprod* 1996;11:1487–91

56. Gosden RG, Baird DT, Wade JC, Webb R. Restoration of fertility to oophorectomized sheep by ovarian autografts stored at –196°C. *Hum Reprod* 1994;9:597–603

57. Salle B, Demirci B, Franck M, *et al.* Normal pregnancies and live births after autograft of frozen–thawed hemi-ovaries into ewes. *Fertil Steril* 2002;77:403–8

58. Sztein J, Sweet H, Farley J, Mobraaten L. Cryopreservation and orthotopic transplantation of mouse ovaries: new approach in gamete banking. *Biol Reprod* 1998;58:1071–4

59. Radford JA, Lieberman BA, Brison DR, *et al.* Orthotopic reimplantation of cryopreserved ovarian cortical strips after high-dose chemotherapy for Hodgkin's lymphoma. *Lancet* 2001;357:1171–5

60. Oktay K, Aydin BA, Economos K. Restoration of ovarian function after autologous transplantation of ovarian tissue in the forearm. *Fertil Steril* 2000;74(Suppl 3):S79

61. Bredkjaer HE, Grudzinskas JG. Cryobiology in human assisted reproductive technology. Would Hippocrates approve? *Early Pregnancy* 2001;5:211–13

62. Elit L. Familial ovarian cancer. *Can Fam Physician* 2001;47:778–84

63. Glenister P, Whittingham D, Lyon M. Further studies on the effect of radiation during storage of frozen 8-cell mouse embryos at –196°C. *J Reprod Fertil* 1984;70:229–34

64. Cohen J, Inge K, Wiker S, *et al.* Duration of storage of cryopreserved human embryos. *J In Vitro Fert Embryo Transf* 1988;5:301–3

65. Machtinger R, Dor J, Levron J, *et al.* The effect of prolonged cryopreservation on embryo survival. *Gynecol Endocrinol* 2002;16:293–8

66. Wada I, Macnamee M, Wick K, *et al.* Birth characteristics and perinatal outcome of babies conceived from cryopreserved embryos. *Hum Reprod* 1994;9:543–6

67. Aytoz A, Van den Abbeel E, Bonduelle M, *et al.* Obstetric outcome of pregnancies after the transfer of cryopreserved and fresh embryos obtained by conventional *in-vitro* fertilization and intracytoplasmic sperm injection. *Hum Reprod* 1999;14:2619–24

68. Sutcliffe A, D'Souza S, Cadman J, *et al.* Minor congenital anomalies, major congenital malformations and development in children conceived from cryopreserved embryos. *Hum Reprod* 1995;10:3332–7

69. Sutcliffe A, D'Souza S, Cadman J, *et al.* Outcome in children from cryopreserved embryos. *Arch Dis Child* 1995;72:290–3

70. Wennerholm U, Albertson-Wikland K, Bergh C, *et al.* Postnatal growth and health in children born after cryopreservation as embryos. *Lancet* 1998;351:1085–90

71. Bielanski A, Nadin-Davis S, Sapp T, *et al.* Viral contamination of embryos cryopreserved in liquid nitrogen. *Cryobiology* 2000;40:110–16

72. Tedder R, Zukerman M, Goldstone A, *et al.* Hepatitis B transmission from a contaminated cryopreservation tank. *Lancet* 1995;346: 137–40

73. Hoffman DI, Zellman GL, Fair C, *et al.* Cryopreserved embryos in the United States and their availability for research. *Fertil Steril* 2003;79:1063–9

74. Fasouliotis SJ, Schenker JG. Ethics and assisted reproduction. *Eur J Obstet Gynecol Reprod Biol* 2000;90:171–80

75. Schuster TG, Hickner-Cruz K, Ohl DA, *et al.* Legal considerations for cryopreservation of sperm and embryos. *Fertil Steril* 2003;80:61–6

Cryopreservation of spermatozoa* 9

M. Morshedi and R. G. Gosden

INTRODUCTION

Low-temperature banking of semen was the first application of reproductive cryotechnology and has been established in clinical practice for 50 years. It should be offered in a timely manner to all young men undergoing potentially sterilizing treatment by chemotherapy, radiotherapy or surgery, because it provides a well-tested, if not wholly reliable, method for fertility preservation. Moreover, it is relatively straightforward and inexpensive and there are no major concerns about the genetic safety of banking male germ cells. Applications have extended from the banking of bulky whole semen samples to the banking of washed and concentrated sperm ready for intrauterine inseminations (IUIs) and to microaspirates of spermatozoa obtained from the testis or epididymis for an *in vitro* fertilization (IVF) or intracytoplasmic sperm injection (ICSI) procedure. Advances in reproductive medicine have made it possible to utilize very-poor-quality cryopreserved semen/sperm containing very few motile sperm and achieve pregnancy rates similar to those obtained using semen samples with excellent quality. However, our understanding of the biological effects of cryoprotectants and thermal change on sperm structure and physiology is still limited, and research is needed so that the valuable technology of sperm banking can be successfully applied to all the individuals who can benefit.

---

*This chapter is abridged and modified from a previous article published by one of the authors[1].

APPLICATIONS FOR PATIENT CARE

Recent advances in reproductive science have created a multitude of assisted reproductive technologies (ART) that are extending the scope of therapeutics to an ever-widening spectrum of fertility disorders. Cryopreservation of the male gamete, either ejaculated sperm or sperm retrieved surgically from the testis or the reproductive tract, has provided a valuable adjunct technology for various assisted conception methods, and ICSI has had a notable impact in extending the reach of this technology. With excellent pregnancy rates resulting from ART, it is possible to utilize cryopreserved samples with very few and/or sluggishly motile sperm, which is reducing the need for patients to resort to repeated retrievals (i.e. surgeries) or donor insemination to have children. Although sperm cryopreservation does not serve a therapeutic purpose by itself, it facilitates other technologies and provides flexibility for various *in vivo* and *in vitro* therapeutic insemination or fertilization techniques. The term 'artificial insemination' (AI) was originally applied in animal husbandry and was (and is) still used in the context of human medicine. However, because of the negative associations of the word 'artificial', a more appropriate term is now widely used, namely 'therapeutic insemination' (TI). At one end of the spectrum of application, TI involves the introduction of semen (or washed sperm) which has been stored by the patient or provided by a donor; at the other end, TI applies to microinsemination procedures involving testicular or epididymal sperm used in IVF and

ICSI settings. In this chapter we focus principally on the former, although the principles of cryopreservation of male gametes apply to them equally.

The range of patients who can benefit from fertility preservation has already been described in other chapters. Here, we principally have in mind patients of reproductive age who are undergoing chemotherapy or radiotherapy or orchiectomy, or indeed a combination of these procedures. Prepubertal boys who cannot produce semen samples are left with the sole option (still experimental) of cryopreserving their immature germ cells. There have been recent advances in the field of immature germ cell cryopreservation, *in vitro* maturation of germ cells, xenografting and auto-transplantation, but these procedures are still in their infancy and require refinement before they can be applied for fertility preservation (see Chapters 10 and 12). Unfortunately, not all patients avail themselves of the opportunities for semen cryopreservation, nor are all offered this option, and those who are cannot completely rely on it. Without gamete banking, those who are irreversibly sterilized cannot have any prospects of genetic parenthood, although they may become a rearing parent through therapeutic donor insemination (TDI). Currently, ejaculated or surgically retrieved sperm from patients (client depositors) for TI and semen/sperm from donors for TDI are cryopreserved similarly. However, the procedure with TDI is complicated by many additional concerns and responsibilities, including donor selection and matching, consent, quarantining semen, psychological factors, legal issues and safeguards against consanguinity (if donors provide specimens for multiple recipients). These issues are not discussed here, but have been reviewed elsewhere[1].

When banking semen samples, timeliness is imperative. They must be collected for storage before the patient starts to undergo rounds of chemotherapy, and not during treatment, especially if he is receiving alkylating agents or other potentially mutagenic compounds. Even so, the pretreatment quality of samples is often poorer than that of young healthy donors, both for those with malignant (e.g. Hodgkin's disease and non-Hodgkin's lymphoma) and non-malignant (e.g. autoimmune) diseases[2–4]. In these cases, sperm motility is impaired and there is more DNA damage as judged by the sperm chromatin structure assay[5]. Yet through the power of ART, including ICSI and sperm aspiration before or after sterilizing treatment from the epididymis (MESA, microsurgical epididymal sperm aspiration) or testis (TESE, testicular sperm extraction), even very small numbers of sperm can be effective. This progress implies a responsibility for health professionals to offer fertility preservation to patients who, little more than a decade ago, could not be helped.

BRIEF HISTORY

The first well-documented case of therapeutic insemination in humans is attributed to the Scottish physician–anatomist, John Hunter, who worked in London during the early 1790s. He advised a patient who had hypospadias to inject his seminal fluid into his wife's vagina using a pre-warmed syringe. Fearing adverse publicity, Hunter never reported the case in the scientific literature during his lifetime, although subsequently it was confirmed that a pregnancy had been achieved[6]. The next report was from France in 1838 when Girault treated a woman with a 'long cervix' using her husband's semen, which was blown into her uterus through a hollow tube. He later treated nine additional patients in the same way and seven were said to have conceived. In the USA, J. M. Sims working in New York City performed 55 intracervical and intrauterine inseminations from the husbands' samples[7]. There was a low pregnancy rate, probably because of the mistaken belief at the time that ovulation occurred during the phase of menstruation. It was not until the 1930s that this error (arising from a mistaken analogy with the estrous cycle of the dog) was corrected and the fertile phase of the menstrual cycle was identified. The credit for introducing therapeutic donor insemination is generally given to Robert Dickinson and one of his students, Sophia Kleegman, also of New York City, and to Margaret Jackson, who worked in England. Under their influence TDI became more acceptable, although resistance to donor insemination continues to this day in some quarters of society.

The preservation of biological specimens using salting and low-temperature storage has been practiced for a long time. As early as 1776, Spallanzani reported that semen samples frozen in the snow contained spermatozoa which could be reanimated after thawing. In the 1820s, John Hunter also began experimentations to cryopreserve specimens, although be did not make any attempts to our knowledge to work with spermatozoa. In 1866, Montegazza claimed some encouraging results after freeze–thawing semen to −15°C, and he suggested the establishment of semen banks for veterinary use and for the production of legitimate offspring for soldiers who were killed on the battlefield. During the late 1930s, Landrum B. Shettles also carried out experiments on human spermatozoa in thin capillary tubes by plunging them into alcohol cooled with liquid nitrogen or other coolants[8]. With these studies, variable but low numbers of cells survived, judging by motility after thawing. Gregory Pincus[9] also obtained motile sperm after freezing semen from rabbits and humans in a bacteriological loop to encourage ultra-rapid freezing – anticipating some modern developments such as the 'cryoloop'[10]. Another breakthrough was Rosthand's discovery that glycerol was a cryoprotectant for frog spermatozoa, and was soon followed by one of greater significance.

The landmark paper was published in 1949[11] after a serendipitous discovery in a laboratory in London, England, showing that glycerol could preserve fowl sperm from freezing damage. The researchers soon found that the protective effect of glycerol, 1,2-propanediol and ethanediol could be applied successfully to bovine spermatozoa, and this has created an industry in which millions of cows have been born after AI of frozen–thawed semen.

Shortly afterwards, similar methods were applied successfully to human spermatozoa, and the first three pregnancies after cryopreservation with glycerol in dry ice were reported in the early 1950s[12]. The sperm samples in these cases were all morphologically 'normal' and the survival rates after freeze–thawing ranged from 53 to 59%. The authors noted that samples with 'good fertility potential' could survive cryopreservation better than those of poor quality, and this shrewd observation is still widely accepted.

In the 1960s, various modifications were introduced to the cryopreservation procedure. First, liquid nitrogen vapor was used to freeze semen samples, and subsequently egg yolk citrate buffer was used to aid preservation. Implementation of these steps dramatically improved the recovery of motile sperm following cryopreservation[13]. But cryopreserved semen/sperm was utilized infrequently until the mid-1980s, when concerns were first raised about the risk of transmission of sexually transmitted diseases, especially human immunodeficiency virus (HIV) and hepatitis, by insemination with fresh donor semen during TDI. Shortly afterwards, the cryopreservation of donor semen/sperm became a matter of necessity. Despite some practical disadvantages, donor semen samples are now normally cryopreserved in almost all countries. Cryopreservation enables quarantining of donor specimens and, hence, avoids the risk of transferring infections. It also facilitates the scheduling of inseminations, which can be performed without making extra demands on the donor's time or the number of days of sexual abstinence. Samples cryopreserved ready for IUI have improved the recovery rate of motile sperm (and the need to wash samples) after thawing. Cryopreservation has also given couples more choice of having siblings with similar genetic backgrounds if they so desire.

PRINCIPLES OF CRYOBIOLOGY AND SPERM CRYOPRESERVATION

Cryobiology involves investigation of the effects of low temperatures on cells and, for mammals, this includes any temperature below 37°C. It is noteworthy that human sperm washed free of seminal fluid and resuspended in a buffered medium supplemented with albumin can survive at ambient temperatures for 2–3 weeks and at refrigeration temperatures for nearly 1 week, although viability is drastically reduced. Human sperm are not as sensitive to cold shock as are sperm from some other species. Although the damage inflicted upon cooling/freezing is less pronounced in human sperm, loss of viability is generally much more pronounced in poor-quality samples than in those of excellent quality. Damage to cells can be inflicted at any stage of the process, and especially during initial cooling, as a result of chemical, thermal and osmotic stress[14]. Fortunately, there is a considerable body of reassuring evidence indicating no significant genetic or epigenetic injury after sperm cryopreservation or association with fetal abnormalities or spontaneous pregnancy loss.

There is no general recipe for cryopreservation of all cell types, or even for the same cell type in different individuals[1,15]. Optimal protocols vary according to the water and solute permeability, surface to volume ratio, type of cryoprotectant, activation energy, cooling and freezing rate, and storage temperature. Spermatozoa are often regarded as ideal cells for cryopreservation because they are small, available in large numbers, readily obtainable, contain little cytoplasm, and have a lower relative and absolute water content than most other cells. The recovery of motility is a useful indicator of sperm viability (although not necessarily of fertility). The first prerequisite of cryopreservation is to reduce the intracellular water content to avoid the formation of intracellular ice crystals, which are normally lethal. Partial removal of water at lower temperatures may also help reduce thermally driven metabolic activities, leading to a stable state and the suspension of most cellular activities. This state is safeguarded by the addition of a cryoprotective agent (CPA), such as glycerol, usually in combination with a buffer-based medium containing phospholipids from egg yolk (extender). Once spermatozoa have been cryopreserved in this manner, they can be stored safely in liquid nitrogen dewars for many years. The only reactions that may proceed are the effects of free radicals and associated low-level background radiation, which would take many decades to be regarded as a significant hazard[16]. Fortunately too, some CPAs actually have free radical scavenging properties.

In general, cryopreservation of semen/sperm involves the reduction of intracellular water content using a buffer-based CPA, transfer of the mixture to a suitable vessel (i.e. cryovials or straws) and cooling the mixture (usually at rates ranging from −0.5 to −2°C/min) to a level at which extracellular ice crystals begin to form (usually at −5 to −10°C). This stage can be reached spontaneously but is preferably induced manually by seeding the mixture (touching the vessel with cooled forceps). The cryopreservation process is completed by controlled cooling to at least −30°C (often to −80°C) and finally plunging the sample into liquid nitrogen for long-term storage.

As noted above, cryopreservation of spermatozoa involves a series of non-physiological events/steps that involve relatively abrupt osmotic changes due to the addition of CPAs to reduce the intracellular water, cooling, freezing, warming and thawing of the sample. To reduce the water content of the cells, both permeable (e.g. glycerol, propanediol, dimethylsulfoxide) and non-permeable (e.g. sucrose, trehalose) CPAs can be used. Glycerol is still the most common CPA used for the cryopreservation of sperm. Upon slow addition of the CPA, an osmotically driven reduction in cell water is the first event to take place. Where the principal CPAs are of the penetrating type, the cell can return to nearly its original volume because of the influx of the CPA (e.g. glycerol). On cooling to −5 to −15°C, ice nucleation begins first in the extracellular space. As the crystals propagate, the extracellular phase becomes solid (with few unfrozen areas high in salt concentration) whereas the intracellular environment remains unfrozen and becomes partially supercooled due to freezing point depression caused by glycerol influx. Supercooled intracellular water has a higher chemical potential and diffuses out as the extracellular water continues to crystallize (first cell volume change). The intact cell membrane provides a barrier to the propagation of extracellular ice crystals. Since the extracellular water freezes with the exclusion of solutes, the medium becomes hypertonic, causing further osmotic withdrawal of water from the cells (second cell volume change). At the same time, the concentration of solutes within the cell increases with potentially adverse consequences, although these are moderated by the influx of glycerol.

Glycerol modifies the physical properties of the solution by lowering its freezing point and allowing less ice to be formed for the specific temperature at which equilibrium is reached. To illustrate with an example, normal saline with an osmolality of about 280 mOsmol/kg has a freezing point of −0.56°C, and at −10°C approximately 90% of the water must be frozen out in order for an equilibrium to be reached between the ice and the remaining saline. Hence, at this temperature the ice in the system is in equilibrium with a 10 times concentrated unfrozen fraction of the saline, with an osmolality of about 5400 mOsmol/kg. Addition of 10% v/v glycerol, with an osmolality of 1500 mOsmol/kg, to the same saline solution requires freezing of only 68% of the water (compared with 90%) in order for the same equilibrium to be reached at −10°C. In this case, ice is at equilibrium with only a 3.4 times concentrated solution rather than 10 times. In addition, by replacing intracellular water, glycerol reduces the harmful effects of excessive cell shrinkage and phase changes (maintains cell volume). Like many other CPAs, glycerol also maintains the structural and functional integrity of regulatory and structural proteins, nucleic acids and phospholipids of the cells by preventing denaturation resulting from the process of freezing and thawing. This protective function is achieved through several mechanisms. Glycerol can enhance the hydrogen bonds in the hydration

shell around the macromolecules and/or stabilize their topology by interacting with them directly and substituting for their hydration shell[17]. Certain precautions must, however, be taken to reduce the damage and improve the effectiveness of CPAs. To minimize osmotic stress, glycerol is added slowly to the cells and the toxicity is reduced by allowing equilibration to take place at lower temperature in a refrigerator[18]. The rate of cooling is also critical for the survival of sperm: if the rate is too rapid, water loss and the CPA influx may be inadequate and intracellular ice could form; if it is too slow, there may be too much water loss leading to excessive cell shrinkage and prolonged exposure to a damaging hypertonic environment and high concentrations of CPA.

Techniques for the cryopreservation of human sperm are diverse. The simplest ones are the freezing of sperm manually in liquid nitrogen vapor, and several protocols have been published[19-21]. Vials containing sperm are positioned about 5 cm above the liquid nitrogen for 20–30 min. The vials can then be transferred into liquid nitrogen storage dewars (see Protocol 1). A number of protocols for use with programable freezers (controlled-rate) have also been proposed[22-24], although an automated system for the cryopreservation of human sperm is not absolutely necessary. With the controlled-rate protocol, commonly the cooling rate is −0.5°C/min from room temperature to −5°C, the freezing rate is −10°C/min from −5 down to −80°C, and followed by plunging into liquid nitrogen (−196°C). The decline in temperature is at a higher rate during the freezing phase than in the preceding cooling phase to counter the release of latent heat, to prevent further water loss and to minimize strain on the cell membrane (see Protocol 2). Several variations of the controlled-rate method have been published. Similar procedures are used for cryopreserving epididymal and testicular sperm/tissue. Ice recrystallization occurs at or above the glass temperature of −130°C and, in consequence, dry ice (approximately −78°C) is not a safe medium for storing or shipping samples[25,26]. Protocols utilized to cryopreserve

Protocol 1. Cryopreservation of Human Semen by Manual Method

Cooling/freezing phase

(1) Allow sample to liquefy at room temperature for approximately 30 min

(2) Determine basic semen parameters manually or using CASA

(3) Slowly add equal volume of Test-Yolk Buffer® containing 12% glycerol (freezing medium; Irvine Scientific, Irvine, CA) to the semen and mix gently each time a portion of the freezing medium is added (10–15 min)

(4) Determine basic parameters of the mixture either manually or using CASA

(5) Place the mixture in a beaker of water at ambient temperature and refrigerated at 4°C for 30–60 min to complete equilibration and slowly cool the mixture (approximately −0.2°C/min)

(6) Aliquot (0.5–0.8 ml/vial) the mixture into pre-cooled and labeled cryovials, place vials into a freezing tray (Taylor-Wharton, Theodore, AL). Smaller volumes/vial may also be cryopreserved

(7) Cryopreserve manually by placing the tray (bottom of tubes) 4–5 cm above liquid nitrogen for 20–30 min

(8) Remove tubes at once, place them on a labeled cane and plunge them into liquid nitrogen

Note: To cryopreserve samples as IUI-ready, semen can be washed and resuspended in a buffer-based medium containing human serum albumin (i.e. HTF®; Irvine Scientific) and cryopreserved as noted above

Thawing phase

Place vials in a water bath at 37°C for 5–7 min. Ensure that the entire portion of the vial containing the sample is submerged in water

CASA, computer-assisted semen analysis; IUI, intrauterine insemination

sperm are less appropriate for oocytes or embryos, which have a higher water content and low permeability (see Chapter 11).

In general, the CPA of choice for semen/sperm cryopreservation is glycerol. Usually a solution of about 6% v/v glycerol is used in a buffered medium containing TES (N-tris (hydroxymethyl) methyl-2-aminoethane-sulfonic acid), TRIS (tris (hydroxymethyl) aminomethane) and citrate buffers mixed with 20% (v/v) egg yolk and antibiotics[19,20]. The concentration of glycerol is initially doubled so that after dilution with an equal volume of semen, the final desired concentration is achieved. After adding the medium to the semen over 10–15 min to allow gradual replacement of cell water, the mixture is placed in a beaker of water at ambient temperature and refrigerated (2–6°C) for 30–60 min to complete equilibration and cool slowly (approximately −0.2°C/min). The mixture is then aliquoted into labeled and refrigerated plastic cryovials in volumes ranging from 0.5 to 0.8 ml (although smaller volumes may also be frozen). The vials are transferred either to a freezing tray for manual freezing or directly into a programable freezer (see Protocols 1 and 2).

Efforts to optimize the freezing phase are wasted, however, unless the thawing phase is also carefully controlled[16,19,27]. If thawing is slow, small ice nuclei may form at the transition temperature and grow into larger ones that can damage cells before they are completely thawed. Thawing is therefore carried out rapidly by placing the vials in a water bath at 37°C.

Protocol 2. Cryopreservation of Human Semen Using a Programable Freezer

Cooling/freezing phase

(1)   Allow sample to liquefy at room temperature for approximately 30 min

(2)   Determine basic semen parameters manually or using CASA

(3)   Slowly add equal volume of Test-Yolk Buffer® containing 12% glycerol (freezing medium; Irvine Scientific, Irvine, CA) to the semen and mix gently each time a portion of the freezing medium is added (10–15 min)

(4)   Determine basic parameters of the mixture either manually or using CASA

(5)   Aliquot the mixture (0.5–0.8 ml/vial) into 2 ml labeled cryovials (Fisher, Pittsburgh, PA)

(6)   Load into the automated freezer and cryopreserve as follows:

   (a)   From room temperature to 5°C at −0.5°C/min

   (b)   From 5°C to 4°C at −1°C/min

   (c)   From 4°C to 3°C at −2°C/min

   (d)   From 3°C to 2°C at −4°C/min

   (e)   From 2°C to 1°C at −8°C/min

   (f)   From 1°C to −80°C at −10°C/min

(7)   Load vials on pre-cooled labeled canes and plunge them into liquid nitrogen

Note: To cryopreserve samples as IUI-ready, semen can be washed and resuspended in a buffer-based medium containing human serum albumin (i.e. HTF®; Irvine Scientific) and cryopreserved as noted above

Thawing phase

Place vials in a water bath at 37°C for 5–7 min. Ensure that the entire portion of the vial containing the sample is submerged in water

CASA, computer-assisted semen analysis; IUI, intrauterine insemination

SUCCESS RATE FOR USING CRYOPRESERVED–THAWED SPERM

There is a widespread belief that the results of TI of cryopreserved sperm are poorer than with fresh semen/sperm. In fact, comparative studies have not consistently supported this view and, while some studies give support to this view, others deny it (see Table 1). Expressed as cumulative insemination cycles, pregnancy rates have been reported to be as high as 70–75%, with a miscarriage rate of 15–16% and a mean number of 3.5 cycles to conception. There are many factors that can affect pregnancy success rates and the effect of cryopreservation *per se* may be small compared with the other variables. It is also important to note that there is considerable variation in tolerance to freeze–thawing between semen specimens, and this is as true of animal species as it is of humans[28]. There is greater consistency between specimens from the same individual than between males[29]. As a rule of thumb, about a third of men produce specimens that cryopreserve very successfully, a third are rather unsuccessful and another third are intermediate (personal experience of 15 years). Thus, frozen banking of sperm

Table 1 Relative success rates per insemination treatment cycle using fresh and cryopreserved semen

Study	Sample type	Number of cycles	Pregnancy rate/cycle
Richter et al., 1984[31]	fresh	676	0.19
	frozen	1200	0.05
Bordson et al., 1986[32]	fresh	165	0.12
	frozen	165	0.10
Keel and Webster, 1989[33]	fresh	67	0.06
	frozen	209	0.05
DiMarzo et al., 1990[34]	fresh	3405	0.11
	frozen	371	0.06
Subak et al., 1992[35]	fresh	102	0.21
	frozen	96	0.09

does not provide assurance for a young cancer sufferer that his semen will cryopreserve successfully, and, of course, his medical condition may prevent him from producing a good or any specimen in time[30]. These differences may be reflected in the plasma membrane susceptibility/properties of the spermatozoa, but at present there is no reliable way of predicting which individuals will be most successful, except on the basis of previous history of cryopreservation and, partially, on the motility of sperm in the semen sample being cryopreserved. In our experience, samples with sperm motilities of > 60% have a better chance of effective cryopreservation than samples with lower motilities. One of the conclusions from such observations is that no single freeze–thaw protocol is ideal for all individuals.

Data obtained from IVF indicate that there is no difference between fresh and cryopreserved sperm samples. In one study of 39 IVF cycles using fresh semen compared with 74 cycles using cryopreserved samples, the pregnancy rates were almost identical at 39.3% and 38.5%, respectively[36]. In our IVF program too, comparable results have been obtained. In a retrospective controlled study, an excellent cumulative pregnancy rate of 83% was obtained after four IVF cycles for patients who had failed with TDI[37]. In a control group

of patients with tubal disease undergoing IVF and matched for age, infertility diagnosis and number of treatment cycle attempts, the corresponding rate was 59%, which was significantly lower. Compared with such important variables as the reproductive history and age of the woman, the problems of sperm cryopreservation are relatively minor (see Chapter 1).

Patients who are younger than 26 years of age had the highest fecundity after TI of 0.20 (conceptions per cycle), compared with 0.10 for those aged 26–35 years and 0.09 for those over 35 years[32]. Unfortunately, many studies have not been designed by randomizing patients or using appropriate controls. In a prospective randomized trial in which each patient served as her own control (alternating fresh and cryopreserved inseminations), fecundity was approximately 0.20 with fresh semen 0.09 for cryopreserved semen[35]. Unexpectedly, a difference was observed with intracervical insemination (ICI), but not with IUI. The results of another larger study[34] produced corresponding rates of monthly fecundity of 0.12 and 0.06, respectively. However, a life table analysis produced a cumulative pregnancy rate for fresh and cryopreserved samples that did not differ significantly. These results indicate that it may take longer to achieve pregnancy using cryopreserved semen, and they have been reviewed in detail elsewhere[1].

A large number of studies have reported the status of sperm cryopreservation for individuals affected by various malignancies. Results of a 22-year experience from an academic center in Sydney, Australia have recently been published[38]. Over this period of time, 930 men sought semen cryopreservation and storage prior to treatment for cancer. Ninety percent of these men had sufficient sperm to cryopreserve and 74% survived their illness. Twenty-one percent of all applicants (28% of survivors) opted to discard their samples and only 7% of all applicants (9% of survivors, 68 men/couples) utilized their cryopreserved samples within 12 to 180 months after storage. Various methods of assisted conception such as IUI (35 cycles), IVF (28 cycles) and ICSI (22 cycles) were utilized. A total of 29 pregnancies and 39 births resulted, with the best results obtained using the ICSI procedure. One infant resulting from an IUI attempt had a non-genetic abnormality, and another from an ICSI procedure had Down's syndrome (the mother of this infant was 38 years old). No obvious association between abnormal pregnancies and the cryopreserved sperm was noted.

There have been few reports about the influence of sperm preparation methods on clinical outcome. However, based on evidence from fresh semen (reviewed by Mortimer[39]), it appears that the protocols may have a significant impact and, if so, are likely to apply to cryopreserved semen also. Ideally, sperm preparation should be rapid, simple, inexpensive and enable the recovery of a maximum number of motile sperm with normal function and morphology. To this end, the 'swim up' method was introduced by Drevious in 1971[40]. The sperm population is heterogeneous and contains many immotile and morphologically abnormal forms. The functionally normal sperm are assumed to be motile, and migration from the washed sperm pellet after gentle centrifugation into a separate phase enables them to be concentrated. Refinements of this method have led to widespread applications for IVF, as well as for TI and TDI[39]. These methods have particular relevance to cases where sperm quality is poor, and even to idiopathic infertility.

Reactive oxygen species (ROS) play important roles in the pathogenesis of infertility, including effects on sperm nuclear DNA and membrane fluidity[41]. Moreover, Aitken and Clarkson[42] have shown that iatrogenic damage can occur during laboratory preparation methods and impair the ability of sperm to fertilize. They pointed out that most semen samples from subfertile patients contain an excess of round cells, including neutrophils, macrophages and round spermatids. Excess production of ROS may occur in this environment and, in some cases, there may be an inability to detoxify these species, or a combination of both. Centrifugation, which concentrates the cells, may increase the risk of damage from superoxide and hydroxyl radicals, as well as from cytokines produced by leukocytes[39,42–44]. To minimize direct contact between different subpopulations of cells, Aitken and Clarkson used Percoll gradient centrifugation, and reported finding a defective subpopulation of sperm with a lower density due to the higher cytoplasmic volume, cytoplasmic droplets and coating envelopes[45]. Originally described by Suarez and colleagues[46], Percoll was first reported for IVF applications in 1986 by Hyne and associates[47] and was applied to cases of unsuccessful IVF attempts by using 'swim up' samples prepared from washed pellets. Significantly higher fertilization rates were obtained[48]. Studies using electron microscopy to assess sperm morphology and chromatin showed that gradient centrifugation produces and also removes a major part of the bacterial contamination from semen[49]. For safety and quality control in clinical practice, Percoll has now been replaced by alternative media in recent years (i.e. ISolate, Pureception, PureSperm, etc.).

Processing of cryopreserved sperm after thawing requires special attention. If spermatozoa are cryopreserved as washed sperm ('IUI-ready'), there is no need to process the sample any further after thawing. However, if whole semen is cryopreserved, it needs to be washed to remove the seminal fluid containing prostaglandins to make it suitable for IUI. If IVF or ICSI is to be attempted using cryopreserved whole semen, post-thaw processing of the sample is also necessary. There is no generally agreed method for washing cryopreserved semen for IUI or other methods of assisted conception, although a number of precautions are recommended. These samples can have an osmolality ranging from 700 to 900 mOsmol/kg, which is approximately three-fold higher than the normal osmolality of $\cong 282$ mOsmol/kg. The sample must be restored after thawing to normal osmolality with a buffer-based medium, and this must be added very slowly to allow gradual osmotic change and minimize stress to the cells.

All of these efforts will be worthless unless there is good synchronization between insemination and ovulation. In a retrospective study over a 2-year period, there was no significant difference between four different methods of ovulation detection and the pregnancy outcome[50]. Insemination carried out several hours before or after presumptive ovulation appeared to have no significant difference on pregnancy outcome. In one study, there was a difference in optimal timing according to whether IUI or ICI was utilized. When the timing of ovulation detection was compared between home kits for detection of urinary luteinizing hormone, or basal body temperature or ultrasound, the results were found to be similar[51,52].

The numbers of inseminations per cycle have also been investigated as another potential variable for pregnancy outcome. In a prospective randomized study, pregnancy rates per cycle with controlled ovarian hyperstimulation of patients receiving one IUI per cycle were compared with those of comparable patients receiving two inseminations per cycle. No significant differences were observed[53]. However, in another study of 25- to 40-year-old patients, there was a three-fold advantage with double insemination, which translated into a two-fold increase in the cumulative probability of conception over six cycles[54]. Another study suggested that the method of insemination (IUI or ICI) affected the outcome[55]. Our evaluation of almost 1330 cycles of TDI revealed no significant differences between one or two IUIs per cycle (unpublished data).

While there must be a threshold number of motile sperm present in a specimen for insemination to be effective, this has not been identified in practice. Using fresh semen with IUI, Dodson and Haney[56] reported that no pregnancies occurred with < 1 million motile sperm for insemination; the pregnancy rates with larger numbers of sperm were similar. Byrd and co-workers[55] reported that pregnancy outcome using cryopreserved semen was, however, dependent on the number of motile sperm present, with a minimum number of 6–15 million for IUI and 50–100 million for

ICI. The same study showed that the post-thaw motility of the sample also affected the pregnancy rate. Samples with motility < 30% had a success rate of 5.5% with IUI, compared with 15.4% with post-thaw motility of 30–50% and 27.2% when motility was > 50%. This is not an exhaustive list of factors that can affect the clinical outcome[57], but other factors have not been as thoroughly investigated or quantified.

RISKS ASSOCIATED WITH THE USE OF CRYOPRESERVED SPERM

The question is often asked whether there is any DNA damage associated with sperm cryopreservation or if insemination increases the risk of an abnormal conceptus and/or spontaneous pregnancy loss. While animal data indicate that cells are genetically stable at liquid nitrogen temperatures, 50% or more of the cells die at some stage of the cryopreservation process itself. Furthermore, studies of human sperm are more equivocal or contradictory and difficult to evaluate; the subject has been reviewed in greater depth by Verp[58]. In many investigations, there was no adequate control group or matching of parental age, genetic history or environmental factors. Full investigation and follow-up of the pregnancies, including stillborns, abortuses and live births, has seldom been carried out, and anomalies that might only manifest later in life (i.e. sex chromosome anomalies, learning disabilities) could have been overlooked. In general, only the most clinically significant and obvious malformations have been reported.

Certainly, the stress of cryopreservation might cause sublethal injury to spermatozoa. Damage could occur to the acrosome, cross fibers, fiber sheaths, mitochondria and axoneme, causing impaired motility[13,58,59]. More importantly, effects on the nuclear genome have not been established. If only the 'hardiest sperm' survive, this could be an explanation for the reduction in the incidence of miscarriage and birth defects after conceiving with cryopreserved sperm as reported by some investigators[60]. On the other hand, another study has reported an increased incidence of trisomy[61]. More reassuringly, the heterologous fertilization technique involving insemination of zona-free hamster oocytes with human sperm has provided evidence for the structural integrity of the chromosomes and a normal ratio after sperm cryopreservation[62]. Studies of bovine spermatozoa have also been a source of confidence, but until genome-wide screening for new mutations can be performed we cannot rule out subtle genetic alterations. While any doubts remain it is important for long-term studies to follow up the children conceived by these techniques. So far, the data regarding offspring conceived using cryopreserved sperm from individuals with malignancies have not shown any sign of genotypic or phenotypic abnormalities above the normal rate observed in the general population[15].

Commonly, cryopreserved samples are kept in liquid nitrogen for long-term storage. Except in isolated cases, most vessels (e.g. cryovials) used for the cryopreservation/ storage of sperm are not leak-proof. Liquid nitrogen easily enters these vessels after they are plunged into the liquid nitrogen. Concerns have surfaced about the risk of cross-contamination between infected and uninfected specimens. Certain viruses and some bacteria can survive in liquid nitrogen, which highlights the need for being cautious about

unscreened specimens[63]. Several measures have been taken to minimize this potential risk. Certain regulatory agencies (e.g. New York State Department of Health) require the storage of cryopreserved sperm from donors separate from those of client depositors (patients). Routinely, donors are tested for various sexually transmitted infectious diseases, but this is not as widely practiced as necessary for the client depositors. Attempts must be made to either test the client depositors for major sexually transmitted diseases (e.g. HIV-1, HIV-2, hepatitis B and C) prior to the deposition of their semen or to store the cryopreserved samples in liquid nitrogen vapor only. However, in this case care must be taken to sustain the temperature of these samples at a minimum of $-130°C$ in order to prevent ice recrystallization and to maintain the integrity of the samples for as long as they are stored.

Finally, it must be recognized that although sperm cryopreservation is a mature technology, continuing vigilance is needed to safeguard specimens and patient health, as well as efforts to improve the effectiveness of services. Recently, live mouse offspring were produced after inseminating oocytes using ICSI with freeze-dried spermatozoa[64]. This opens a new avenue for research, although it remains questionable whether this technique will prove safer than existing ones for human reproduction.

References

1. Morshedi M. Artificial insemination 1: using a donor's sperm. In Acosta A, Kruger T, eds. *Human Spermatozoa in Assisted Reproduction*, 2nd edn. Carnforth, UK: Parthenon Publishing, 1996:367–98
2. Hallak J, Mahran AM, Agarwal A. Characteristics of cryopreserved semen from men with lymphoma. *J Assist Reprod Genet* 2000;17:591–4
3. Hallak J, Mahran A, Chae J, Agarwal A. Poor semen quality from patients with malignancies does not rule out sperm banking. *Urol Res* 2000;28:281–4
4. Ranganathan P, Mahran AM, Hallak J, Agarwal A. Sperm cryopreservation from men

with nonmalignant, systemic diseases: a descriptive study. *J Androl* 2002;23:71–5
5. Kobayashi H, Larson K, Sharma RK, *et al.* DNA damage in patients with untreated cancer as measured by the sperm chromatin structure assay. *Fertil Steril* 2001;75:469–75
6. Kleegman JS. Therapeutic donor insemination. *Fertil Steril* 1954;5:7–31
7. Arny M, Quagliarello JR. History of artificial insemination. A tribute to Sophi Kleegman, MD. *Semin Reprod Endocrinol* 1987;5:1–3
8. Shettles LB. The respiration of human spermatozoa and their response to various gases and low temperatures. *Am J Physiol* 1940;128:408–15

9. Hoagland H, Pincus G. Revival of mammalian sperm after immersion in liquid nitrogen. *J Gen Physiol* 1942;25:337–44

10. Lane M, Bavister BD, Lyons EA, Forest KT. Containerless vitrification of mammalian oocytes and embryos. *Nat Biotechnol* 1999;17:1234–6

11. Polge C, Smith AU, Parkes AS. Revival of spermatozoa after vitrification and dehydration at low temperatures. *Nature* 1949;169:626–7

12. Bunge RG, Keettel WC, Sherman JK. Clinical use of frozen semen. Report of four cases. *Fertil Steril* 1954;5:520–9

13. Brotherton J. Cryopreservation of human semen. *Arch Androl* 1990;25:181–95

14. Hammerstedt RH, Graham JJ, Nolan JP. Cryopreservation of mammalian sperm: what we ask them to survive. *J Androl* 1990;11:73–87

15. Anger JT, Gilbert BR, Goldstein M. Cryopreservation of sperm: indications, methods and results. *J Urol* 2003;170:1079–84

16. Mazur P. Freezing of living cells: mechanisms and implications. *Am J Physiol* 1984;247:25–142

17. Karow MA. Pharmacological interventions *in vitro*. In Karow MA, Critser JK, eds. *Reproductive Tissue Banking*. New York: Academic Press, 1997:201–5

18. Wolf DP, Patton PE. Sperm cryopreservation: state of the art. *J In Vitro Fert Embryo Transf* 1989;6:315–17

19. Duru NK, Morshedi MS, Schuffner A, Oehninger S. Cryopreservation–thawing of fractionated spermatozoa is associated with membrane phosphatidylserine externalization and not DNA fragmentation. *J Androl* 2001;22:646–51

20. Mahony MC, Morshedi M, Scott RT, *et al*. Role of spermatozoa cryopreservative in assisted reproduction. In Acosta AA, Kruger TF, eds. *Human Spermatozoa in Assisted Reproduction*. Baltimore, MD: Williams and Wilkins, 1989:310–18

21. Jouannet P, Frydman R, Van Steirteghem A, *et al*. Cryopreservation and infertility. In Seibel MM, ed. *Infertility, A Comprehensive Text*. Norwalk, CT: Appleton and Lange, 1990:525–38

22. Sherman JK. Cryopreservation of human semen. In Keel BA, Webster BW, eds. *Handbook of the Laboratory Diagnosis and Treatment of Infertility*. Boca Raton, FL: CRC Press, 1990:224–59

23. Serafini P, Marrs RP. Computerized staged-freezing technique improves sperm survival and preserves penetration of zona-free hamster ova. *Fertil Steril* 1986;5:854–8

24. Critser JK, Huse-Benda AR, Aaker DV, *et al*. Cryopreservation of human spermatozoa. I. Effects of holding procedure and seeding on

25. motility, fertilizability, and acrosome reaction. *Fertil Steril* 1987;47:656–63

25. Karow AM. Biophysical and chemical consideration in cryopreservation. In Karow AM, Pegg DE, eds. *Organ Preservation for Transplantation*. New York: Dekker, 1981:113–41

26. Walker RH. Pilot surveys for proficiency testing of semen analysis. Comparison of dry ice versus liquid nitrogen shipments. *Arch Pathol Lab Med* 1992;116:423–4

27. Schneider U. Cryobiological principles of embryo freezing. *J In Vitro Fertil Embryo Transf* 1986;3:3–9

28. Leibo SP, Picton HM, Gosden RG. Cryopreservation of human spermatozoa. In Vayena E, Rowe PJ, Griffin PD, eds. *Current Practices and Controversies in Assisted Reproduction*. Report of a WHO meeting; WHO Technical Reports. Geneva: World Health Organization, 2002:152–65

29. Heuchel V, Schwartz D, Czyglik F. Between and within subject correlations and variances for certain semen characteristics in fertile men. *Andrologia* 1983;15:171–6

30. Lass A, Akagbosu F, Abusheikha N, *et al*. A programme of semen cryopreservation for disease in a tertiary infertility centre: lessons from 8 years' experience. *Hum Reprod* 1998;13:3256–61

31. Richter MA, Haning RV Jr, Shapiro SS. Artificial donor insemination: fresh versus frozen semen; the patient as her own control. *Fertil Steril* 1984;41:277–80

32. Bordson BL, Ricci E, Dunaway H, *et al*. Comparison of fecundability with fresh and frozen semen in therapeutic donor insemination. *Fertil Steril* 1986;46:466–9

33. Keel BA, Webster BW. Semen analysis data from fresh and cryopreserved donor of cryoprotectants and pregnancy rates. *Fertil Steril* 1989;52:100–5

34. DiMarzo SJ, Huang J, Kennedy JF, *et al*. Pregnancy rates with fresh versus computer-controlled cryopreserved semen for artificial insemination by donor in a private practice setting. *Am J Obstet Gynecol* 1990;102:1483–90

35. Subak LL, Adamson C, Boltz NL. Therapeutic donor insemination: a prospective randomized trial of fresh versus frozen sperm. *Am J Obstet Gynecol* 1992;166:1597–604

36. Yavetz H, Hessing JB, Niv Y, *et al*. The efficacy of cryopreserved semen versus fresh semen for *in vitro* fertilization/embryo transfer. *J In Vitro Fertil Embryo Transf* 1991;8:145–8

37. Robinson JN, Lockwood GM, Dokras A, *et al*. A controlled study to assess the use of *in vitro* fertilization with donor semen after failed therapeutic donor insemination. *Fertil Steril* 1993;59:353–8

38. Kelleher S, Wishart SM, Liu PY, *et al*. Long-term outcome of elective human sperm cryostorage. *Hum Reprod* 2001;16:2632–9

39. Mortimer D. Sperm preparation techniques and iatrogenic failures of *in vitro* fertilization. *Hum Reprod* 1991;6:173–6

40. Drevius LO. The 'sperm rise' test. *J Reprod Fertil* 1971;24:427–32

41. Moustafa MN, Sharma RK, Thornton J, *et al*. Relationship between ROS production, apoptosis and DNA denaturation in spermatozoa from patients examined for infertility. *Hum Reprod* 2004;19:129–38

42. Aitken RJ, Clarkson JS. Significance of reaction oxygen species and antioxidants in defining the efficacy of sperm preparation techniques. *J Androl* 1988;9:367–76

43. Buch JP, Kolon TF, Maulik N, *et al*. Cytokines stimulate lipid membrane peroxidation of human sperm. *Fertil Steril* 1994;62:186–8

44. Saleh RA, Agarwal A, Kandirali E, *et al*. Leukocytospermia is associated with increased reactive oxygen species production by human spermatozoa. *Fertil Steril* 2002;78:1215–24

45. Tanphaichitr N, Millette CF, Agulnick A, Fitzgerald LM. Egg penetration ability and structural properties of human sperm prepared by Percoll-gradient centrifugation. *Gamete Res* 1988;20:67–81

46. Suarez SS, Wolf DP, Meizel S. Induction of the acrosome reaction in human spermatozoa by a fraction of human follicular fluid. *Gamete Res* 1986;14:107–21

47. Hyne RV, Stojanoff A, Clarke GN, *et al*. Pregnancy from *in vitro* fertilization of human eggs after separation of motile spermatozoa by density gradient centrifugation. *Fertil Steril* 1986;45:93–6

48. Guerin JF, Mathieu C, Lornage J, *et al*. Improvement of survival and fertilizing capacity of human spermatozoa in an IVF programme by selection of discontinuous Percoll gradients. *Hum Reprod* 1989;4:798–804

49. Bolton VN, Warner RE, Braude P. Removal of bacterial contaminants from semen for *in vitro* fertilization or artificial insemination by the use of buoyant density centrifugation. *Fertil Steril* 1986;46:1128–32

50. Brook PF, Barratt CL, Cooke ID. The more accurate timing of insemination with regard to ovulation dos not create a significant improvement in pregnancy rates in a donor insemination program. *Fertil Steril* 1994;61:308–13

51. Robinson JN, Lockwood GM, Dalton JD, *et al*. A randomized prospective study to assess the effect of the use of home urinary luteinizing hormone detection on the efficiency of donor insemination. *Hum Reprod* 1992;7:63–5

52. Odem RR, Durso NM, Long CA, *et al*. Therapeutic donor insemination: a prospective randomized study of scheduling methods. *Fertil Steril* 1991;55:976–82

53. Ransom MX, Blotner MB, Bohrer M, *et al*. Does increasing frequency of intrauterine insemination improve pregnancy rates significantly during superovulation cycles? *Fertil Steril* 1994;61:303–7

54. Centola GM, Mattox JH, Raubertas RF. Pregnancy rates after double versus single insemination with frozen donor sperm. *Fertil Steril* 1990;54:1089–92

55. Byrd W, Bradshaw K, Carr B, *et al*. A prospective randomized study of pregnancy rates following intrauterine and intracervical insemination using frozen donor sperm. *Fertil Steril* 1990;53:521–7

56. Dodson WC, Haney AF. Controlled ovarian hyperstimulation and intrauterine insemination for treatment of infertility. *Fertil Steril* 1991;55:457–67

57. Oehninger S. Assessment of sperm cryodamage and strategies to improve outcome. *Mol Cell Endocrinol* 2000;169:3–10

58. Verp MS. Genetic issues in artificial insemination by donor. *Semin Reprod Endocrinol* 1987;5:59–68

59. Mahadevan MM, Trounson AO. Relationship of fine structure of sperm head to fertility of frozen human semen. *Fertil Steril* 1984;41:287–93

60. Sanger WG, Schwartz MB, Housel G. The use of frozen–thawed semen for therapeutic insemination (donor). *Int J Fertil* 1979;24:267–9

61. Fédération Française des CECOS, Mattei JF, Le Mare CB. Genetic aspects of artificial insemination by donor (AID). Indications, surveillance, and results. *Clin Genet* 1983;23:132–8

62. Martin RH, Chernos JE, Rademaker AW. Effect of cryopreservation on the frequency of chromosomal abnormalities and sex ratio in human sperm. *Mol Reprod Dev* 1991;30:159–63

63. Clarke GN. Sperm cryopreservation: is there a significant risk of cross-contamination? *Hum Reprod* 1999;14:2941–3

64. Ward MA, Kaneko T, Kusakabe H, *et al*. Long-term preservation of mouse spermatozoa after freeze-drying and freezing without cryoprotection. *Biol Reprod* 2003;69:2100–8

A surgical strategy using spermatogonial stem cells for restoring male fertility

10

M. C. Nagano

INTRODUCTION

Spermatogonial stem cells (SSCs) are the stem cells of the male germ line and the foundation of spermatogenesis[1,2]. These stem cells have a dual biological function: to reproduce themselves (self-renewal) and concurrently to generate progenitors that are committed to differentiation. While the self-renewal activity of stem cells sustains the stem cell pool, the generation of progenitor spermatogonia triggers the germ cell differentiation cascade that leads to the final product of spermatogenesis, spermatozoa. SSCs are present in the seminiferous tubules at birth and continuously perform their dual function throughout adult life, conferring life-long reproductive activity to a male. This shows a remarkable contrast to female gametogenesis. Since all female germ cells enter meiosis and lose self-renewal potential before birth, stem cells do not exist in the postnatal female germ line and the reproductive life of females is significantly limited. SSCs are thus the only cell population in the human body that can continuously self-renew and transmit genetic information to the next generation.

Because of this unique dual function, SSCs are an important target cell population for strategies aimed at restoring fertility in men after radio/chemotherapy for cancer[1,3]. Since spermatogenesis is an active cell proliferation process, it is sensitive to anticancer treatments and can be lost permanently in cancer survivors. In fact, infertility occurs more often in male than female patients following cancer therapies[4,5]. Since SSCs are the mother cell population of spermatogenesis, however, the regeneration of spermatogenesis and the subsequent restoration of male fertility can be achieved if SSCs conduct their dual function in the testes of cancer survivors. Therefore, the manipulation of SSCs is a promising approach toward restoring male fertility after sterilizing cancer therapies.

Although SSC manipulation has hardly been realized in clinical settings, it is well established in experimental animals and is expected to be applicable in humans. To restore fertility in male cancer survivors, the manipulation of SSCs can be approached using two potential strategies. The first strategy is to encourage the activity of SSCs that have survived anticancer treatments. In this case, pharmacological manipulations of hormone levels after treatment stimulate the functional recovery of the somatic environment and the activity of surviving SSCs to reinitiate their dual function and to maintain spermatogenesis. This non-invasive strategy is discussed in Chapter 5 and elsewhere[6]. The second strategy is to surgically manipulate SSCs in the following three steps (Figure 1):

(1) Harvest testis biopsies and SSCs before the therapy;

(2) Cryopreserve SSCs;

(3) Autologously transfer SSCs to the patient after the therapy.

This surgical strategy is further divided into two approaches: transplantation of SSCs and implantation of testicular biopsies (Figure 1).

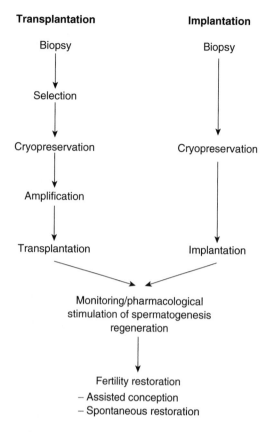

Transplantation

Biopsy

↓

Selection

↓

Cryopreservation

↓

Amplification

↓

Transplantation

Implantation

Biopsy

↓

Cryopreservation

↓

Implantation

Monitoring/pharmacological
stimulation of spermatogenesis
regeneration

↓

Fertility restoration
– Assisted conception
– Spontaneous restoration

Figure 1 A simplified flow chart illustrating the surgical strategy (transplantation of testis cells and implantation of testis pieces) for male fertility restoration based on spermatogonial stem cells (SSCs). The fundamental steps in these strategies are: (1) harvesting testis biopsies; (2) cryopreservation; and (3) autologous transfer. The biopsy specimens are made into single-cell suspensions in the transplantation approach, whereas whole specimens are used in the implantation approach. These cells/tissues are harvested prior to anticancer treatments and cryopreserved until transfer. In the transplantation approach, SSCs included in a single-cell suspension could be selected and amplified to ensure the absence of cancer cells in the cell preparation and to enable efficient recovery of male fertility after transplantation. In future clinical applications, cryopreservation of SSCs may need to be done before and/or after SSC selection and amplification. In the implantation approach, frozen–thawed biopsies are implanted into a patient's testes or ectopically under the skin. Following these surgical procedures, spermatogenesis can be regenerated in the patient's seminiferous tubules or in testis implants. The restoration of male fertility can be accomplished using assisted conception or even spontaneously. The regeneration of spermatogenesis may be monitored on the basis of serum hormone levels and can be stimulated by pharmacological treatments of the patient

In the transplantation approach, SSCs are injected into the seminiferous tubules and regenerate spermatogenesis in the testes of cancer survivors. In the implantation approach, testis biopsies are grafted into patients' testes or ectopically under the skin, and spermatogenesis is re-established from SSCs in the implants. After both of these procedures, a patient can regain fertility either spontaneously or through assisted conception using sperm produced from regenerated spermatogenesis. Although both approaches are invasive, their advantage over the pharmacological strategy is that SSCs are not exposed to sterilizing or mutagenic agents, because they are harvested before cancer therapies. Unless affected by the disease itself, therefore, genetically and physiologically intact stem cells are the source of regeneration of spermatogenesis and restoration of male fertility.

The transplantation and implantation approaches are expected to be beneficial for prepubertal cancer patients who do not produce sperm at the time of treatment and for adult patients whose attempts at assisted conception were unsuccessful or who did not have an opportunity to cryopreserve sperm prior to cancer therapies. As discussed below, both approaches are technically feasible at present in selected cases, although they are still experimental and involve several problems that need to be solved before they are safely and efficiently applied in clinical settings. For example, both approaches can be used for patients with non-metastatic brain cancers, but not for those with leukemias and lymphomas, due to the possibility that testis specimens obtained before cancer therapy may include tumor cells (see p. 129). However, most of the techniques required in the surgical strategy, including cryopreservation and assisted conception, are currently available (Figure 1), and the technological developments related to spermatogonial transplantation and testicular biopsy implantation have been remarkably rapid in recent years. Thus, cancer patients should now be provided with the opportunity to at least cryopreserve testis cells and/or tissues, allowing a majority of cancer patients the possibility of regaining fertility in the near future.

This chapter, which focuses on fertility restoration for male cancer survivors, first describes the current status of the transplantation and implantation techniques, which have been achieved largely in studies using experimental animals. Then the advantages and disadvantages of each approach are considered, and some issues that future studies must address to apply these techniques clinically are discussed. Finally, further issues to be considered for both approaches are addressed. The discussions presented in this chapter are intended to summarize the potential of the surgical strategy for male fertility restoration, not only for immediate use but also for future application, and thus include various hypothetical scenarios.

CURRENT STATUS OF TECHNOLOGICAL DEVELOPMENTS OF THE SURGICAL STRATEGY

Spermatogonial transplantation

Spermatogonial transplantation was developed in 1994 by Brinster using the mouse as a model species[7,8]. In this procedure, a suspension of single cells obtained from the testes of donor mice is injected into the lumen of seminiferous tubules (directly[7-9] or via efferent ducts[9]) of recipient infertile mice. SSCs contained in the suspension of donor testis cells colonize the recipient's seminiferous epithelium and regenerate donor-derived spermatogenesis. The regeneration of spermatogenesis can be accomplished using donor cells obtained from both adult and immature mice[7,8]. Recipient mice subsequently produce spermatozoa and sire offspring carrying the donor haplotype[8]. Donor cells injected into recipient testes are a crude preparation of testis cells at present, including germ cells at various differentiation stages and somatic cells. However, long-term and complete spermatogenesis can be established only by SSCs after transplantation, because

spermatogenesis is a one-way differentiation cascade and thus, even if advanced (i.e. non-stem) spermatogonia are injected into recipient testes, they are exhausted during differentiation. Hence, spermatogonial transplantation is a novel approach based strictly on SSCs to restore male fertility.

In spermatogonial transplantation in the mouse model, donor testes are first digested using collagenase followed by trypsin and DNase to prepare the suspension of testis cells[9,10]. While these cells can be transplanted immediately, they can also be cryopreserved[11]. Donor cells stored for a long time in liquid nitrogen retain the activity of SSCs to regenerate complete spermatogenesis upon transplantation. Donor cells are frozen in tissue culture medium with 10% dimethyl sulfoxide and 10% serum[11], which is a routine method developed for cryopreservation of somatic cells. Partly because they are diploid cells, SSCs may be as robust as somatic cells and such a simple solution is effective for their cryopreservation. Thus, the three steps (harvest, cryopreserve and transplant SSCs; Figure 1) required for male fertility restoration based on transplantation have been well established in the mouse model.

Recent progress in SSC studies indicates that male fertility restoration by transplantation could also be realistic in humans. Of the three steps essential to the surgical strategy, the first step, harvesting testis biopsies, is a routine procedure. Preparation of a single-cell suspension has been shown to be feasible from human testis biopsies[12]. As demonstrated with mouse testes, a cocktail of multiple enzymes is also effective in digesting human testis biopsies, although the optimal conditions for enzymatic digestion (e.g. type and concentration of enzymes) have not been verified. These single-cell preparations can be cryopreserved without the apparent loss of SSC activity using the simple cryopreservation fluid employed for mouse testis cells[12]. The final step, transplantation, is under development in humans. Attempts have been made to transplant testis cells into the testes of farm animals and non-human primates, and ultrasound has played an important role in monitoring such transplantation procedures[13-15]. The technique of transplanting human testis cells should thus not be a significant obstacle; in fact, clinical trials to transplant human germ cells into human testes are under way[16].

This progress demonstrates that spermatogonial transplantation is applicable to restore fertility in cancer survivors. Regeneration of spermatogenesis arising from transplanted SSCs may allow spontaneous recovery of fertility or may at least facilitate subsequent procedures using assisted reproductive technologies (ART).

Implantation of testis pieces

The other approach to surgical restoration of male fertility is to harvest testis pieces before cancer therapy and implant them in patients following cryopreservation (Figure 1). This approach has been developed and applied in clinical settings for female fertility restoration using ovarian tissues, as discussed in Chapter 12. Although clinical application of the same method has not been reported for male fertility restoration, studies using experimental animals (mice, hamsters, rabbits, pigs, goats and marmosets) have shown that spermatogenesis can be established in testis pieces implanted in the testis or under the skin of immuno-deficient mice[17-20]. Furthermore, microinsemination using spermatozoa obtained from the implants results in the production of offspring of donor mice and rabbits[18,20]. Thus, studies using experimental animals indicate a promising future of the implantation approach for male fertility restoration.

In this approach, testis biopsies are used without further manipulations such as the enzymatic digestion required in the transplantation approach. It appears that these biopsies can readily be cryopreserved. One study has shown that testes biopsies obtained from mice and rabbits are successfully cryopreserved in the same freezing solution as used for single-cell preparations of testis cells[18]. These testis biopsies were cryopreserved for 10 days and implanted into the testis of immuno-deficient recipient mice through small incisions made in the tunica albuginea. Spermatozoa were harvested from the implants 2 months later, and were subsequently frozen for 3 days. Microinsemination using these spermatozoa followed by culture led to live birth of 50% of the embryos transferred to foster mothers[18]. The successful cryopreservation may have resulted from the small size of the testis pieces, which measured ∼ 3.4 mm^3 (mouse) and 8–16 mm^3 (rabbit). Thus, it is reasonable to be optimistic about successful cryopreservation of human testicular biopsies if they fall within this size range. More detailed discussions on the cryopreservation of testis pieces are presented in Chapter 12.

Testis tissue can also be implanted ectopically under the skin. Spermatogenesis has been observed in testis pieces derived from mice, hamsters, pigs, goats and marmosets, when implanted under the skin of immuno-deficient mice[17,19,20]. Spermatozoa retrieved from the ectopic implants can fertilize eggs (in mice, goats and pigs)[17], whereby the live birth of offspring (in mice) can be achieved[20]. Although live birth after ectopic implantation has not been confirmed using frozen–thawed testis pieces (mouse offspring were obtained after implantation of fresh biopsies[20]), we can be optimistic about its eventual success, because the fertilization of eggs can be induced following implantation of frozen–thawed specimens and microinsemination[17].

Implantation of testis pieces is expected to be applicable even when the biopsies are obtained from prepubertal males, as all four studies described above used testis pieces of immature animals[17-20]. Although no spermatogenesis was initially present in the biopsies of immature testes, spermatogenesis was regenerated and spermatozoa were produced after implantation into the testis or under the skin. These results indicate the possibility of fertility restoration for male survivors of childhood cancer. Particularly in the ectopic implantation, the regeneration of spermatogenesis is more likely to be successful if testis pieces are obtained from prepubertal boys. A study using mice showed that complete spermatogenesis was established in ectopic grafts of immature testes, whereas the regeneration of spermatogenesis was limited in adult ectopic grafts[19] (see p. 131).

Regarding application of the implantation strategy in clinical settings, harvesting testis biopsies and microinsemination are already routinely performed. Therefore, given the development of cryopreservation techniques of testis biopsies, this approach could be readily applied for male fertility restoration in humans. Although it would not allow spontaneous fertility recovery even when testis pieces are implanted into the testis (anastomosis of seminiferous tubules between implants and host testis has not been reported) and requires assisted conception, owing to its simple and less invasive procedure, the implantation of testis biopsies is technically feasible at present for cancer patients.

ADVANTAGES AND DISADVANTAGES OF TRANSPLANTATION AND IMPLANTATION APPROACHES FOR CLINICAL APPLICATIONS

Spermatogonial transplantation

In the clinical application of transplantation and implantation techniques, it is essential that transmission of cancer cells back to the patient does not occur. Since the target cells/tissues are obtained before anticancer treatments, these specimens may include malignant cells and, thus, surgical procedures without cell separation are highly risky. In fact, a study using rats has shown that as few as 20 leukemic cells included in a testis cell preparation can result in the recurrence of leukemia after spermatogonial transplantation[21]. There is certainly no reason to believe that the implantation of testis pieces is free of such a risk either. Since germ cells are dispensable for the life of cancer survivors after successful treatment, such a risk cannot be taken in clinical settings.

Probably the most significant advantage of spermatogonial transplantation over implantation of testis pieces is that it allows the selection of SSCs. Since testicular biopsies are

made into a suspension of single cells for transplantation, cell-sorting processes can be integrated in the transplantation-based approach (Figure 1). In this regard, it is encouraging that a set of identification markers for mouse SSCs has been determined in recent studies[22–24]. On the basis of the expression of cell-surface antigens, a single-cell suspension obtained from mouse testes can be immunologically enriched for SSCs up to 670-fold using fluorescent-activated cell sorting[23,24]. At present, positive markers identified are α_6-integrin, β_1-integrin, CD24 and Thy-1, whereas negative markers are α_V-integrin, c-kit and MHC-I. It is likely that more markers will be discovered for mouse SSCs, which will enable the purification of SSCs in future. Such immunological cell sorting is thus expected to be a powerful method to purge cancer cells from testis cell preparations.

Although this progress is encouraging, the selection of human SSCs is not feasible at present. First of all, there is no information about identification markers of human SSCs, and it is not guaranteed that mouse SSC markers can also be used to identify human SSCs. For example, in the case of hematopoietic stem cells, cell-surface markers are not commonly shared in mice and humans[25]. Furthermore, since SSCs represent only 0.01% of the total testis cells in mice[26], even the maximum enrichment that can be achieved to date (670-fold[24]) does not allow the purification of mouse SSCs, leaving the possibility that tumor cells could still exist in a cell preparation. Intensive investigations to determine human SSC markers are thus needed to purify SSCs and to apply spermatogonial transplantation safely in clinical settings. An alternative approach to purge cancer cells, however, could make the purification of SSCs unnecessary. Kubota and colleagues have shown that mouse SSCs can be negatively enriched using the MHC-I molecule (β_2-microglobulin light chain) as a marker[24]. Although MHC-I molecules are expressed on almost all nucleated cells, it is believed that spermatogonia do not express MHC-I proteins[24,27]. Thus, the elimination of cells expressing MHC-I molecules may be effective to purge cancer cells, except those arising from spermatogonia, while retaining SSC activity in the testis cell preparation.

To efficiently restore male fertility by transplantation, it is important to recover a sufficient number of SSCs after cryopreservation. Although SSCs of a wide range of animal species[28–31], including humans[12], can be cryopreserved, we currently do not know the percentage of SSCs that survive and remain functional after cryopreservation. It is also unknown whether SSCs should be cryopreserved before or after cell separation; in some cases, cryopreservation both before and after cell separation may be necessary. Considering that the quantity of testis biopsies may well be limited, the recovery of a sufficient number of functional SSCs following cryopreservation is an important parameter for the efficient restoration of fertility by transplantation.

The efficiency of male fertility restoration by transplantation is also influenced by the transplantation itself. It has recently been reported that when adult mouse testis cells are transplanted into the testes of adult recipient mice, the efficiency of spermatogenesis regeneration is ∼ 10%[26]. In other words, only one in ten SSCs transplanted can successfully migrate, survive and re-establish spermatogenesis in the seminiferous epithelium of adult recipient mice. The same study has further shown that ∼ 75% of SSCs are lost within one day after transplantation[26], suggesting that SSCs do not efficiently attach Sertoli cells, migrate and survive during the early post-transplantation period under the current conditions. The efficiency of colonization appears to be much higher when recipients are immature mice. Approximately nine times more colonies of donor-derived spermatogenesis can be formed after transplantation into the testes of immature mice than into those of adult mice[32]. It has been proposed that this higher colonization efficiency occurs because intercellular junctions between Sertoli cells are not established in the seminiferous epithelium of immature mice[32]. Assuming that this situation is applicable in human SSCs, fertility recovery by transplantation

could be inefficient in clinical settings when transplantation is performed into adult testes. Considering the rarity of SSCs[26], this may present a problem when the testis cells are obtained from a limited amount of biopsies followed by cell sorting and cryopreservation. Therefore, improvements in the transplantation technique itself are necessary, and the early processes of SSC colonization could be a prime target for such investigations.

On the other hand, this low colonization efficiency could be compensated for if SSCs were amplified *ex vivo* before transplantation (Figure 1). Studies during the past several years have led to the *ex vivo* amplification of SSCs in mice, although not on a consistent basis at present. First, it was shown that not only can SSCs be cultured for a long time (∼ 4 months)[33] but they can also self-renew *in vitro*[34,35]. Further studies then demonstrated that SSCs derived from immature mouse testes exhibit a significantly higher proliferation activity than those of adult testes *in vitro*[34,36]. These studies suggested the possibility of amplifying SSCs *ex vivo*, particularly those derived from immature testes. Finally, a recent study has shown that immature SSCs can be amplified significantly in a long-term culture (> 10^{14}-fold over 5 months) supplemented with a cocktail of growth factors, including glial cell line-derived neurotrophic factor (GDNF), epidermal growth factor, basic fibroblast growth factor and leukemia inhibitory factor[37]. These results show a remarkably rapid achievement in *ex vivo* manipulation of SSCs. It should be noted, however, that even the best culture system to amplify SSCs is not without drawbacks, as the efficacy of SSC amplification is dependent on mouse strains. Immature SSCs derived from DBA, DBA × C57BL/6 (B6) F_1, or ICR strains proliferate actively *in vitro*, whereas those from B6 or 129 strains do not[37]. Another study using SSCs derived from B6 × 129 mice has shown that GDNF alone encourages the *in vitro* maintenance of SSCs but does not induce a net amplification of SSCs[38]. Taken together, it appears that there are genetic mechanisms specific to mouse strains that regulate the proliferation potential of SSCs, and thus the success of human SSC amplification could involve significant individual differences. These studies collectively indicate that although the *ex vivo* amplification of SSCs cannot consistently be achieved at present, it is certainly not impossible. It is expected that our continued efforts will facilitate the development of an effective culture system to amplify SSCs *ex vivo* in mice that could be applied in humans in future. Such a culture system will enhance the efficiency of male fertility restoration using spermatogonial transplantation.

When spermatogonial transplantation is applied in clinical settings, it may be desirable to be able to monitor the regeneration of spermatogenesis in a non-invasive manner (Figure 1). In mice, complete spermatogenesis with spermatozoa can be observed as early as 2 months after transplantation[39–41], and spontaneous fertility recovery can be achieved as early as 8 months after transplantation when the recipients are adult mice, and 4–8 months when the recipients are immature or genetically infertile mice[8,35,42]. Since one cycle of spermatogenesis takes ~ 35 days in mice and ~ 64 days in humans[43], proportional extrapolation of these data suggests that human male fertility recovery could be achieved in 7–15 months after transplantation ($4–8/35 \times 64$). However, the validity of this hypothetical calculation is unknown. On the other hand, spontaneous fertility recovery is not an absolute requirement in clinical settings: as long as spermatozoa are recovered after transplantation, ART will support the conception. In this case, the issue is when male gametes should be retrieved. Monitoring serum hormone levels after transplantation may provide the basis to decide on the optimal timing for the retrieval of spermatozoa or sperm. Unfortunately, temporal changes in serum hormone levels after transplantation have not been examined, and thus, further studies are necessary to develop a monitoring system of spermatogenesis regeneration after transplantation.

Implantation of testis pieces

As mentioned earlier, the advantage of implantation over transplantation approaches is that it is technically feasible at present, at least in selected cases. The implantation procedure is simple and less invasive, and most, if not all, of the other techniques involved in this approach are well established. In addition, the implantation approach allows SSCs to remain in their most favored microenvironment in the seminiferous epithelium (so-called stem cell niches), and thus all SSCs present in the implants can be intact and fully functional. Furthermore, because Sertoli and Leydig cells in the implants are not exposed to anticancer reagents, the function of these somatic cells should also be left almost intact. In contrast, transplantation requires removal of SSCs from the stem niches and exposure of SSCs to enzymes during the preparation of the singlecell suspension, and is performed into the testis with Sertoli and Leydig cells that have been exposed to anticancer reagents.

However, there are three important issues to be considered in the clinical application of the implantation of testis pieces. The first and most important issue is that the approach does not provide the opportunity to purge cancer cells. The elimination of cancer cells is possible using transplantation because testis biopsies are made into a single-cell suspension, which allows immunological cell separation; however, this would be very difficult, if not impossible, when whole pieces of testis are the source of fertility restoration. Therefore, implantation should be applied on a case-by-case basis in clinical settings: it cannot be used if tumor cells are likely to be included in testis pieces (e.g. leukemias and lymphomas), but it can be used for patients of more restricted types of cancer (e.g. non-metastatic brain cancer).

Second, the number of biopsy specimens is a significant limiting factor in the implantation approach. Although multiple biopsies can be harvested or a single biopsy can be divided into multiple pieces, they cannot be amplified before implantation. Thus, it can be said that the implantation approach does not fully take advantage of the self-renewal activities of SSCs, analogous to the situation in adult ovaries where a limited number of ovarian follicles determines the reproductive life of a female. Even though this disadvantage may not be highly significant, it is certainly an issue to be considered in clinical settings, particularly for prepubertal boys from whom a large quantity of biopsy specimens could not be harvested.

Third, spermatogenesis established in implants might not continue for a long time. Animal studies have shown that spermatogenesis is not quantitatively complete when testis pieces are ectopically implanted under the skin of castrated mice[19,20], although it appears to be normal when they are implanted into testes[18]. In one study, when immature testis pieces were ectopically implanted, nearly all tubules in the grafts contained meiotic germ cells at 12 and 16 weeks after implantation[20]. However, only 40% of these tubules included spermatids, and the number of spermatozoa remained low[20]. Furthermore, intratubular fluid accumulated in the seminiferous tubules of ectopic implants by 4 weeks, which continued until at least 16 weeks[20]. As a consequence, many tubules showed damage to the seminiferous epithelium and became devoid of germ cells. Another study showed that when adult testis pieces were implanted under the skin, the recovery of spermatogenesis was limited; interestingly, germ cells at less advanced stages were often lost, suggesting that primitive germ cells arising from SSCs were not continuously replenished[19]. These results indicating disadvantages of the implantation strategy may have in part resulted from the fact that spermatogenesis is sensitive to ischemia and temperature[44,45]. Thus, ectopic implantation under the skin may not be optimal for long-term maintenance of spermatogenesis, and spermatozoa

need to be obtained before the adverse effects become evident in implants.

To identify the timing of spermatozoa retrieval, Schlatt and associates examined serum levels of follicle stimulating hormone and testosterone after implantation of testis pieces under the skin of castrated host mice, and analyzed the relationship between the hormone levels and the development of spermatogenesis[20]. Based on the increase in serum levels of these hormones, they concluded that 2 months after ectopic implantation is the best time to retrieve spermatozoa. Therefore, monitoring of hormone levels may be necessary when the ectopic implantation is performed in clinical settings.

On the other hand, it might be possible to induce and maintain complete spermatogenesis in ectopic implants if an appropriate hormonal treatment is given to the host. In three of the studies described above[17,19,20], the hosts of ectopic grafts were castrated before implantation, implying that these grafts were exposed to a limited amount of testosterone produced by Leydig cells contained in the grafts. It has been shown that the normal concentration of intratesticular testosterone (ITT) is significantly higher than that of serum testosterone in intact rats (1080 vs. 5.9 nmol/l)[46]. Since ectopic testis grafts are not structurally restricted by the tunica albuginea and are exposed to the subcutaneous space, germ cells in these grafts may not be supplied with a sufficient level of testosterone. Therefore, given an appropriate environment that provides the grafts with a proper blood supply and the optimum temperature[44,45], a testosterone supplement may be beneficial to maintain spermatogenesis after ectopic implantation of testis pieces.

In the case of implantation into the testis, similar data are not available. However, if transplantation of testis cells into infertile mouse testes results in a long-term regeneration of spermatogenesis, it is likely that the same can be accomplished in the grafts in the testis. However, it should be noted that the procedure for implanting testis pieces into the testes is very different in mice and humans.

The mouse testis is encapsulated by only a thin membrane of the tunica albuginea, rendering implantation of the testis piece a simple and easy procedure. However, the tunica albuginea is considerably thicker in humans and, consequently, the implantation procedure becomes more invasive than in mice. As described previously[44,45], the surgical manipulation of human testes often causes calcification/fibrosis of seminiferous tubules, due at least in part to ischemia. Considering the limited amount of precious testis biopsies, it can be said that implantation of testis pieces into testes still involves some technical and physiological risks.

FURTHER ISSUES TO BE CONSIDERED IN BOTH TRANSPLANTATION AND IMPLANTATION APPROACHES

Conditions of host testes exposed to anticancer reagents

When SSCs are transplanted or implanted into a patient's testes after cancer therapy, the improvement of intratesticular conditions may be required. Currently, a major cause of the failure of spermatogenesis regeneration after cancer therapy is believed to be a high level of ITT[6]. Although a certain level of ITT apparently needs to be maintained[46], an abnormally high ITT level blocks spermatogenesis from proceeding beyond the spermatogonia stage[6]. Therefore, hormone treatments to reduce ITT levels (Chapter 5) are expected to be beneficial for efficient recovery of male fertility in the surgical strategy. Animal studies have shown that, following transplantation, treatment of recipient mice with gonadotropin releasing hormone (GnRH) analogs, which reduce ITT levels[6], stimulates the regeneration of spermatogenesis[47,48]. Similarly, such treatments should be beneficial in implantation of testis pieces into the testes. Although the positive effects of GnRH administration on the regeneration of spermatogenesis have not definitively been confirmed in humans, such a treatment could

be a prerequisite for efficient male fertility restoration in the surgical strategy.

In relation to the condition of host testes after cancer therapies, it may be useful to consider the activity of SSCs that survived the therapies. Transplantation of SSCs will provide a stem cell population additional to the surviving SSCs in a patient's testes. If the condition of the testes is improved pharmacologically after anticancer treatments, the regeneration of spermatogenesis from surviving SSCs may further be facilitated by the addition of presumably healthy SSCs. Then, both sets of SSCs will produce spermatozoa, and a greater number of spermatozoa may result in spontaneous recovery of male fertility. Therefore, the transplantation approach, when combined with the pharmacological strategy, could be a powerful approach to facilitate the spontaneous restoration of male fertility.

In addition, the reason that adverse conditions persist in the testes after cancer therapies may be that the SSC population is too small to activate the somatic environment, especially Sertoli cells, for the regeneration of spermatogenesis. Although Sertoli cells are an important regulator of spermatogenesis, their function is apparently permissive in nature, rather than inducing, and these cells may need to be stimulated through the communication with germ cells to support spermatogenesis. For example, when rat SSCs are transplanted into mouse testes, complete spermatogenesis of rat origin is re-established, and the cycle of spermatogenesis follows the pattern specific to rat spermatogenesis, even though it is supported by mouse Sertoli cells[49]. These results indicate that germ cells dominate the control of the spermatogenic cycle and that Sertoli cells provide the permissive environment for germ cells to conduct their functions. It is also known that when germ cells are added to Sertoli cell culture, Sertoli cells rapidly change their gene expression patterns[50], indicating that signals sent by germ cells promptly modulate Sertoli cell functions. Thus, the addition of SSCs by transplantation may affect the pattern of communication between germ cells and Sertoli cells. Subsequent modulations of Sertoli cell functions could further influence the activity of other somatic cells in the testis (e.g. Leydig cells) through the intercellular communications, which might improve the condition of the whole testis. Similarly, implantation of rather healthy testis pieces into testes that have been exposed to anti-cancer reagents may also lead to an improved condition of host testes, and spermatogenesis and male fertility could be spontaneously restored from surviving SSCs.

These scenarios are highly hypothetical but may still be worth considering for future clinical applications of the surgical strategy. For example, following implantation of testis pieces into a patient's testes, it may not be necessary to retrieve the implants promptly to obtain spermatozoa. Leaving the implants in the testis might improve the testicular conditions, and fertility could be spontaneously recovered from SSCs that survived anticancer treatments.

Xenogeneic transplantation and implantation

Xenogeneic transplantation and implantation could be a powerful assay system to ensure the absence of tumor cells in testis cells/tissues. In this system, human testis specimens are injected or implanted into immuno-deficient mice, in which cancer cells proliferate and are detected using human-specific markers. Kim and co-workers have applied this safety assessment method based on xenogeneic transplantation of ovarian tissue for female lymphoma patients[51]. They implanted tissues obtained from lymphoma patients into immuno-deficient NOD/SCID (non-obese diabetic/severe combined immunodeficiency) mice. The presence or absence of human cancer cells in mice was analyzed by histology and the polymerase chain reaction using human microsatellite DNA as a marker. Using this method, they clearly distinguished ovarian tissues contaminated with cancer cells from those not contaminated[51]. A similar approach should be feasible using testis cells/tissues, and

xenogeneic transfer of human testis specimens will provide the safety assessment system.

Xenogeneic transplantation/implantation can also be used for studies of human SSCs and spermatogenesis, and for development of human male germ cell manipulation techniques. The studies of human SSCs and spermatogenesis have been hampered because appropriate experimental systems have not been available and the manipulation of germ cells is an ethically sensitive issue. Xenogeneic transplantation/implantation using immuno-deficient mice as hosts now provides a novel approach to study and manipulate human SSCs and spermatogenesis with minimal ethical conflict.

As an attempt to establish a human SSC assay system, human testis cells were transplanted into the testes of immuno-deficient nude mice[12]. Following transplantation, human germ cells partially proliferated for short periods and survived for at least 6 months in mouse testes. Human germ cells remaining in mouse testes showed a morphology indicative of primitive, so-called undifferentiated, spermatogonia (single cell or two cells connected by cytoplasmic bridge). Thus, xenogeneic transplantation of human testis cells into the testis of immuno-deficient mice can be an assay system for primitive spermatogonia, including SSCs, of human origin and may also provide a diagnostic tool to evaluate their quality and quantity[12].

A drawback of current xenogeneic human spermatogonial transplantation is that it is not yet a definitive assay specific for SSCs. Following xenogeneic transplantation, human germ cells apparently stay dormant for long periods as undifferentiated spermatogonia and do not undergo any further differentiation process. Since SSCs are defined by their activity to regenerate long-term complete spermatogenesis, the inability of human germ cells to do so in mouse testes precludes the unequivocal detection of human SSCs. Thus, further improvement of this assay system is necessary. Two immediate targets can be suggested for such an attempt. First, the methods of host mouse preparation need to be explored. For example, human hematopoiesis can be reconstituted from transplanted stem cells in immuno-deficient mice following bone marrow transplantation. In this case, host mice are either treated with human cytokines[52] or implanted with human fetal liver, bone marrow and thymus[53–55]. Similar manipulations of host mice may thus be beneficial for human SSC transplantation. Second, other animal species may be preferred to mice as hosts for the function of SSCs and the reconstitution of human spermatogenesis. Primates are an immediate candidate as optimal hosts. Alternatively, Sertoli cells in host mice could be replaced with primate Sertoli cells to provide a better environment for human SSCs and their functions[56].

As an approach to study human spermatogenesis, implantation of human testis pieces into immuno-deficient mice may be more appropriate than transplantation. In xenogeneic implantation, human SSCs and germ cells are encapsulated by human Sertoli cells and, thus, are provided with a desirable environment to exhibit their functions. Then, the administration of human growth factors and hormones may facilitate the regeneration of human spermatogenesis in mice, as was the case with human hematopoiesis in mice.

Harvesting spermatogonial stem cells after anticancer treatments

Finally, it may be worth considering the possibility of applying the surgical strategy using testis specimens obtained after cancer therapy. While it is ideal to harvest SSCs before cancer therapy, such an approach may not always be feasible in clinical settings, and a considerable number of cancer survivors may not have had the opportunity to cryopreserve testis specimens before therapy. In such cases, SSCs harvested after therapy could still be of some use, even though SSCs were exposed to sterilizing treatments. At first glance, transplantation or implantation of SSCs recovered after therapies appears to have no advantage over the pharmacological strategy. However, compared

to the pharmacological strategy, two unique aspects can be considered.

First, ectopic implantation may allow SSCs to escape from an undesirable environment with abnormally high ITT levels after cancer therapy. While the pharmacological strategy attempts to improve the testicular environment by reducing ITT levels, if testis pieces are ectopically implanted under the skin, the adverse effects of high ITT levels could be avoided. Then, the regeneration of spermatogenesis may be more readily achieved following precise regulation of testosterone levels supplied to the implants. Second, if the majority of SSCs are damaged or killed by anticancer reagents, the pharmacological strategy may not be effective. Following administration of an alkylating reagent (busulfan) at a dose of 15 mg/kg in mice, the number of SSCs per testis decreased rapidly within 3 days to ~4% of the pretreatment level[57], suggesting the death of SSCs. Although SSC numbers recovered somewhat in the long term, they were still ~60% of the pretreatment level even 70 days after the treatment. Thus, in addition to high ITT levels, a diminished population size of SSCs may also be the cause of inefficient regeneration of spermatogenesis after cancer therapies. Since SSCs remaining after busulfan treatment sustain their self-renewal activity[57], these cells could be amplified *ex vivo* in future and transplanted into a patient's testes. Then, an expanded SSC population would encourage the regeneration of spermatogenesis, overcoming the adverse effects of high ITT levels.

When the regeneration of spermatogenesis is attempted surgically or pharmacologically based on SSCs exposed to anticancer reagents, an unknown issue is the genetic integrity of the SSCs. It is possible that anticancer reagents damage the genome of SSCs and cause defects in offspring. A particular concern is a long-term effect that emerges generations later. Although spontaneous fertility recovery can occur in cancer survivors with no apparent increase in defects of their children (see Chapter 17), there are reasons to be cautious

Table 1 Comparison of two approaches in the surgical strategy based on spermatogonial stem cells (SSCs) for male fertility restoration following cancer therapies

Parameter	Transplantation	Implantation
Operation procedure	available	available
Cryopreservation	yes	yes
Cell selection	possible	no
Ex vivo amplification of stem cells[*]	possible	no
Number of stem cells[*]	potentially unlimited	limited
Repeated procedures[†]	possible	limited
Microinsemination	yes	yes
Spontaneous fertility recovery	possible	no
Time to fertility restoration	unknown	unknown
Sertoli cells[‡]	exposed to treatments	not exposed to treatments
Effects of testis conditions[§]	unknown	unknown
Ectopic transfer[¶]	no	yes
Use after treatment[‖]	possible	possible

*The number of SSCs can be unlimited in the transplantation approach due to the possibility to amplify them *ex vivo*, which would be very difficult or nearly impossible in the implantation approach; †SSC amplification would allow multiple trials in the transplantation approach whereas the number of biopsies limits the frequency of implantation; ‡regeneration of spermatogenesis is supported by Sertoli cells exposed to anticancer reagents in the transplantation approach, but by unexposed Sertoli cells in the implantation approach; §regeneration of spermatogenesis can be affected by the post-treatment condition of host testes and may need to be assisted by pharmacological manipulation of hormone levels after SSC transfer in the transplantation approach and the implantation into the testes; ¶ectopic transfer is possible in the implantation approach (e.g. subcutaneous implantation); ‖both procedures can be performed using testis biopsies harvested after anticancer treatments

about this issue. For example, a study using knockout mice showed that the lack of functional telomerase RNA in mice did not cause any apparent defects in offspring up to the fifth generation[58]. However, no offspring were obtained from the descendants at the sixth generation due to defective gonadal function in both males and females, demonstrating an extremely long latency period of the genetic defect in the germ line[58]. Therefore, more intensive studies are necessary to evaluate the genetic effects on SSCs of cancer therapies and their long-term consequences.

CONCLUDING REMARKS

As summarized in Table 1, the approaches to male fertility restoration based on spermatogonial transplantation and implantation of testis pieces have unique advantages and disadvantages. It is important to point out that these two approaches are complementary, and both are feasible at this time or are expected to be so in the near future. Therefore, patients should now be provided with the opportunity to cryopreserve testis cells and/or testis pieces, and to autologously transfer these specimens after successful anticancer treatments in the future. Although procedures remain to be established for eliminating cancer cells, the surgical strategy can now be applied in some cases (e.g. brain tumors) as long as the absence of metastasis is confirmed. Following these procedures, the regeneration of spermatogenesis may be stimulated by pharmacological treatment of patients (Chapter 5). Fertility in men can then be restored spontaneously or by using assisted conception. Therefore, the development of effective procedures based on transplantation and implantation will provide an important safeguard for restoring male fertility and will particularly be beneficial for survivors of childhood cancer.

ACKNOWLEDGMENTS

I am grateful to Dr Peter Chan (McGill University) and F. Clerk for their critical reading and valuable comments, and to the editors for giving me the opportunity to contribute to this book. Studies carried out in my laboratory were supported financially by the Canadian Institutes of Health Research and the Canada Foundation for Innovation.

References

1. Brinster RL. Germline stem cell transplantation and transgenesis. *Science* 2002;296:2174–6
2. Meistrich ML, van Beek MEAB. Spermatogonial stem cells. In Desjardins C, Ewing LL, eds. *Cell and Molecular Biology of the Testis*. New York: Oxford University Press, 1993:266–95
3. Gosden RG, Nagano M. Preservation of fertility in nature and ART. *Reproduction* 2002;123:3–11
4. Chapman RM, Sutcliffe SB, Malpas JS. Cytotoxic-induced ovarian failure in women with Hodgkin's disease. *J Am Med Assoc* 1979;242:1877–86
5. Schilsky RL, Lewis BJ, Sherins RJ, Young RC. Gonadal dysfunction in patients receiving chemotherapy for cancer. *Ann Intern Med* 1980;93:109–14
6. Meistrich ML, Shetty G. Inhibition of spermatogonial differentiation by testosterone. *J Androl* 2003;24:135–48
7. Brinster RL, Zimmermann JW. Spermatogenesis following male germ cell transplantation. *Proc Natl Acad Sci USA* 1994;91:11298–302
8. Brinster R, Avarbock MR. Germline transmission of donor haplotype following spermatogonial transplantation. *Proc Natl Acad Sci USA* 1994;91:11303–7
9. Ogawa T, Arechaga JM, Avarbock MR, Brinster RL. Transplantation of testis germinal cells into mouse seminiferous tubules. *Int J Dev Biol* 1997;41:111–22
10. Bellve AR, Cavicchia JC, Millette CF, et al. Spermatogenic cells of the prepuberal mouse. Isolation and morphological characterization. *J Cell Biol* 1977;74:68–85
11. Avarbock MR, Brinster CJ, Brinster RL. Reconstitution of spermatogenesis from frozen spermatogonial stem cells. *Nat Med* 1996;2:693–6
12. Nagano M, Patrizio P, Brinster RL. Long-term survival of human spermatogonial stem cells in mouse testes. *Fertil Steril* 2002;78:1225–33
13. Schlatt S, Foppiani L, Rolf C, et al. Germ cell transplantation into X-irradiated monkey testes. *Hum Reprod* 2002;17:55–62
14. Honaramooz A, Megee SO, Dobrinski I. Germ cell transplantation in pigs. *Biol Reprod* 2002;66:21–8
15. Honaramooz A, Behboodi E, Blash S, et al. Germ cell transplantation in goats. *Mol Reprod Dev* 2003;64:422–8
16. Radford JA, Shalet SM, Lieberman B. Fertility after treatment for cancer. Questions remain over ways of preserving ovarian and testicular tissue. *Br Med J* 1999;319:935–6
17. Honaramooz A, Snedaker A, Boiani M, et al. Sperm from neonatal mammalian testes grafted in mice. *Nature* 2002;418:778–81
18. Shinohara T, Inoue K, Ogonuki N, et al. Birth of offspring following transplantation of cryopreserved immature testicular pieces and *in vitro* microinsemination. *Hum Reprod* 2002;17:3039–45
19. Schlatt S, Kim SS, Gosden R. Spermatogenesis and steroidogenesis in mouse, hamster and monkey testicular tissue after cryopreservation and heterotopic grafting to castrated hosts. *Reproduction* 2002;124:339–46
20. Schlatt S, Honaramooz A, Boiani M, et al. Progeny from sperm obtained after ectopic grafting of neonatal mouse testes. *Biol Reprod* 2003;68:2331–5
21. Jahnukainen K, Hou M, Petersen C, et al. Intratesticular transplantation of testicular cells from leukemic rats causes transmission of leukemia. *Cancer Res* 2001;61:706–10
22. Shinohara T, Avarbock MR, Brinster RL. β_1- and α_6-integrin are surface markers on mouse spermatogonial stem cells. *Proc Natl Acad Sci USA* 1999;96:5504–9
23. Shinohara T, Avarbock MR, Brinster RL. Spermatogonial stem cell enrichment by multiparameter selection of mouse testis cells. *Proc Natl Acad Sci USA* 2000;97:8346–51
24. Kubota H, Avarbock MR, Brinster RL. Spermatogonial stem cells share some, but not all, phenotypic and functional characteristics

with other stem cells. *Proc Natl Acad Sci USA* 2003;100:6487–92

25. Weissman IL. Translating stem and progenitor cell biology to the clinic: barriers and opportunities. *Science* 2000;287:1442–6

26. Nagano MC. Homing efficiency and proliferation kinetics of male germ line stem cells following transplantation in mice. *Biol Reprod* 2003;69:701–7

27. Klein J. *Natural History of Major Histocompatibility Complex.* New York: Wiley, 1986:152–75

28. Clouthier DE, Avarbock MR, Maika SD, *et al.* Rat spermatogenesis in mouse testis. *Nature* 1996;381:418–21

29. Ogawa T, Dobrinski I, Avarbock MR, Brinster RL. Xenogeneic spermatogenesis following transplantation of hamster germ cells to mouse testes. *Biol Reprod* 1999;60:515–21

30. Dobrinski I, Avarbock MR, Brinster RL. Transplantation of germ cells from rabbits and dogs into mouse testes. *Biol Reprod* 1999;61: 1331–9

31. Dobrinski I, Avarbock MR, Brinster RL. Germ cell transplantation from large domestic animals into mouse testes. *Mol Reprod Dev* 2000; 56:1–10

32. Shinohara T, Orwig KE, Avarbock MR, Brinster RL. Remodeling of the postnatal mouse testis is accompanied by dramatic changes in stem cell number and niche accessibility. *Proc Natl Acad Sci USA* 2001;98:6186–91

33. Nagano M, Avarbock MR, Leonida EB, *et al.* Culture of mouse spermatogonial stem cells. *Tissue Cell* 1998;30:389–97

34. Nagano M, Shinohara T, Avarbock MR, Brinster RL. Retrovirus-mediated gene transfer into male germline stem cells. *FEBS Lett* 2000;475:7–10

35. Nagano M, Brinster CJ, Orwig KE, *et al.* Transgenic mice produced by transduction of male germ line stem cells. *Proc Natl Acad Sci USA* 2001;98:13090–5

36. Nagano M, Watson DJ, Ryu BY, *et al.* Lentiviral vector transduction of male germ line stem cells in mice. *FEBS Lett* 2002;524:111–15

37. Kanatsu-Shinohara M, Ogonuki N, Inoue K, *et al.* Long-term proliferation in culture and germline transmission of mouse male germline stem cells. *Biol Reprod* 2003;69:612–16

38. Nagano M, Ryu BY, Brinster CJ, *et al.* Maintenance of mouse male germ line stem cells *in vitro*. *Biol Reprod* 2003;68:2207–14

39. Parreira GG, Ogawa T, Avarbock MR, *et al.* Development of germ cell transplants in mice. *Biol Reprod* 1998;59:1360–70

40. Nagano M, Avarbock MR, Brinster RL. Pattern and kinetics of donor mouse spermatogonial stem cell colonization in recipient testes. *Biol Reprod* 1999;60:1429–36

41. Ohta H, Yomogida K, Yamada S, *et al.* Real-time observation of transplanted 'green germ cells'; proliferation and differentiation of stem cells. *Dev Growth Differ* 2000;42:105–12

42. Ogawa T, Dobrinski I, Avarbock MR, Brinster RL. Transplantation of male germ line stem cells restores fertility in infertile mice. *Nat Med* 2000;6:29–34

43. Russell LD, Ettlin RA, SinhaHikim AP, Clegg ED. *Histological and Histopathological Evaluation of the Testis.* Clearwater: Cache River Press, 1990: 41–58

44. Schlegel PN, Su L-M. Physiological consequences of testicular sperm extraction. *Hum Reprod* 1997;12:1688–92

45. Schlegel PN. Testicular sperm extraction: microdissection improves sperm yield with minimal tissue excision. *Hum Reprod* 1999;14: 131–5

46. Sharpe RM, Donachie K, Cooper I. Reevaluation of the intratesticular level of testosterone required for quantitative maintenance of spermatogenesis in the rat. *J Endocrinol* 1988;117:19–26

47. Ogawa T, Dobrinski I, Avarbock MR, Brinster RL. Leuprolide, a gonadotropin-releasing hormone agonist, enhances colonization after spermatogonial transplantation into mouse testes. *Tissue Cell* 1998;30:583–8

48. Dobrinski I, Ogawa T, Avarbock MR, Brinster RL. Effect of the GnRH-agonist leuprolide on colonization of recipient testes by donor spermatogonial stem cells after transplantation in mice. *Tissue Cell* 2001;33:200–7

49. Franca LR, Ogawa T, Avarbock MR, *et al.* Germ cell genotype controls cell cycle during spermatogenesis in the rat. *Biol Reprod* 1998; 59:1371–7

50. Vidal F, Lopez P, Lopez-Fernandez LA, *et al.* Gene trap analysis of germ cell signaling to Sertoli cells: NGF-TrkA mediated induction of Fra1 and Fos by post-meiotic germ cells. *J Cell Sci* 2001;114:435–43

51. Kim SS, Radford J, Harris M, *et al.* Ovarian tissue harvested from lymphoma patients to preserve fertility may be safe for autotransplantation. *Hum Reprod* 2001;16:2056–60

52. Nolta JA, Kohn DB. Haematopoietic stem cells for gene therapy. In Potten CS, ed. *Stem Cells.* San Diego: Academic Press, 1997: 447–62

53. McCune JM, Namikawa R, Kaneshima H, *et al.* The SCID-hu mouse: murine model for the analysis of human hematolymphoid differentiation and function. *Science* 1988;241:1632–9

54. Lapidot T, Pflumio F, Doedens M, *et al.* Cytokine stimulation of multilineage hematopoiesis from immature human cells engrafted in SCID mice. *Science* 1992;255:1137–41

55. Fraser CC, Kaneshima H, Hansteen G, *et al.* Human allogeneic stem cell maintenance and differentiation in a long-term multilineage SCID-hu graft. *Blood* 1995;86:1680–93

56. Shinohara T, Orwig KE, Avarbock MR, Brinster RL. Restoration of spermatogenesis in infertile mice by Sertoli cell transplantation. *Biol Reprod* 2003;68:1064–71

57. Kanatsu-Shinohara M, Toyokuni S, Morimoto T, *et al.* Functional assessment of self-renewal activity of male germline stem cells following cytotoxic damage and serial transplantation. *Biol Reprod* 2003;68:1801–7

58. Lee HW, Blasco MA, Gottlieb GJ, *et al.* Essential role of mouse telomerase in highly proliferative organs. *Nature* 1998;392:569–74

NOTE

A recent study reported the recovery and activity of spermatogonial stem cells after cryopreservation. *See* Kanatsu-Shinohara M, Ogonuki N, Inoue K, *et al.* Restoration of fertility in infertile mice by transplantation of cryopreserved male germline stem cells. *Hum Reprod* 2003;18:2660–7

Cryopreservation of mammalian oocytes

11

S. P. Leibo

INTRODUCTION

An effective method to cryopreserve human oocytes will have an important clinical impact on present and future methods of assisted reproduction. It will reduce or eliminate the necessity to use drugs for follicular recruitment and maturation. If cryopreserved oocytes could also be induced to undergo *in vitro* maturation (IVM), this might permit oocytes to be aspirated directly from the ovary regardless of the stage of the patient's menstrual cycle. Reduction of the use of such fertility drugs would avoid ovarian hyperstimulation syndrome, a potentially serious iatrogenic condition arising from ovarian over-responsiveness to gonadotropin stimulation. Preservation of oocytes may provide an option for treatment of anovulation that is resistant to drugs in certain cases of polycystic ovarian disease. Reduction or elimination of fertility drugs would obviate the controversy surrounding possible increased risks of ovarian cancer caused by pharmacological agents used to induce oocyte development.

Oocyte cryopreservation would permit female patients facing radiation or chemotherapy as treatment for certain types of cancer to avoid the risk of sterility or potential genetic damage to their offspring by allowing them to store their oocytes in liquid nitrogen (LN$_2$). This would be analogous to the option already available to men, for example those with Hodgkin's disease, to store their semen in LN$_2$ while they undergo treatment. The ability to cryopreserve oocytes from voluntary donors would facilitate the ability of women with premature ovarian failure to conceive through donor-oocyte programs. A 'bank' of cryopreserved oocytes collected from women having voluntary tubal ligation would drastically ease the logistics of matching oocyte donors and recipient patients. In addition, oocyte cryopreservation would permit retrospective analysis of the health status of the egg donor at 6 months post-donation, analogous to the testing of sperm donors that is currently and routinely done with males. Once perfected and fully reliable, oocyte cryopreservation could be used by young women who wish to delay childbearing until their professional careers are established, yet avoid the increased risk of chromosomal anomalies associated with older maternal age, such as Down's syndrome.

The clinical efficacy of various methods of assisted reproduction to treat human infertility is well known. Since the birth of the first child conceived by *in vitro* methods[1], it is estimated that more than one million children have been born as a result of *in vitro* fertilization (IVF), culture of resultant zygotes, and transfer of pronuclear-stage or cleavage-stage embryos into the genetic mothers or their surrogates. In animals, all aspects of analogous techniques have long since involved cryopreservation of gametes (oocytes and spermatozoa), zygotes or developing embryos. This is beginning to be true in human medicine as well. The first successful cryopreservation of mammalian embryos resulting in the live birth of mice was reported more than 30 years ago[2]. Four years later, the birth of mice derived by IVF of frozen–thawed oocytes was also reported[3]. Since then, embryos of at least 22 other mammalian species have been successfully cryopreserved, as tabulated in recent reviews[4,5]. Success in those cases means that live offspring have been produced. As an example of how widespread embryo cryo-preservation has become throughout the world, in the year 2001, 235 900 bovine embryos, ~ 15 000 of which had been produced by IVF and culture, were transferred after having been cryopreserved; approximately 50% of these transferred embryos resulted in preg-nancy[6]. The relevance of this fact to human oocyte cryopreservation is that almost all human embryos are currently frozen by a procedure first described by Willadsen[7] for the freezing of ovine and bovine embryos. And this same method, with only slight modi-fications, has also been used to cryopreserve many human oocytes. According to this method, embryos suspended in a permeating cryoprotective additive (CPA) are cooled and seeded to induce ice formation at about −6°C, cooled slowly at 0.3°C/min to −30°C or so, and then plunged into LN_2 for storage. Frozen embryos are warmed at a moderately rapid rate of ~ 250°C/min, and the CPA is removed either by stepwise dilution with isotonic medium or with a hypertonic solution of a sac-charide (usually sucrose or galactose) acting as an osmotic buffer to prevent osmotic shock[8].

The first human pregnancy from a cryo-preserved embryo was reported by Trounson and Mohr[9], although this pregnancy aborted spontaneously at 24 weeks of gestation because of septic chorion amnionitis after premature membrane rupture. The first human preg-nancies resulting in births were reported by Zeilmaker and colleagues[10]. Since then, cryo-preservation of human embryos has become an integral part of assisted reproduction to treat human infertility (summarized in refer-ence[11]). As an example, data tabulated by the Society for Assisted Reproductive Technology (SART) indicates that the number of children born each year in the USA as a result of the transfer of cryopreserved embryos is close to 2400. The results in Figure 1, based on the final tabulation by SART for 1998, show that almost 20% of 10 058 cryopreserved human embryos (Cryo ET) resulted in deliveries of

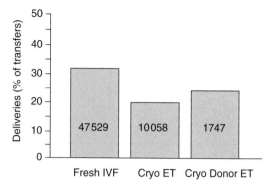

Figure 1 Results of assisted reproductive technologies in the USA in 1998. Each bar shows the number of deliv-eries of children as a percentage of the total number of transfers, categorized according to the status of the embryos transferred. The embryos were transferred straight after *in vitro* fertilization (Fresh IVF), after having been cryopreserved (Cryo ET), or after having been derived from a donated oocyte that was frozen before being transferred (Cryo Donor ET). The data are adapted from reference 12

children. Furthermore, transfer of more than 1700 cryopreserved embryos derived from oocytes donated by the genetic mothers to other women (Cryo Donor ET) also resulted in live births.

Evolving policies in many countries stipu-late that no more than two (or perhaps only one) embryos may be transferred into a single patient to prevent high-risk pregnancies with multiple fetuses. Since a growing number of countries will not permit destruction of a human embryo once conceived by IVF, this inevitably means that more human embryos will be cryopreserved[13]. Thus, there is increas-ing urgency to improve methods to cryopre-serve oocytes and embryos of the human. In general, cryopreservation of human gametes is viewed as posing few, if any, risks other than those resulting from the procedures of IVM, IVF and *in vitro* culture (IVC), although serious challenges to this attitude have been raised[14].

There have been occasional indications that cryopreservation of oocytes might induce mutagenic effects in resultant embryos[15,16]. Several years ago, based on 'morphophysio-logical and behavioral' studies of mice which

Table 1 Results of cryopreservation of human oocytes reported in the literature

Study	Cryopreservation method	Fertilized by	Oocytes (n)	Pregnancies	Live-born babies
Chen, 1986[25]	slow cool	IVF	40		1
Van Uem et al., 1987[26]	slow cool	IVF	28		1
Al-Hasani et al., 1987[27]	slow & rapid cool	IVF	182		2
Siebzehnrübl et al., 1986[28]	slow cool	IVF	38		1
Tucker et al., 1996[38]	slow cool, PG + S	ICSI	81	3	0
Porcu et al., 1997[39]	slow cool, PG + S	ICSI	12	1	1
Tucker et al., 1998[40]	slow cool, PG + S	ICSI	13	1	1
Borini et al., 1998[41]	slow cool, PG + S	ICSI	129	3	—
Porcu et al., 1998[42]	slow cool, PG + S	ICSI	709	9	6
Young et al., 1998[43]	slow cool, PG + S	ICSI	9	1	(3)
Polak de Fried et al., 1998[44]	slow cool, PG + S	ICSI	10	1	1
Kuleshova et al., 1999[45]	vitrification, EG + S	ICSI	17	1	1
Kuwayama and Kato, 2000[46]	vitrification, EG + S	ICSI	?	1	1
Donaldson et al., 2000[47]	slow cool, PG + S	ICSI	18	2	—
Yoon et al., 2000[48]	vitrification, EG + S	ICSI	90	3	2
Porcu et al., 2000[20]	slow cool, PG + S	ICSI	1840	19	12
Winslow et al., 2001[49]	slow cool, PG + S	ICSI	324	—	16
Wu et al., 2001[50]	vitrification, EG + S	IVF		1	—
Chen et al., 2002[51]	slow cool, PG + S	ICSI	8	1	—
Porcu et al., 2002[52]	slow cool, PG + S	ICSI	124	—	3
Yang et al., 2002[53]	slow cool, PG + S	ICSI	158	11	14
Quintans et al., 2002[54]	slow cool, PG + S	ICSI	109	5	2
Katayama et al., 2003[55]	vitrification, EG + S	ICSI	46	2	—
Yoon et al., 2003[56]	vitrification, EG + S	ICSI	474	—	7
Fosas et al., 2003[57]	slow cool, PG + S	ICSI	88	—	5
Boldt et al., 2003[58]	slow cool, PG + S	ICSI	90	—	5

PG, propylene glycol; S, sucrose; EG, ethylene glycol; IVF, *in vitro* fertilization; ICSI, intracytoplasmic sperm injection

developed from cryopreserved embryos, it was suggested that embryo freezing 'may not be completely neutral' and that delayed consequences of cryopreservation 'justify a more limited use of this technique in clinical practice'[17]. This view has become a focus of public concern, whether justified or not, and highlights the need for improved understanding of the effects of cryopreservation on human embryos and especially oocytes. On the other hand, a recent analysis of children born from cryopreserved embryos concluded that the available data indicate that cryopreservation has no apparent negative effect on perinatal outcome and early infant development[18]. That report also noted that there are several potential advantages of oocyte cryopreservation, although it must still be regarded as a research procedure, since the number of children produced from cryopreserved

oocytes is still limited: fewer than 100 in the entire scientific literature (see Table 1 above, and other reviews[19–21]). Oocytes are especially difficult to freeze successfully since their meiotic spindles, microtubules and microfilaments may be damaged by cooling and exposure to CPAs[22,23]. For ethical and practical reasons, and because some consequences of cryopreservation may be extremely subtle and difficult to discern, prudence suggests that human studies ought to be coupled with informative experimentation with gametes and embryos of other mammalian species.

CURRENT STATUS OF OOCYTE CRYOPRESERVATION

As mentioned above, the first children that developed from cryopreserved embryos were born in 1984. Shortly after that, other investigators began to introduce modifications of the original method, most notably the use of propylene glycol (PG; or 1,2-propanediol, as it is often termed) as a CPA, as was first described by Lassalle and associates[24]. Shortly afterwards, the first child resulting from cryopreservation of a human oocyte was conceived[25]. Over the next few years, others also began to freeze human oocytes with limited success, and the births of more children were reported [26-28]. However, disturbing questions began to be raised when it was discovered that oocytes of all species, including those of the human, are susceptible to damage from several of the steps used for their cryopreservation[29]. Among the steps found to be deleterious were cooling to temperatures near 0°C and exposure to CPAs[30-32]. Consequently, it was as if an informal moratorium had been declared and efforts to cryopreserve human oocytes came to a halt.

In the early 1990s, other important advances in assisted reproduction were made, notably the use of intracytoplasmic sperm injection (ICSI) to fertilize oocytes by direct injection of a single spermatozoon into an oocyte[33]. Although only limited success with this procedure had been achieved with animal oocytes, ICSI yielded remarkable results with human oocytes[34]. Advances in the field of cryobiology had also been made, notably the use of high concentrations of CPAs coupled with high cooling and warming rates to cryopreserve embryos without actually freezing them[4,35]. Furthermore, studies with mouse and human oocytes suggested that the deleterious effects might not be as serious as first thought[36,37]. As a consequence, efforts to cryopreserve human oocytes were renewed, but now after being warmed and thawed, the oocytes were fertilized by ICSI. Many of these efforts have been published in full experimental reports but some have been described only in abstract form. A list of these reports, as well as the first ones of oocyte freezing cited above, is given in Table 1. Although inevitably this list may not be complete, it does give a reasonably comprehensive summary of the current status of clinical applications of human oocyte cryopreservation. It should

also be understood that there were many differences among the various reports as to the specific procedures of oocyte handling, fertilization and transfer of resultant embryos, as well as the details of the cryopreservation procedures themselves. Furthermore, not all articles presented the results in the same format or with similar details. Where there are missing values, it is because these were either not stated or the specific number was ambiguous. Nevertheless, the list does provide useful information.

In the past 8 years, the cryopreservation of more than 4300 human oocytes has been described in 22 articles or abstracts. The births of 80 children derived from cryopreserved oocytes have been reported. Since not all of the reports contained the same information, it is not possible to calculate an overall live-birth rate for the total number of preserved oocytes. Furthermore, in some studies multiple embryos were transferred into patients, whereas in others single embryo transfers were performed. Despite these ambiguities, it is informative to consider these data from several perspectives. In most of these studies, the oocytes were frozen by 'standard' equilibrium cooling. With this method, oocytes, usually at the metaphase II (MII) stage of maturation, are suspended in a 1.5 mol/l solution of PG, often supplemented with 0.1 to 0.3 mol/l sucrose. Thereafter, the sample is cooled and frozen under conditions similar to the procedure of Willadsen[7] described above. Samples cooled to about −6 or −7°C are seeded to induce crystallization and to prevent the highly variable supercooling that would otherwise occur. The frozen samples are cooled to about −30 to −35°C, and then cooled at ~150°C/min to below −100°C or plunged directly into LN_2 for long-term storage. As can be seen from the list, since 1996, all human oocytes cryopreserved by slow freezing have been fertilized by ICSI. A total of 3598 oocytes cryopreserved by slow cooling and subjected to ICSI has resulted in 57 pregnancies, or a 1.6% pregnancy rate. In those cases in which full-term pregnancies have been described, a total of 3576 oocytes were frozen and thawed; 74 babies were born from these oocytes, a 2.1% live-birth rate.

For reasons that will be explained more fully below, there has been growing application of various rapid cooling methods applied to oocyte cryopreservation. Descriptions of the vitrification by rapid cooling of a total of 153 oocytes have been published; 11 children have been born from these vitrified oocytes. As more experience and understanding of such non-equilibrium cryopreservation is gained, there will almost certainly be an increased use of these methods for human oocytes.

One final note regarding storage of cryopreserved gametes and embryos must be made. Surprisingly, there have been occasional anecdotal reports that human oocytes and embryos may deteriorate while stored at −196°C. Such deterioration can almost certainly be ascribed to accidental or inadvertent mishandling of frozen samples, since human pregnancies have been reported for embryos stored for more than 8 years[59,60]; sheep and mouse embryos have been successfully stored for at least 13 years, developing into live young after being thawed and transferred into suitable recipients[61]. The tabulated results clearly demonstrate that children can be conceived by fertilization of cryopreserved oocytes. However, those results also show that considerable research needs to be done to improve the overall efficiency of human oocyte cryopreservation. Improvements will undoubtedly come from collaborative efforts of basic scientists and physicians to identify and optimize conditions of oocyte handling and fertilization, methods of cryopreservation, and also clinical aspects of embryo transfer and patient care. One purpose of this chapter is to describe the cryobiological aspects of this problem; a good place to begin is with basic cryobiology. A recent review has summarized some aspects of this subject as it applies to mammalian oocytes in general[62].

BASIC ASPECTS OF CRYOBIOLOGY

Reduced to its fundamentals, cryopreservation involves exposing cells to three non-physiological conditions:

(1) Exposure to molar concentrations of CPAs;

(2) Cooling to subzero temperatures;

(3) Removal and conversion of all liquid cell water into the solid state.

Any one or all of these conditions may damage cells, especially oocytes. Among the characteristics that render oocytes especially sensitive to damage is their large size, their low permeability to water and to permeating compounds, their sensitivity to temperature fluctuations, especially to cooling, and the presence of the meiotic spindle, at least within the mature oocyte at the MII stage.

However carefully practiced, current techniques of cryopreservation must be assumed to inflict an 'insult' on gametes or embryos. There are numerous reasons for supposing that the results of an insult inflicted upon a gamete or embryo during its development may not become apparent until much later in embryogenesis or even postnatally. For example, abnormalities of sperm decondensation occur when immature human oocytes are fertilized prematurely[63]. Furthermore, cytogenetic analyses of oocytes, zygotes and embryos made available during human IVF procedures have revealed that 35% of oocytes and up to 40% of embryos display chromosomal anomalies[64]. Cryopreservation further complicates the analysis. For example, after being cryopreserved, human oocytes were found to be abnormally penetrated by sperm at the germinal vesicle (GV) stage, rather than at MII stage as mature oocytes; although fertilized, their development was arrested and their cleavage patterns were abnormal[65].

When aqueous solutions are frozen, water is removed in the form of ice, causing the solutions to become increasingly concentrated with decreasing temperature; the reverse occurs during thawing. Because of their low molecular weight and high solubility, solutions of many low-molecular-weight compounds that act to protect cells against freezing damage exhibit such sequential concentration and dilution when frozen and thawed. Depending on their initial concentration, solutions of

CPAs may become 15- to 30-fold more concentrated during freezing. When a concentrated solution in which cells are suspended is abruptly diluted, the rapid decrease in osmotic pressure of the solution can cause osmotic shock of the cells. Rapid warming and melting of a frozen cell suspension is equivalent to rapid dilution of the CPA that became concentrated during freezing, and thus can also cause osmotic shock. Sensitivity to osmotic shock is a function of a cell's permeability to water and solutes and of the temperature dependence of these permeability coefficients, all of which are fundamental properties of membranes and directly reflect membrane composition. When frozen and thawed, embryos of mice[66], cattle[67] and sheep[68] are damaged by osmotic shock resulting from rapid dilution of extracellular solutions. However, as first described in 1978[69], osmotic shock of embryos can be prevented by the use of an impermeant sugar as an osmotic buffer to prevent the rapid change in osmotic pressure of the solution[8]. Various mono- and disaccharides are equally effective as osmotic buffers for both mouse zygotes and human oocytes, and osmotic shock of zygotes and oocytes can be prevented by dilution of CPAs with such osmotic buffers[70]. Prevention of osmotic shock has made it possible to use cryopreserved hamster oocytes for the sperm penetration assay to assess the fertilizing capability of human spermatozoa[71]. The same procedure to prevent osmotic shock has been used to cryopreserve human embryos[72].

Analysis of possible causes of freezing injury has revealed that mouse zygotes can be damaged by osmotic shock when the concentrated cryoprotectant solutions in which they are suspended are diluted rapidly[73]. The extent of time-dependent volumetric responses of mouse zygotes to various solutions of CPAs determines their survival when rapidly frozen. Attempts to adapt rodent cryopreservation procedures to bovine embryos demonstrated that bovine embryos produced by *in vitro* maturation and fertilization of ovarian oocytes are considerably more sensitive both to chilling and to freezing than their normal *in vivo*-derived counterparts. This sensitivity

to cryopreservation of embryos produced by IVF is highly stage-dependent[67].

In an attempt to reduce osmotic injury of human oocytes that might occur during cryopreservation, several investigations have been conducted to determine their permeability characteristics[74–77]. The rationale of these experiments is that a key to successful cryopreservation may be to reduce osmotic injury from volume excursions that occur during the addition or removal of CPAs. Therefore, knowledge of the permeability coefficients might yield an optimized method to expose human oocytes to CPAs. Construction of a Boyle–van't Hoff plot has revealed that human oocytes, like those of several other species, have a non-osmotic volume of approximately 19%[75]. In several of these studies, osmotic responses of oocytes exposed to 1.5 mol/l solutions of dimethylsulfoxide (DMSO) or PG were determined. These studies revealed that human oocytes have a hydraulic conductivity of approximately 0.8 µm/atm/min, although there have been some differences reported by the various groups. The permeability of the human oocyte to DMSO has been found to be about 3×10^{-5} cm/s, although again some differences among these studies have been noted.

Cryopreservation inevitably exposes oocytes to subzero temperatures. Therefore, it is important to consider the effects of low temperatures on oocytes. The chilling sensitivity of oocytes of many species at either the GV stage or the MII stage has been studied. As early as 1948, Chang reported that oocytes and zygotes of the rabbit are damaged when cooled and held at 0°C. An important observation regarding oocyte sensitivity to cold and freezing was the finding that the second meiotic spindle of mouse oocytes became disorganized and the microtubules underwent depolymerization[78]. The effects of chilling were at least partially reversible when the oocytes were incubated at 37°C for more than 15 min. Since then, there have been many investigations of the effects of cooling and chilling on the structure and function of oocytes of several species (reviews in references 22 and 23).

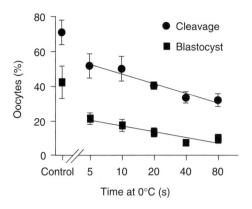

Figure 2 Effect of cooling *in vitro*-derived bovine oocytes. After having been cooled directly to 0°C and held for various times, the oocytes were then warmed to 37°C and subjected to *in vitro* fertilization (IVF) and culture. Development was calculated as a percentage of the total oocytes that were chilled before IVF. Time is shown as a $\log_{10}$ scale on the *x*-axis. Each point represents data pooled from three replicates and shows the mean ± SEM. The figure is adapted from reference 82, and is used with permission of the publisher and authors

Because of their agricultural importance, there has been a rapidly expanding use of *in vitro*-produced bovine embryos for commercial applications. Consequently, it is also important to determine the effects of various treatments and conditions that influence the overall production of bovine embryos. Among such studies, there have been several analyses of the effects of chilling on bovine oocytes[79–81]. These studies demonstrate that the developmental capacity of *in vitro*-matured bovine oocytes is adversely affected when they are cooled to 0°C. An example of these findings from Martino and co-workers[82] is shown in Figure 2. Even a 5-s exposure to 0°C is sufficient to decrease the percentage of oocytes that will cleave into two-cell embryos after IVF from 70% to ~ 50%; extending the exposure at 0°C to 80 s causes a further decrease in their cleavage rate. The effects of chilling on blastocyst development are even more severe. Oocytes at the GV stage exhibit time-dependent sensitivities to chilling to 0°C very similar to those of oocytes at the MII stage[79]. This means that chilling injury cannot be entirely explained as

resulting from disassembly of the meiotic spindle, since this structure has not yet formed in the oocyte at GV stage. Even after *in vitro*-matured oocytes have been fertilized and have cleaved, their development, both in terms of blastocyst-formation rate and the number of cells per blastocyst, can be adversely affected as a result of exposure to a non-physiological temperature of +20°C[83]. The relevance of chilling sensitivity is that conventional equilibrium methods of cryopreservation inevitably expose oocytes to temperatures at or near 0°C for 10 min or longer.

Detailed analyses have also been performed to determine the effects of chilling and freezing on the ultrastructure, cytoskeleton and spindle morphology of human oocytes[31,36,84]. Recognizing that standard methods of oocyte recovery as practiced in many clinics might expose oocytes to non-physiological temperatures, Pickering and colleagues[31] found that cooling human oocytes to room temperature for as little as 10 min causes irreversible damage to the meiotic spindle. Warming the oocytes afterwards resulted in only partial recovery of normal morphology. Chilling oocytes to 0°C in the presence of a CPA only exacerbates the abnormalities[32]. These and other recent studies provide at least a partial explanation of the fact that the number of full-term pregnancies achieved by IVF of cryopreserved oocytes remains only about 2 to 4% as a percentage of the total number of oocytes warmed and recovered after cryopreservation (see Table 1). Although the percentage of human oocytes scored morphologically as 'survivors' in some cases may exceed 75 or 80%, the percentage that actually undergoes development after fertilization remains rather variable and low.

A recent study has been made to determine the kinetics of chilling injury of human oocytes[85]. To do this, mature oocytes were abruptly cooled from 37°C to 0°C in fine glass capillaries for times ranging from 1 to 10 min. The rationale of this experiment was to determine how quickly human oocytes might be damaged by chilling injury. Oocytes were warmed to 37°C and then fixed and subjected

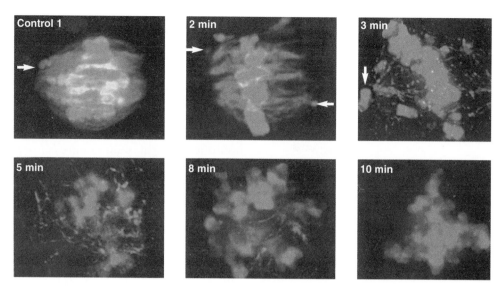

Figure 3 Fluorescent micrographs of meiotic spindles in human oocytes that had been cooled rapidly to 0°C and held for the times indicated. The panel labeled control 1 is an untreated oocyte. The micrographs were made with an optical sectioning microscope together with deconvolution software. Chromosomes are stained red and spindles are stained green. The figure is adapted from reference 85, and is used with permission of the publisher and authors. See Color Plate I

to immunostaining. The effects on spindle morphologyp were determined by examining the oocytes with an epifluorescence microscope. Some oocytes from each time point were also imaged on a deconvoluted microscope, analogous to a confocal microscope. Selected images to illustrate the kinetics of chilling injury are shown in Figure 3. The control oocyte exhibits a rather typical meiotic spindle with the chromosomes aligned along the metaphase plate. However, in the chilled oocytes, it is clear that the microtubules have undergone disassembly and the chromosomes have become disorganized. Within 10 min, there is little left of the microtubules. In light of these observations, it is not too surprising that many human oocytes subjected to slow freezing may undergo fertilization yet they do not develop normally after IVF. Analogous findings of spindle and chromosome configurations after cryopreservation of human oocytes at the GV and MII stages have recently been published[84].

As a model for human oocytes, the effects of chilling on the organization and distribution of tubulin and chromosomes in rhesus monkey oocytes have also been studied[86]. Among the advantages of this experimental approach is that oocytes may be collected repeatedly from the same female. Exposure of rhesus oocytes to 0°C for only 1 min resulted in complete depolymerization of tubulin. Although incubation of chilled oocytes at 37°C for 60 min caused partial restoration of tubulin, most oocytes exhibited abnormal alignment of chromosomes and disorganized meiotic spindles. Curiously, there were significant differences in the sensitivity of oocytes from different females to chilling injury. If true for humans as well, this might explain why it has been difficult to achieve high survival of oocytes in a reproducible fashion.

RATIONALE OF CRYOPRESERVATION BY RAPID COOLING METHODS

Because of the extreme sensitivity of mammalian oocytes to chilling injury, attempts have been made to derive cryopreservation methods by cooling the oocytes at very high rates so as to circumvent chilling injury. This rationale was first applied to cryopreservation of embryos of the fruit fly, *Drosophila*. All attempts to cryopreserve eggs and embryos of this insect by standard methods failed because of their extreme sensitivity to chilling. Working independently, two groups of investigators did derive successful methods to cryopreserve *Drosophila* embryos by very rapid cooling methods[87,88]. A similar rationale was first applied to bovine oocytes, and has now been extended to the oocytes of several other species.

To try to improve survival after cryopreservation of bovine oocytes, Martino and associates[82] suspended matured bovine oocytes in two versions of a vitrification solution (either 4 mol/l ethylene glycol (EG) supplemented with 0.5 mol/l sucrose or 5.5 mol/l EG supplemented with 1.0 mol/l sucrose). The novel feature of this method was that bovine oocytes, after a very brief exposure to the vitrification solutions, were placed on a fine copper electron microscope (EM) grid and plunged directly into LN_2. The vitrified oocytes were warmed and liquefied by being transferred directly from LN_2 into 0.5 mol/l sucrose at 37°C. Given the small volume of medium containing the oocytes, it was estimated from published literature that the resultant cooling rate might approach 180 000°C/min. In any case, of 150 oocytes suspended in 5.5 mol/l EG + 1.0 mol/l sucrose and cooled ultra-rapidly on grids, close to 60% exhibited morphological survival, 40% of them cleaved and 15% developed into blastocysts after warming and IVF. This was ten times higher than the survival of oocytes cooled rapidly in plastic straws. In other words, increasing the cooling rate significantly improved the functional survival of bovine oocytes. The development rate was the same regardless of the vitrification solution used, and was the same for control oocytes that were only exposed to the solutions but were not cryopreserved. These results suggest that one important key to improving oocyte cryopreservation will require reducing deleterious effects of CPAs.

Other recent results suggest that chilling and freezing injury of mammalian oocytes may depend on the properties of their membranes, particularly the relative proportions of cholesterol, lipids and phospholipids within them, characteristics which vary with maturational stage, species and specific culture conditions, including both supplemental hormones and proteins. The membranes of most mammalian cells are ordered domains of double-leaflet, dynamic structures composed primarily of lipids, proteins, phospholipids, glycolipids, glycoproteins, cholesterol, water, sugars and metal ions[89–91]. Interactions of these components determine the function and properties of the membranes of different types of cell. From the perspective of cryobiology, two important characteristics of a membrane are its permeability and its fluidity, both of which vary with cholesterol content[92–95]. Fluidity, the reciprocal of viscosity, refers to the mobility of molecular components of the membrane within the plane of the membrane, perpendicular to that plane and across the membrane. The rotational and lateral diffusion of proteins and lipids within membranes reflect their composition, structure and function[93], as do other changes in membranes. The osmotic properties of erythrocytes of newborn animals of many species, including human, differ significantly from those of erythrocytes of mature individuals[96], presumably reflecting age-dependent changes in membrane composition.

Membranes may also be altered by various CPAs; glycerol or DMSO, for example, causes redistribution of intramembranous particles in lymphocytes[97] or in tissue-culture cells[98]. The domains of submembranous microfilaments in rabbit oocytes are affected differently by PG and DMSO[99]. It may be relevant to consider that several CPAs, including glycerol, PG and sucrose, have recently been shown to stabilize bull sperm membranes[100].

METHODS TO CRYOPRESERVE OOCYTES

Since chilling injury to oocytes is time-dependent, the rationale is to prevent injury by cooling the oocytes at very high rates through the damaging temperature zone to 'outrace' injury before it can occur. Once the entire system has solidified at subzero temperatures, no further change can occur. This rationale was first used to improve the survival and development of bovine oocytes[82]. It has now been used by many others to cryopreserve the oocytes and embryos of cattle[101–103], mice[104] and humans[45,46,48,50,55,56].

Nevertheless, as mentioned above, oocytes of many species have also been cryopreserved by slow, 'equilibrium' cooling as well. In fact, the first human pregnancies resulting from standard IVF of cryopreserved oocytes were achieved with oocytes frozen by such methods[25–28]. As also described above, many more human pregnancies have resulted from the transfer of zygotes or embryos derived from oocytes cryopreserved by a freezing procedure very similar to that first described for cattle embryos[20,38,105–107]. In all of these latter cases, however, fertilization was achieved by ICSI. Although full-term pregnancies resulted, the use of ICSI for fertilization suggests that the zona pellucida is likely to have been altered by the various steps of cryopreservation.

An innovative alternative has recently been described for cryopreservation of mouse oocytes by slow cooling methods, and very recently the same method has been successfully applied to human oocytes as well. Recognizing that oocyte membranes may be damaged by exposure to high salt concentrations resulting during freezing, Stachecki and co-workers[107] replaced sodium in the basic salt solution with the organic osmolyte, choline, and achieved high rates of survival and fertilization of mouse oocytes cryopreserved by slow freezing. More recently, these same investigators have produced live mouse pups from oocytes cryopreserved by slow cooling in a choline-based solution[108]. Here again, however, fertilization was accomplished by opening the zona with a laser, again suggesting that oocytes cryopreserved by this method are not completely equivalent to unfrozen oocytes.

Oocytes can be cryopreserved as either (i) denuded individual oocytes or (ii) cumulus-enclosed oocytes. The approach selected usually depends on the stage of nuclear maturity of the oocyte prior to cryopreservation. For example, when mature MII oocytes are collected for cryopreservation, they are commonly denuded prior to freezing to confirm nuclear status. In contrast, it is physiologically far more appropriate to leave fully grown GV-stage oocytes enclosed within their cumulus cells during the freezing process for optimal IVM after thawing. Each approach has advantages and limitations.

RECENT INNOVATIONS

Several novel procedures for cryopreservation of oocytes and embryos have been described during the past few years. All offer distinct improvements compared to more traditional methods. Some of these have already been applied to human oocytes with encouraging results. Notable among these new methods are various ways to achieve vitrification of human oocytes. This subject has recently been reviewed in considerable detail[109]. As mentioned above, it has been shown that functional survival of animal oocytes can be improved significantly by use of an EM grid to achieve high cooling rates[82]. This approach has now been used both with human embryos and oocytes. Blastocysts have been produced by IVF of oocytes that were cryopreserved on EM grids[110,111]. Recently, two children have been born as a result of IVF of oocytes vitrified on EM grids; a third pregnancy was continuing[56].

An equally novel method of achieving vitrification by cooling a very small sample at very high rates was described by Vajta's group[101,102]. With this method, plastic straws are heated and pulled to produce a thin wall and a small diameter. These 'open-pulled straws' (OPS) have been used to cryopreserve oocytes and embryos from various species with excellent results[112]. This method has now also been used to cryopreserve human oocytes, one of which developed into a child after IVF and embryo transfer[45].

Yet another approach to rapid cooling has been the introduction of a very small plastic device to cryopreserve oocytes and embryos referred to as a 'Cryotop'. The rationale of this device is the same as others: to provide a holder for extremely small volumes of media containing the oocytes so that they may be cooled at very high rates. This device has already been used to cryopreserve human oocytes that have subsequently been fertilized; the resultant zygotes have developed into blastocysts in culture. Furthermore, pregnancies have resulted from transfer of some of these embryos and a child has already been born[46,55].

One other device that has been used to cryopreserve both embryos and oocytes is the cryoloop. This very small nylon loop can be used to hold oocytes in a thin film of CPA before plunging it directly into LN_2. It has been used to cryopreserve oocytes or embryos of various species, which have developed into blastocysts in culture and into live young after transfer. Its use was pioneered by Lane and colleagues[113], who have used it to cryopreserve embryos of various species, including the human[104,114].

As mentioned, one of the more novel approaches to oocyte cryopreservation has been to modify the basic isotonic solution used to prepare the cryoprotectant solution. This approach of substituting choline chloride in place of NaCl has been described in several publications by Stachecki and co-workers[107,108]. This method has now been used successfully to cryopreserve human oocytes and has resulted in the birth of two children[54].

Yet another novel approach has been to modify the oocyte itself. In these experiments, Eroglu and associates[115,116] injected 0.15 mol/l trehalose as a CPA directly into human oocytes before freezing them in a solution of 0.5 mol/l trehalose. They have shown that the oocytes can tolerate the injection and will survive after having been cooled to –60°C at 1°C/min. In contrast, uninjected control oocytes are killed by being cooled to only –30°C. They have also shown that mouse oocytes will develop after having been injected with trehalose[117]. The significance of this approach is that oocytes are impermeable to trehalose. Only by injection can it be introduced intracellularly. Evidence suggests that this may be an effective method of conferring protection to oocytes.

PROSPECTS FOR THE FUTURE

A number of considerations point to the likelihood that there will continue to be improvements in methods to cryopreserve human oocytes. This is an extremely important and, one might even say, urgent matter for patients requiring fertility preservation, as well as for reproductive medicine more generally. As methods to perform human IVF continue to improve, there is a growing consensus that multiple embryos ought not be transferred so as to avoid the risk of pregnancy with multiple fetuses. One way to avoid this is to transfer only single embryos into each patient. From a logistical point of view, the easiest way to achieve this is to cryopreserve oocytes. Another factor that will likely contribute to improvements is that efforts to improve the cryopreservation of animal oocytes, especially those of cattle, will also continue to increase. Nevertheless, given the fact that the overall success rates with cryopreserved oocytes are still rather low, caution must be exercised before recommending this option to patients.

References

1. Steptoe PC, Edwards RG. Birth after the reimplantation of a human embryo. *Lancet* 1978; 2:366
2. Whittingham DG, Leibo SP, Mazur P. Survival of mouse embryos frozen to –196° and –269°C. *Science* 1972;178:411–14
3. Parkening TA, Tsunoda Y, Chang MC. Effects of various low temperatures, cryoprotective agents and cooling rates on the survival, fertilizability and development of frozen–thawed mouse eggs. *J Exp Zool* 1976;197: 369–74

4. Rall WF. Cryopreservation of mammalian embryos, gametes, and ovarian tissues. In Wolf DP, Zelinski-Wooten M, eds. *Contemporary Endocrinology: Assisted Fertilization and Nuclear Transfer in Mammals*. Towata, NJ: Humana Press, 2001:173–87

5. Leibo SP, Songsasen N. Cryopreservation of gametes and embryos of non-domestic species. *Theriogenology* 2002;57:303–26

6. Thibier M. The 2001 embryo transfer statistics from around the world: a data retrieval committee report. *Embryo Transfer Newsletter* 2002;20:13–19

7. Willadsen SM. Factors affecting the survival of sheep embryos during deep-freezing and thawing. In *The Freezing of Mammalian Embryos*. Ciba Foundation, Symposium 52 (New Series). Amsterdam: Elsevier Excerpta Medica/North-Holland, Amsterdam, 1977:175–201

8. Leibo SP. Cryobiology: preservation of mammalian embryos. In: Genetic Engineering of Animals. JW Evans, A Hollaender, eds. Plenum Publishing Corp, 1986:251–72

9. Trounson A, Mohr L. Human pregnancy following cryopreservation, thawing and transfer of an eight-cell embryo. *Nature* 1983;305:707–9

10. Zeilmaker GH, Alberda AT, van Gent I, *et al.* Two pregnancies following transfer of intact frozen–thawed embryos. *Fertil Steril* 1984;42:293–6

11. Shaw JM, Oranratnachai A, Trounson A. Cryopreservation of oocytes and embryos. In Trounson A, Gardner DK, eds. *In Vitro Fertilization*. Boca Raton, FL: CRC Press, 1993:213–36

12. SART/ASRM (Society for Assisted Reproductive Technology/American Society for Reproductive Medicine). Assisted reproductive technology in the United States: 1998 results generated from the American Society for Reproductive Medicine/Society for Assisted Reproductive Technology Registry. *Fertil Steril* 2002;77:18–31

13. Van der Elst J, Camus M, Van den Abbeel E, *et al.* Prospective randomized study on the cryopreservation of human embryos with dimethylsulfoxide or 1,2-propanediol protocols. *Fertil Steril* 1995;63:92–100

14. Marina F, Marina S. Comments on oocyte cryopreservation. *Reprod Biomed Online* 2003; 6:401–2

15. Bouquet M, Selva J, Auroux M. Cryopreservation of mouse oocytes: mutagenic effects in the embryo? *Biol Reprod* 1993;49:764–9

16. Bouquet M, Selva J, Auroux M. Effects of cooling and equilibration in DMSO, and cryopreservation of mouse oocytes, on the rates of *in vitro* fertilization, development, and chromosomal abnormalities. *Mol Reprod Dev* 1995;40:110–15

17. Dulioust E, Toyama K, Busnel MC, *et al.* Long-term effects of embryo freezing in mice. *Proc NatlAcad Sci USA* 1995;92:589–93

18. Wennerholm UB. Cryopreservation of embryos and oocytes: obstetric outcome and health in children. *Hum Reprod* 2000;15(Suppl 5):18–25

19. Lüdwig M, Al-Hasani S, Felberbaum R, *et al.* New aspects of cryopreservation of oocytes and embryos in assisted reproduction and future perspectives. *Hum Reprod* 1999;14(Suppl 1):162–85

20. Porcu E, Fabbri R, Damiano G, *et al.* Clinical experience and applications of oocyte cryopreservation. *Mol Cell Endocrinol* 2000;169:33–7

21. Chen SU, Lien YR, Chao KH, *et al.* Effects of cryopreservation on meiotic spindles of oocytes and its dynamics after thawing: clinical implications in oocyte freezing – a review article. *Mol Cell Endocrinol* 2003;202:101–7

22. Vincent C, Johnson, JH. Cooling cryoprotectants and the cytoskeleton of the mammalian oocyte. *Oxford Rev Reprod Biol* 1992;14:73–100

23. Parks JE, Ruffing NA. Factors affecting low temperature survival of mammalian oocytes. *Theriogenology* 1992;37:59–73

24. Lassalle B, Testart J, Renard JP. Human embryo features that influence the success of cryopreservation with the use of 1,2 propanediol. *Fertil Steril* 1985;44:645–51

25. Chen C. Pregnancy after human oocyte cryopreservation. *Lancet* 1986;ii:884–6

26. Van Uem JFHM, Siebzehnrübl ER, Schuh B, *et al.* Birth after cryopreservation of unfertilized oocytes. *Lancet* 1987;i:752–3

27. Al-Hasani S, Diedrich K, van der Ven H, *et al.* Cryopreservation of human oocytes. *Hum Reprod* 1987;2:695–700

28. Siebzehnrübl E, Trotnow S, Weigel M, *et al.* Pregnancies after *in vitro* fertilization, cryopreservation and embryo transfer. *J In Vitro Fertil Embryo Transf* 1986;3:261–3

29. Trounson A. Cryopreservation of human eggs and embryo. *Fertil Steril* 1986;46:1–12

30. Pickering SJ, Johnson MH. The influence of cooling on the organization of the meiotic spindle of the mouse oocyte. *Hum Reprod* 1987;2:207–16

31. Pickering SJ, Braude PR, Johnson MH, *et al.* Transient cooling to room temperature can cause irreversible disruption of the meiotic spindle in the human oocyte. *Fertil Steril* 1990;54:102–8

32. Sathananthan AH, Trounson A, Freeman L, *et al.* The effects of cooling human oocytes. *Hum Reprod* 1988;3:968–77

33. Palermo G, Joris H, Devroey P, et al. Pregnancies after intracytoplasmic injection of single spermatozoon into an oocyte. Lancet 1992;340:17–18

34. Van Steirteghem A, Tournaye H, Van der Elst J, et al. Intracytoplasmic sperm injection three years after the birth of the first ICSI child. Hum Reprod 1995;10:2527–8

35. Rall WF, Fahy GM. Ice-free cryopreservation of mouse embryos at –196°C by vitrification. Nature 1985;313:573–5

36. Gook DA, Osborn SM, Johnston WI. Cryopreservation of mouse and human oocytes using 1,2–propanediol and the configuration of the meiotic spindle. Hum Reprod 1993;8:1101–9

37. Gook DA, Osborn SDM, Bourne H, et al. Fertilization of human oocytes following cryopreservation; normal karyotypes and absence of stray chromosomes. Hum Reprod 1994;9:684–91

38. Tucker M, Wright G, Morton P, et al. Preliminary experience with human oocyte cryopreservation using 1,2-propanediol and sucrose. Hum Reprod 1996;11:1513–15

39. Porcu E, Fabbri R, Seracchioli R, et al. Birth of a healthy female after intracytoplasmic sperm injection of cryopreserved human oocytes. Fertil Steril 1997;68:724–6

40. Tucker MJ, Wright G, Morton PC, et al. Birth after cryopreservation of immature oocytes with subsequent in vitro fertilization. Fertil Steril 1998;70:578–9

41. Borini A, Bafaro MG, Bonu MA, et al. Pregnancies after oocyte freezing and thawing. Hum Reprod 1998;13(Abstract Book 1):124–5

42. Porcu E, Fabbri R, Seracchioli R, et al. Birth of six healthy children after intracytoplasmic sperm injection of cryopreserved human oocytes. Hum Reprod 1998;13(Abstract Book 1):124

43. Young E, Kenny A, Puigdomenech E, et al. Triplet pregnancy after intracytoplasmic sperm injection of cryopreserved oocytes: case report. Fertil Steril 1998;70:360–1

44. Polak de Fried E, Notrica J, Rubinstein M, et al. Pregnancy after human donor oocyte cryopreservation and thawing in association with intracytoplasmic sperm injection in a patient with ovarian failure. Fertil Steril 1998;69:555–7

45. Kuleshova L, Gianaroli L, Magli C, et al. Birth following vitrification of a small number of human oocytes. Hum Reprod 1999;14:3077–9

46. Kuwayama M, Kato O. Successful vitrification of human oocytes. Fertil Steril 2000;74:549

47. Donaldson MJ, Quintans CJ, Rocha M, et al. Pregnancies achieved after the transfer of embryos obtained by IVF of human oocytes cryopreserved in low sodium medium: report of two cases. Hum Reprod 2000;15(Abstract Book 1):152

48. Yoon TK, Chung HM, Lim JM, et al. Pregnancy and delivery of healthy infants developed from vitrified oocytes in a stimulated in vitro fertilization–embryo transfer program. Fertil Steril 2000;74:180–1

49. Winslow KL, Yang D, Blohm PL, et al. Oocyte cryopreservation: a three year follow up of sixteen births. Fertil Steril 2001;76:S28

50. Wu J, Zhang L, Wang X. In vitro maturation, fertilization and embryo development after ultrarapid freezing of immature human oocytes. Reproduction 2001;121:389–93

51. Chen SU, Lien YR, Tsai YY, et al. Successful pregnancy occurred from slowly freezing human oocytes using the regime of 1.5 mol/l 1,2-propanediol with 0.3 mol/l sucrose. Hum Reprod 2002;17:1412

52. Porcu E, Fabbri R, Ciotti PM, et al. Oocytes or embryo storage? Fertil Steril 2002;78:S15

53. Yang D, Winslow KL, Blohm PL, et al. Oocyte donation using cryopreserved donor oocytes. Fertil Steril 2002;78:S14–15

54. Quintans CJ, Donaldson MJ, Bertolino MV, et al. Birth of two babies using oocytes that were cryopreserved in a choline-based freezing medium. Hum Reprod 2002;17:3149–52

55. Katayama KP, Stehlik J, Kuwayama M, et al. High survival rate of vitrified human oocytes results in clinical pregnancy. Fertil Steril 2003;80:223–4

56. Yoon TK, Kim TJ, Park SE, et al. Live births after vitrification of oocytes in a stimulated in vitro fertilization–embryo transfer program. Fertil Steril 2003;79:1323–6

57. Fosas N, Marina F, Torres PJ, et al. The births of five Spanish babies from cryopreserved donated oocytes. Hum Reprod 2003;18:1417–21

58. Boldt J, Cline D, McLaughlin D. Human oocyte cryopreservation as an adjunct to IVF–embryo transfer cycles. Hum Reprod 2003;18:1250–5

59. Go KJ, Corson SL, Batzer FR, et al. Live birth from a zygote cryopreserved for 8 years. Hum Reprod 1998;13:2970–1

60. Quintans CJ, Donaldson MJ, Bertolino MV, et al. Birth of a healthy baby after transfer of embryos that were cryopreserved for 8.9 years. Fertil Steril 2002;77:1074–6

61. Glenister PH, Thornton CE. Cryoconservation – archiving for the future. Mamm Genome 2000; 11:565–71

62. Critser JK, Agca Y, Gunasena KT. The cryobiology of mammalian oocytes. In Karow AM, Critser JK, eds. Reproductive Tissue Banking. San Diego, CA: Academic Press, 1997:329–57

63. Zenzes MT, de Geyter C, Bordt J, et al. Abnormalities of sperm chromosome condensation in the cytoplasm of immature human oocytes. Hum Reprod 1990;5:842–6

64. Zenzes MT, Casper RF. Cytogenetics of human oocytes, zygotes, and embryos after in vitro fertilization. Hum Genet 1992;88:367–75

65. Van Blerkom J, Davis PW. Cytogenetic, cellular, and developmental consequences of cryopreservation of immature and mature mouse and human oocytes. Microsc Res Tech 1994;27:165–93

66. Leibo SP, Mazur P, Jackowski SC. Factors affecting survival of mouse embryos during freezing and thawing. Exp Cell Res 1974;89:79–88

67. Leibo SP, Martino A, Kobayashi S, et al. Stage-dependent sensitivity of oocytes and embryos to low temperatures. Anim Reprod Sci 1996;42:45–53

68. Songsasen N, Buckrell BC, Plante C, Leibo SP. In vitro and in vivo survival of cryopreserved sheep embryos. Cryobiology 1995;32:78–91

69. Leibo SP, Mazur P. Methods for the preservation of mammalian embryos by freezing. In Daniel JC Jr, ed. Methods in Mammalian Reproduction. New York: Academic Press, 1978:179–201

70. McWilliams RB, Gibbons WE, Leibo SP. Osmotic and physiological responses of mouse and human ova to mono- and disaccharides. Hum Reprod 1995;10:1163–71

71. Leibo SP, Giambernardi TA, Meyer TK, et al. The efficacy of cryopreserved hamster ova in the sperm penetration assay. Fertil Steril 1990;53:906–12

72. Freedman M, Farber M, Farmer L, et al. Pregnancy resulting from cryopreserved human embryos using a one-step in situ dilution procedure. Obstet Gynecol 1988;72:502–5

73. Oda K, Gibbons WE, Leibo SP. Osmotic shock of fertilized mouse ova. J Reprod Fertil 1992;95:737–47

74. McGrath JJ, Fuller BJ, Hunter JE, et al. The permeability of fresh pre-ovulatory human oocytes to dimethylsulfoxide at 3°C. Cryo Letters 1995;16:79–84

75. Newton H, Pegg DE, Barrass R, et al. Osmotically inactive volume, hydraulic conductivity, and permeability to dimethyl sulphoxide of human mature oocytes. J Reprod Fertil 1999;117:27–33

76. Paynter SJ, Cooper A, Gregory L, et al. Permeability characteristics of human oocytes in the presence of the cryoprotectant dimethylsulphoxide. Hum Reprod 1999;14:2338–42

77. Paynter SJ, O'Neil L, Fuller BJ, et al. Membrane permeability of human oocytes in the presence of the cryoprotectant propane-1,2-diol. Fertil Steril 2001;75:532–8

78. Magistrini M, Szöllösi D. Effects of cold and isopropyl-N-phenylcarbamate on the second meiotic spindle of mouse oocytes. Eur J Cell Biol 1980;22:699–707

79. Martino A, Pollard JW, Leibo SP. Effect of chilling bovine oocytes on their developmental competence. Mol Reprod Dev 1996;45:503–12

80. Wu B, Tong J, Leibo SP. Effects of cooling germinal vesicle-stage bovine oocytes on meiotic spindle formation following in vitro maturation. Mol Reprod Dev 1999;54:388–95

81. Saunders KM, Parks JE. Effects of cryopreservation procedures on the cytology and fertilization rate of in vitro-matured bovine oocytes. Biol Reprod 1999;61:178–87

82. Martino A, Songsasen N, Leibo SP. Development into blastocysts of bovine oocytes cryopreserved by ultra-rapid cooling. Biol Reprod 1996;54:1059–69

83. Loskutoff NM, Johnson WH, Betteridge KJ. The developmental competence of bovine embryos with reduced cell numbers. Theriogenology 1993;39:95–107

84. Boiso I, Marti M, Santalo J, et al. A confocal microscopy analysis of the spindle and chromosome configurations of human oocytes cryopreserved at the germinal vesicle and metaphase II stage. Hum Reprod 2002;17:1885–91

85. Zenzes MT, Bielecki R, Casper RF, et al. Effects of chilling to 0°C on the morphology of meiotic spindles in human metaphase II oocytes. Fertil Steril 2001;75:769–77

86. Songsasen N, Yu IJ, Ratterree MS, et al. Effect of chilling on the organization of tubulin and chromosomes in rhesus monkey oocytes. Fertil Steril 2002;77:818–25

87. Mazur P, Cole KW, Hall JW, et al. Cryobiological preservation of Drosophila embryos. Science 1992;258:1932–5

88. Steponkus PL, Myers SP, Lynch DV, et al. Cryopreservation of Drosophila melanogaster embryos. Nature 1990;345:170–2

89. Kleinfeld AM. Current views of membrane structure. Current Topics in Membranes and Transport 1987;29:1–27

90. Jain MK. Introduction to Biological Membranes. New York: John Wiley & Sons, 1988:423 pp.

91. Gennis RB. Biomembranes. New York: Springer-Verlag, 1989:553 pp.

92. Cooper RA. Influence of increased membrane cholesterol on increased membrane fluidity and cell function in human red blood cells. J Supramol Struct 1978;8:413–30

93. Yeagle PL. Cholesterol and the cell membrane. Biochim Biophys Acta 1985;822:267–87

94. Edidin M. Rotational and lateral diffusion of membrane proteins and lipids: phenomena and function. Current Topics in Membranes and Transport 1987;29:91–127

95. Edidin M. In Glaser R, ed. *Biophysics of the Cell Surface*. Berlin: Springer-Verlag, 1990: 45–59

96. Perk K, Frei YF, Herz A. Osmotic fragility of red blood cells of young and mature domestic and laboratory animals. *Am J Vet Res* 1964; 25:1241–8

97. McIntyre JA, Gilula NB, Karnovsky MJ. Cryoprotectant-induced redistribution of intramembranous particles in mouse lymphocytes. *J Cell Biol* 1974;60:192–203

98. Furcht LT, Scott RE. Modulation of the distribution of plasma membrane intramembranous particles in contact-inhibited and transformed cells. *Biochim Biophys Acta* 1975; 401:213–20

99. Vincent C, Garnier V, Heyman Y, *et al.* Solvent effects on cytoskeletal organization and *in vivo* survival after freezing of rabbit oocytes. *J Reprod Fertil* 1989;87:809–20

100. De Leeuw FE, De Leeuw AM, Den Daas JH, *et al.* Effects of various cryoprotective agents and membrane-stabilizing compounds on bull sperm membrane integrity after cooling and freezing. *Cryobiology* 1993;30:32–44

101. Vajta G, Booth PJ, Holm P, *et al.* Successful vitrification of early stage bovine *in vitro* produced embryos with the open pulled straw (OPS) method. *Cryo Letters* 1997;18:191–5

102. Vajta G, Holm P, Kuwayama M, *et al.* Open pulled straw (OPS) vitrification: a new way to reduce cryoinjuries of bovine ova and embryos. *Mol Reprod Dev* 1998;51:53–8

103. Le Gal F, De Roover R, Verhaeghe B, *et al.* Development of vitrified matured cattle oocytes after thawing and culture *in vitro*. *Vet Rec* 2000;146:469–71

104. Lane M, Gardner DK. Vitrification of mouse oocytes using a nylon loop. *Mol Reprod Dev* 2001;58:342–7

105. Fabbri R, Porcu E, Marsella T, *et al.* Technical aspects of oocyte cryopreservation. *Mol Cell Endocrinol* 2000;169:39–42

106. Fabbri R, Porcu E, Marsella T, *et al.* Human oocyte cryopreservation: new perspectives regarding oocyte survival. *Hum Reprod* 2001;16:411–16

107. Stachecki JJ, Cohen J, Willadsen SM. Cryopreservation of unfertilized mouse oocytes: the effect of replacing sodium with choline in the freezing medium. *Cryobiology* 1998;37:346–54

108. Stachecki JJ, Cohen J, Schimmel T, *et al.* Fetal development of mouse oocytes and zygotes cryopreserved in a nonconventional freezing medium. *Cryobiology* 2002;44:5–13

109. Liebermann J, Nawroth F, Isachenko V, *et al.* Potential importance of vitrification in reproductive medicine. *Biol Reprod* 2002;67: 1671–80

110. Hong SW, Chung HM, Lim JM, *et al.* Improved human oocyte development after vitrification: a comparison of thawing methods. *Fertil Steril* 1999;72:142–6

111. Yoon HJ, Moon JH, Son WY, *et al.* The survival and fertilization of human MII-stage oocytes cryopreserved by vitrification. *Fertil Steril* 2002;78:S14

112. Vajta G. Vitrification of the oocytes and embryos of domestic animals. *Anim Reprod Sci* 2000;60–61:357–64

113. Lane M, Bavister BD, Lyons EA, *et al.* Containerless vitrification of mammalian oocytes. *Nat Biotechnol* 1999;17:1234–6

114. Reed ML, Lane M, Gardner DK, *et al.* Vitrification of human blastocysts using the cryoloop method: successful clinical application and birth of offspring. *J Assist Reprod Genet* 2002;19:304–630

115. Eroglu A, Russo MJ, Bieganski R, *et al.* Intracellular trehalose improves the survival of cryopreserved mammalian cells. *Nat Biotechnol* 2000;18:163–7

116. Eroglu A, Toner M, Toth TL. Beneficial effect of microinjected trehalose on the cryosurvival of human oocytes. *Fertil Steril* 2002;77:152–8

117. Eroglu A, Lawitts JA, Toner M, *et al.* Quantitative microinjection of trehalose into mouse oocytes and zygotes, and its effect on development. *Cryobiology* 2003;46:121–34

Cryobanking of ovarian and testicular tissue for children and young adults

12

S. S. Kim, H. Yin and R. G. Gosden

INTRODUCTION

In recent decades, advances in cancer treatment have resulted in a dramatic increase in the long-term survival and cure of many children and young adult patients. Aggressive treatment can, however, cause premature gonadal failure and sterility. Indeed, most patients undergoing bone marrow transplantation lose fertility as a result of destruction of germ cells by alkylating agents at high doses and/or ionizing radiation[1] (see Chapter 3). According to a mathematical model, a 90% reduction of the germ cell population before the age of 14 years would result in permanent ovarian failure by 27 years of age[2]. Male germ cells are also highly susceptible to chemotherapy and irradiation, although a few surviving spermatogonia are theoretically sufficient to repopulate the testes and restore sperm production. Where the risks of gonadal failure after intensive cancer therapy are high, timely consideration of all the options for safeguarding fertility is advisable.

Semen banking is a relatively robust and effective safeguard for male fertility[3] but, although this option is routinely offered, it does not guarantee success. Disease processes *per se* may affect sperm numbers and quality, and some men are unable to produce semen before cancer treatment commences. What is more, semen banking is not an option for prepubertal boys. Intracytoplasmic sperm injection (ICSI) has substantially improved the fertility potential of poor-quality or oligospermic specimens. In the future, germ cell transplantation[4,5] and/or testicular tissue

transplantation after cryopreservation[6,7] may prove to be practicable strategies for preserving fertility in boys. Further ahead, it may be possible to produce enough spermatozoa for ICSI by culturing germ cells after low-temperature storage.

Although there are several options for preserving female fertility, none are as reliable as sperm banking in men and all require invasive procedures and/or drugs. Cryopreservation of embryos is a well-established technique with a relatively good efficiency, but requires ovarian stimulation followed by *in vitro* fertilization (IVF), which is a lengthy protocol. This choice may delay cancer treatment, and could be risky for some patients. It is definitely not an option for prepubertal girls, and is often unacceptable to women who do not want to use donor spermatozoa to fertilize their eggs. In addition, exposure to a high estrogen milieu during ovarian stimulation is undesirable when patients have estrogen-sensitive tumors. Ethical and legal issues with embryo storage generate additional concerns, not least the disposal of embryos should the patient die. Nevertheless, it is prudent to consider embryo freezing as a primary option for fertility conservation in women who have a partner and enough time to undergo an IVF cycle (see Chapter 8).

Cryopreservation of mature oocytes is an alternative to embryo storage, but the prospects of pregnancy are low if only one treatment cycle is available[8]. Mature human oocytes are extremely sensitive to temperature

Table 1 Ovarian tissue cryobanking

Advantages	Disadvantages
Abundant germ cells	Requires grafting or follicle
Smaller, dormant, less	culture to produce
differentiated oocyte	mature gametes
Lack of spindle and zona	Optimal freezing
pellucida	conditions may differ
Opportunity for repairing	between constituent
damage during growth	cell types
No delay in cancer	Requires surgical
treatment	procedures

changes (even chilling above 0°C) and have limited capacity for repairing cytoplasmic damage. Cryoprotective agents (CPAs) and/or ice crystal formation during a freeze–thaw procedure can lead to depolymerization of the meiotic spindle and, consequently, to aneuploidy in oocytes and embryos[9,10]. Zona hardening can also occur as a result of premature release of cortical granules from the ooplasm when oocytes are chilled or exposed to certain types of CPA[11], although this problem is circumvented using ICSI. Of course, this strategy requires ovarian stimulation and follicle aspiration which can delay cancer therapy.

Cryopreservation of ovarian tissue has several advantages and carries fewer ethical dilemmas (Table 1). In this procedure, hundreds of immature oocytes can be cryopreserved *in situ* without the necessity for ovarian stimulation. Immature oocytes are small, relatively quiescent and lack a zona pellucida or cortical granules[12], as well as possessing other characteristics which make them more tolerant to freezing and thawing than mature oocytes. In addition, autografting of frozen–thawed tissue can restore endocrine as well as gametogenic functions of the ovary.

The efficacy of treatment with gonadotropin releasing hormone analogs to protect the gonads from cytotoxic cancer therapy is controversial and is discussed elsewhere (see Chapter 5). Another possible *in vivo* strategy for preserving female fertility is the use of anti-apoptotic agents, such as sphingosine-1-phosphate, whose protective effects on irradiated female germ cells have been demonstrated in mice[13,14] (see Chapter 4). At present,

ovarian tissue cryobanking is a more practical strategy for fertility preservation for children and young adults, and is already being tested in a few centers on an experimental basis. Testicular tissue cryobanking is the complementary strategy for males, but will not be discussed in as much depth because it is at an earlier stage of development.

HISTORICAL BACKGROUND

The potential of gonadal tissue banking for fertility conservation has only recently been fully realized. Although gonadal tissue transplantation has been performed for more than a century in Europe and China, it was not practicable to cryopreserve tissue until the discovery of CPAs in 1948. Credit for the first successful testicular transplant should probably go to the Göettingen biologist, A. Berthold, in the mid-nineteenth century. Paul Bert pioneered ovarian transplantation experiments with rabbits in 1863. Although initial results were disappointing, other investigators refined the technique and, in 1895, the first human ovarian transplant was reported by a New York surgeon in a woman suffering from ovarian failure[15]. Today, scientific hindsight reveals the futility of allotransplants, which are rapidly rejected in animals[16]. In an era when long-term organ frozen storage was not feasible, auto-transplantation was hardly considered, but has now entered center stage.

The first studies of gonadal cryopreservation were performed in London some 50 years ago and proved successful despite crude freezing techniques by today's standards. Alan Parkes and his colleagues succeeded in restoring estrous cycles in rats that had been oophorectomized and grafted with frozen–thawed ovarian tissue[17,18]. These studies were all the more remarkable (and lucky) because the donors and recipients were not genetically matched from a highly inbred strain. The authors were able to demonstrate that small follicles were not only capable of surviving freezing, thawing and grafting, but could also grow to the Graafian stage, secrete estrogen and ovulate. In 1960, the same group reported that orthotopic isografting of frozen– thawed ovarian tissue in two strains of oophorectomized mice could restore fertility[19]. However, because there were no obvious applications at the time, interest in this technology waned and there was no further progress until the 1990s.

Two developments have rekindled interest in ovarian tissue banking. First, advances in cancer treatment have increased long-term cancer survivorship and, second, improvements in reproductive technology and cryotechnology. Ovarian cryobanking as a strategy to preserve fertility became perceived as a novel option after promising results using the sheep model[20]. This model was selected because the size and structure of ewe ovaries are much more comparable to human than rodent organs. In the first study, frozen–thawed strips of ovarian cortical tissue were autografted to the ovarian pedicles of six ovariectomized yearling lambs. The animals were mated and two pregnancies resulted in healthy lambs (one conceived after ovarian cryopreservation). Subsequently, the same group reported that normal estrous cycles were restored for at least 2 years after this procedure[21]. Recently, restoration of endocrine function after auto-transplantation of fresh or frozen and thawed ovarian tissue has been demonstrated in humans[22–25] (see Chapter 13). Follicles in frozen–thawed human ovarian tissue have also been grown to small antral sizes in SCID (severe combined immuno-deficient) mice by xenotransplantation[26,27].

TECHNICAL CHALLENGES OF TISSUE BANKING

Although gonadal tissue banking appears to hold promise for clinical application, there are many problems that need to be resolved (Table 2). This chapter discusses these problems, including freeze–thaw injury, CPA toxicity, ischemic injury, and safety for the woman and future child.

Optimization of freeze–thaw protocol

Unlike a uniform population of isolated cells, the heterogeneity of tissue presents a

Table 2 Unresolved issues in human ovarian transplantation

Patient selection and exclusion criteria
Optimization of freeze–thaw protocols
Optimal graft site(s)
Quality of oocytes matured in a graft
Efficacy of transplantation for restoration of fertility
Safety issues
Ischemia–reperfusion injury
Advantages of vitrification compared to conventional equilibrium cooling methods
Prospects for *in vitro* follicle culture

challenge for optimizing freezing and thawing. The physical parameters that determine viability after the freezing and thawing process, such as hydraulic conductivity, permeability to CPAs and activation energies, vary between cell types in a given tissue. Thus, a compromise has to be struck between the optimal dehydration time, cooling and thawing rates for each cell type in the tissue. Furthermore, tissue slices are rarely uniform in size, and their composition changes with age and other factors. Despite all these problems, gonadal tissue cryopreservation has been remarkably successful. The main danger is intracellular ice crystal formation and salt concentration[28]. Potentially the most damaging phase of freezing is during cooling between −10 and −40°C, especially when the liquid phase is supercooled. To minimize cryoinjury, cooling rates need to be fast enough to reduce exposure of cells to high intracellular concentrations of electrolytes, but they should be slow enough to dehydrate cells and avoid intracellular ice formation. For thawing, significantly more pregnancies were achieved in mice after orthotopic ovarian transplantation when fast thawing was used rather than slow warming, in line with theoretical predictions[29]. Currently, the best follicular survival rate obtained in frozen–thawed human ovarian tissue is approximately 70–80%, with the majority of follicles morphologically normal by light microscopy[30,31]. However, distinctive ultrastructural changes can be observed in frozen–thawed tissue by electron microscopy (Figure 1) even when tissue damage is undetectable by

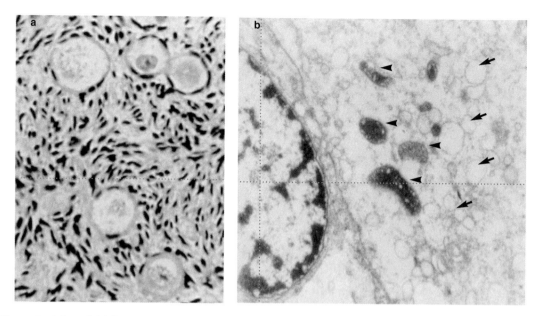

Figure 1 Primordial follicles and stromal cells in frozen–thawed ovarian tissue appeared to be relatively intact by light microscopy (a). However, transmission electron microscopy revealed extensive vacuolation throughout the cytoplasm as well as mitochondrial damage (b) Arrow, vacuolation; arrowhead, mitochondria

light microscopy[12,32]. These findings indicate the need to investigate structural and molecular consequences of the freezing and thawing process using techniques to reveal finer structural details than can be seen using conventional microscopy.

Liquids can solidify under conditions of high viscosity without ice crystal formation if ultra-rapid cooling and very high concentrations of CPAs are used[33]. Vitrification (glass formation) has some theoretical advantages for cryopreserving tissues and organs because it avoids intracellular and extracellular ice formation regardless of cell types and sizes. However, the concentrations of CPAs needed to achieve vitrification are potentially toxic (usually > 5 mol/l) and osmotically challenge the integrity of living cells. Toxicity can be reduced by minimizing the duration of exposure to CPAs and by low temperatures above the freezing point. Vitrification of ovarian tissue has achieved some success, although it is unclear whether this method is superior to conventional slow cooling–rapid thawing protocols[34]. Various methods have been proposed to reduce cryoinjury, including

choline substitution[35], intracellular trehalose[36] and antifreeze glycoproteins[37], but, while these strategies have merits for oocytes and embryos, application to intact tissue may be more problematic.

Toxicity of cryoprotectants

Permeability and toxicity are the two main factors affecting the efficacy of CPAs. It has been suggested that the optimum time of exposure to a CPA depends on its permeation and that detrimental effects after prolonged exposure are mainly a consequence of chemical toxicity[38]. As no CPA is totally free of toxicity, it is important to understand the physical properties of these agents. Although glycerol is perhaps the least toxic CPA, dimethyl-sulfoxide (DMSO), 1,2-propanediol (PROH) and ethylene glycol (EG) have proved to be effective and have superseded glycerol for many applications[39] (Figure 2).

The effects of CPAs on cellular viability and the character of toxicity are still largely unknown. Some CPAs promote increased intracellular $[Ca^{2+}]$ in oocytes[40], possibly by

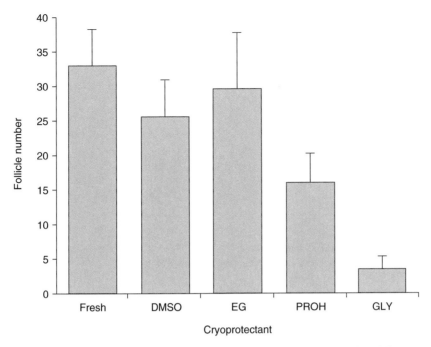

Figure 2 Comparison of the number of follicles in human ovarian tissue frozen–thawed in different cryoprotective solutions and grafted into SCID mice. $n = 23$–28 grafts per group. DMSO, dimethyl sulfoxide; EG, ethylene glycol; PROH, 1,2-propanediol; GLY, glycerol. Reproduced from reference 30, with permission

stimulating the release of $[Ca^{2+}]$ from storage sites in the mitochondria and endoplasmic reticulum. This effect could, in turn, activate intracellular phospholipases, proteases, ATPases and endonucleases, resulting in altered plasma membrane integrity, denaturation of cystolic proteins and leading to irreversible cell injury and apoptosis[41]. In addition to chemical effects, volume changes from osmotic stress may contribute to cytogenetic damage during cryopreservation of mature oocytes and, in extreme cases, cause cellular lysis[42]. As a rule of thumb, volume excursions should be restricted to < 30% for mammalian cells, although the tolerance of oocytes is not well-defined.

Rapid permeation of cells with cryoprotectants at low temperatures is desirable to minimize CPA toxicity. Multicellular tissues, however, require longer incubation times to reach equilibrium and, consequently, have a greater risk of toxic effects (especially for cells at the periphery). Balancing permeation

against CPA toxicity remains a major challenge for bulky tissues and organs.

Ischemic tissue damage

Ischemia–reperfusion injury is a major cause of compromised organ function after transplantation. In rodents, ovarian tissue slices are revascularized within 2–3 days after transplantation[43], but this process is likely to be more lengthy with human ovarian grafts, which are more bulky, fibrous and have a lower follicle density. Hence, human ovarian grafts are potentially more vulnerable to ischemia than murine grafts, and prolonged hypoxia causes follicular loss. In fact, more primordial follicles die during this phase than from freezing and thawing injury, but their survival after transplantation is highly variable and ranges from 5 to 50%[21,30,44]. Primordial follicles were surprisingly more resistant to ischemia than growing follicles or cortical stromal cells[45]. In theory, there are two ways to protect grafted tissue from

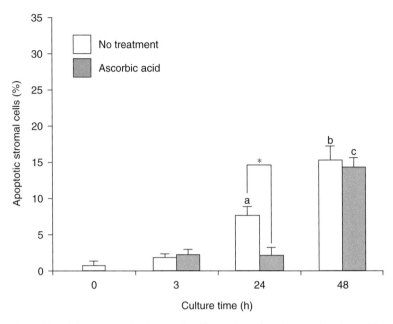

Figure 3 Effect of ascorbic acid on apoptosis of stromal cells in cultured bovine ovarian tissue. The apoptotic rate of stromal cells increased significantly after 24 h incubation compared to 0 h (a, b, c: $p < 0.05$). However, ascorbic acid treatment (50 µg/ml) reduced apoptosis of stromal cells in the 24 h incubation group (*$p < 0.05$). Reproduced with permission

ischemic injury: to alleviate hypoxic tissue damage by the use of antioxidants or anti-apoptotic agents, and to facilitate angiogenesis by manipulating the expression of angiogenic factors.

Nugent and colleagues[46] demonstrated that antioxidant treatment using vitamin E improved the survival of follicles in ovarian grafts by reducing ischemic injury. In a recent study, we used ascorbic acid as an antioxidant to study the protection of bovine ovarian grafts during ischemia[45] (Figure 3). Quantitative assessment of ischemic tissue damage was made by measuring the rates of oxygen consumption and apoptosis after incubating ovarian tissue at 37°C for different time periods ('ischemia time') with or without ascorbic acid. The results showed that the severity of tissue damage was correlated with the duration of ischemia regardless of ascorbic acid treatment. However, the treatment group showed significantly less apoptosis in ovarian cortical stroma after 24 hours of ischemia.

There are numerous angiogenic factors, such as vascular endothelial growth factors (VEGF), transforming growth factors (TGF), fibroblast growth factors and angiopoietin, all of which promote neovascularization. It is recognized that transcriptional regulation of key angiogenic growth factors is linked to the HIF (hypoxia inducible factor) system[47]. Angiogenesis is also stimulated directly or indirectly by gonadotropic hormones[48], and the ovary is particularly rich in angiogenic factors. Vascular invasion is accompanied by a 40- to 60-fold increase in the expression of mRNA for VEGF and TGF-β[43], which are probably stimulated by a combination of hypoxia and rising concentrations of gonadotropins after oophorectomy.

Exogenous gonadotropin administration may, therefore, upregulate endogenous VEGF and increase vascular ingrowth to influence graft survival. A recent murine study showed that gonadotropins given to either the donor or the recipient could increase the surviving number of developing follicles, but the magnitude was influenced by the timing of hormone stimulation[49]. The best result was obtained when the recipient was treated with gonadotropins (follicle stimulating hormone and luteinizing hormone) within 2 days before or after transplantation surgery. In contrast, administration of VEGF failed to promote graft survival or function in a primate study[50].

The ultimate strategy for preventing ischemic tissue injury is to use intact gonad transplantation with vascular anastomosis. The surgical technique is less of an obstacle than the technical challenge of freezing whole organs. As a step towards this goal, we reported limited success in rats in which the ovary and proximal reproductive tract were frozen–thawed before transplantation by vascular anastomosis[16,51]. A subsequent study of transplanted frozen–thawed rat testes was less successful[16]. Efforts are also under way using the sheep model[52], which, if successful, will provide much encouragement for application to the larger human ovary.

Risks of tissue banking and grafting

As gonadal tissue banking often requires long-term storage, it is necessary to use liquid nitrogen ($-196°C$) to halt biological deterioration. During storage, there is a very small risk that infectious agents, such as viruses, can be spread from sample to sample and cause contamination[53], although the risk is probably higher with gonad tissue than with embryos or oocytes. Double-bagging and/or storage in liquid nitrogen vapor potentially avoid this problem. Freeze-drying is unlikely to find applications for tissue, although it has been successful for mouse spermatozoa[54].

A more serious risk for cancer patients is if tissue harbors any malignant cells that can be transmitted back to the patient in an auto-transplant. Shaw and associates[55] reported that healthy AKR strain mice with fresh or cryo-banked grafted ovarian tissue from donor mice with lymphoma died of the disease within 2 to 3 weeks. Clinically, however, ovarian metastases are rare in 'common' cancers of young people, such as Wilms' tumor and Hodgkin's disease. The risk of transferring cancer cells depends on the disease type, activity, stage and the mass of malignant cells transferred. Kim and co-workers[56] reported

Table 3 Methods for detecting minimal residual disease (MRD)

MRD assay	Detection sensitivity*
Conventional cytology	$1–5 \times 10^3$
Immunohistochemistry	1×10^5 to 1×10^6
Flow cytometry	1×10^4 to 1×10^7
In vitro culture	Variable
Polymerase chain reaction (PCR)	1×10^5 to 1×10^7

*Each MRD assay has its respective limits of detection sensitivity. For example, cytology may not detect MRD if there are fewer than 1–5 cancer cells in 10^3 hematopoietic cells, but PCR can, even if only one tumor cell exists in 10^6 hematopoietic cells (because of its high detection sensitivity)

that ovarian tissue harvested from lymphoma patients with high-grade disease might be safe for auto-transplantation. They tested the safety of frozen–thawed human ovarian tissue from 18 lymphoma patients by xenografting to NOD (non-obese diabetic)/SCID mice. None of the animals grafted with ovarian tissue from lymphoma patients developed disease, whereas all positive control animals receiving lymph node tissue containing non-Hodgkin's lymphoma cells developed human B-cell lymphoma. Xenotransplantation of gonadal tissue from cancer patients could eliminate this risk of cancer transmission, but there is a theoretical risk of transmitting animal viruses or prions to patients. Wherever possible, it is important to prescreen for metastatic cancer cells in stored tissue, for which a number of techniques are available[57] (Table 3). A tumor-purging method using specific antibodies to clear cancer, which has been developed for hematopoietic stem cell transplantation, may be useful for safeguarding gonadal tissue transplants[58,59].

TECHNICAL ASPECTS OF OVARIAN TISSUE CRYOBANKING

Since growing follicles are lost during freezing and thawing, surviving follicles in frozen–thawed human ovarian tissue are predominantly at the primordial follicle stage. As

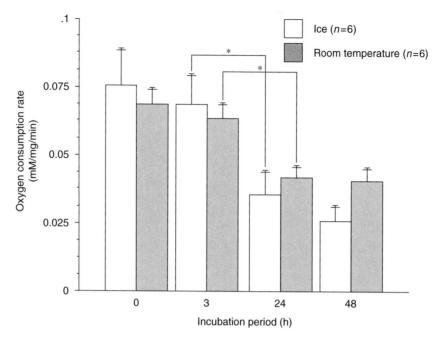

Figure 4 Comparison of ischemic tissue damage at two different transportation temperatures. There was no significant difference in oxygen metabolism when specimens were transported in 2 h either on ice or at room temperature. When comparing the oxygen consumption rates between each incubation period (ischemia time), a significant decrease after 24 h incubation was noticed (*p < 0.001)

already noted, primordial follicles have many advantages for ovarian tissue cryobanking.

Tissue collection

A major advantage of ovarian cryopreservation is that tissue can usually be collected with little delay, although the patient has to undergo a surgical procedure. In most cases, ovarian tissue can be collected using a laparoscopic technique, either oophorectomy or multiple ovarian biopsy. For an experienced laparoscopic surgeon, there is little difference between these two procedures in terms of either operation time or surgical difficulty. The choice of the surgical procedure can be determined by the risk of premature ovarian failure and the prognosis after cytotoxic cancer treatment. The density of primordial follicles varies between ovarian biopsies because primordial follicles are non-randomly distributed in the cortex[60]. A random biopsy may miss primordial follicle-dense areas, but

there are no external markers to guide the surgeon's choice. Some follicular loss also occurs during freezing and thawing, especially after grafting[12], and it is not possible to predict how long frozen–thawed ovarian tissue will function after transplantation. Certainly, the removal of a whole ovary offers a greater prospect of success because of the relatively larger number of follicles that can be stored and replaced.

Transportation time needs to be considered because of ischemia. Once the ovary is removed, it should be transported to the laboratory immediately in a buffered salt solution, such as Leibovitz L-15 medium. We found no difference in oxygen consumption when bovine ovarian tissue was transported on ice ($\sim 0°C$) or at room temperature ($\sim 20°C$) for 2 h, and respiratory activity was not compromised even after 3 h of additional incubation at 37°C[61] (Figure 4). However, if transportation time exceeds 4–5 h, it may be prudent to keep the specimen on ice.

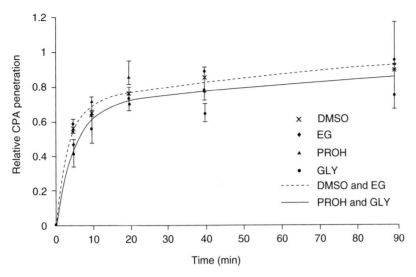

Figure 5 The rate of penetration of dimethyl sulfoxide (DMSO), ethylene glycol (EG), 1,2-propanediol (PROH) and glycerol (GLY) into human ovarian tissue at 4°C. Reproduced from reference 39, with permission

Choice of cryoprotective agent

CPAs are mandatory for successful cryopreservation. These agents protect cells from damage by ice crystals and high concentrations of solutes. They must be water-soluble, highly permeable to cell membranes (to minimize osmotic stress) and relatively non-toxic[62]. While many compounds have these properties, DMSO, PROH, EG and glycerol are most commonly used. The efficiency of these four CPAs has been compared by freeze–thawing and subsequently xenografting human ovarian tissue to immuno-deficient mice[30]. Based on histological criteria, DMSO, PROH and EG were much more effective than glycerol, which, although chemically less toxic, penetrates tissue slowly and causes large osmotic excursions. In a proton nuclear magnetic resonance spectroscopy study to compare the permeation rates of different CPAs, the best protocol for equilibrating human ovarian cortex was to incubate the tissue in 1.5 mol/l EG or DMSO for approximately 30 min at 4°C[39] (Figure 5). Alternatively, Gook and colleagues[31] have recommended a single step dehydration in PROH for 90 min at room temperature for the same type of tissue.

Compounds that do not penetrate cells (such as sugar molecules or proteins) can also help to protect against freeze–thaw damage. For ovarian tissue cryopreservation, sucrose and human serum albumin are commonly used as non-permeable CPAs. It appears that their addition enhances the cryoprotective effects of permeable CPAs, and sugar molecules can buffer osmotic stress during freezing and thawing. Macromolecules, such as albumin, antifreeze glycopeptide and polyvinylpyrrolidone, bind water and have a thermal hysteresis effect, and some proteins can stabilize cell membranes against denaturation by solutes.

Although PROH and EG are effective CPAs for ovarian tissue banking, DMSO has been widely used, but there are little data identifying the best CPA. For preparing the cryopreservation solution, the CPA is dissolved in a medium (e.g. Leibovitz L-15 medium, phosphate-buffered saline (PBS) or other culture medium buffered with HEPES (*N*-2-hydroxyethyl piperazine-*N*′-2-ethanesulfonic acid)) and non-permeable CPAs (e.g. sugar and macromolecules) are added. To reduce osmotic stress the tissue is taken up and down the osmotic gradient in equimolar steps.

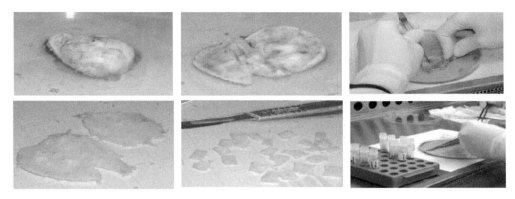

Figure 6 The human ovary was bisected and processed to make thin cortical sections before cryopreservation

Preparation of ovarian tissue

In the laboratory, the ovary is placed in a large Petri dish containing Leibovitz L-15 medium. The ovary is bisected and medullary tissue is removed with a scalpel. The ovarian tissue is usually prepared as thin sheets of ovarian cortex (1–2 mm in thickness), which are then cut into square sections of dimensions 5 mm × 5 mm to 10 mm × 10 mm (Figure 6). The cortical sections are transferred to the freezing medium in 1.8 ml cryovials with one or two sections per vial (or, preferably, larger volumes) and gently agitated for 30 min at 4°C to promote equilibration. Equilibration time can be reduced at higher temperatures, but this may increase the risk of toxicity.

Freezing and thawing of ovarian tissue

To date, the highest proportion of surviving primordial and primary follicles has been obtained by slow freezing/rapid thawing methods[29,63]. Here we summarize two protocols commonly used for ovarian tissue cryopreservation, although it should be recognized that other protocols exist and none has been fully optimized.

Modified Gosden's protocol[20]

As a freezing solution, 1.5 mol/l DMSO or EG is dissolved in Leibovitz L-15 medium with 0.1 mol/l sucrose and 1% human serum albumin. The equilibrated tissue in cryovials is cooled in an automated programmable freezer as follows:

(1) Start at 0°C and cool at 2°C/min to −7°C;

(2) Soak for 5 min before manual seeding;

(3) Seed manually at −7°C and hold for 5 min;

(4) Continue to cool at 0.3°C/min to −40°C;

(5) Cool at faster rate of 10°C/min to −120°C;

(6) Plunge into liquid nitrogen (−196°C) for storage.

When required, the frozen tissue is thawed rapidly (~100°C/min) and rehydrated gradually:

(1) Hold cryovials for 30 s in air at room temperature (to evaporate any liquid nitrogen in the tube and avoid an explosion);

(2) Place cryovials in a water bath at 30°C for 2–3 min and agitate vigorously;

(3) Wash tissue stepwise using prepared thawing solutions (TS1: 1.0 mol/l DMSO with 0.1 mol/l sucrose, TS2: 0.5 mol/l DMSO with 0.1 mol/l sucrose, TS3: 0.1 mol/l sucrose);

(4) Transfer to MEM medium containing 500 IU/ml penicillin G and 382 IU/ml streptomycin for 30 min at 37°C in the incubator (5% CO_2 in air).

The tissue is now ready for transplantation, and is held at 37°C. A piece of frozen–thawed ovarian tissue is usually saved for histological examination to confirm the presence of follicles and normal morphology.

Gook's protocol[31]

(1) Ovarian cortical slices are rinsed briefly in PBS and then dehydrated in 1.5 mol/l PROH and 0.1 mol/l sucrose for 90 min at room temperature. All freezing and thawing solutions contain 10 mg/ml human serum albumin in PBS.

(2) Slices are frozen at a slow rate (2°C/min from room temperature to −8°C, at which temperature ice nucleation is induced manually, followed by a further reduction of temperature to −30°C at a rate of 0.3°C/min and, finally, to −150°C at 50°C/min). The tube is plunged into liquid nitrogen.

(3) For thawing, the vials are placed in a water bath at 37°C for 2–3 min. CPA is removed by a stepwise reduction of PROH concentrations.

Guidelines for ovarian tissue banking

Considering the golden rule of medical practice, 'Do no harm', and that ovarian tissue banking is still in its infancy, the benefits and risks must be weighed carefully. All patients should be provided with counseling in which the current status of the technology is fully and accurately explained. At the same time, some details about ovarian tissue banking should be discussed, including the medical risks and the surgical procedure for tissue retrieval, efficacy of freezing and storage, and options for future use of the tissues. In addition, it is imperative to communicate with the patient's oncologist before and after the procedure.

Follicle numbers *in vivo* fall continuously after birth, and the rate of loss accelerates during the fourth decade of life. At a threshold of less than 1000 follicles, cyclic ovulations cease[62]. We presume that the functional life-span of ovarian grafts varies over time according to follicular status, except that the initial numbers are much lower than in an intact ovary of the same age. Considering these facts and that a majority of follicles is likely to be lost by ischemia[21], the prospects of successful auto-transplantation are low for women of advanced reproductive age or after treatment with gonadotoxic chemotherapy, as well as for those who are genetically predisposed to early menopause. In view of individual differences, it is perhaps inappropriate to have a fixed cut-off age before menopause, but it is helpful to assess ovarian reserve with routine endocrine tests (e.g. FSH, estradiol) as well as pelvic ultrasound to guide clinical decision-making. A complete blood count and platelet count must be obtained before the surgical procedure.

The safety of auto-transplantation of human ovarian tissue is crucial and, although there is some reassurance for lymphoma patients[56], the risks for other cancer patients have not been investigated. At present, the type of malignancy and the prognosis are two prime considerations determining which patients are suitable for this procedure.

In childhood, the uterus is very vulnerable to high-dose irradiation, which can cause uterine damage and lead to infertility, miscarriage and preterm labor[64]. Therefore, the uterine factor should be considered before storing ovarian tissue for children who need to undergo high-dose radiotherapy. The physical and psychological conditions of the patient are also important factors to consider. Until there is a consensus about ovarian tissue cryobanking, it should be offered selectively and only to women who are at highest risk of losing fertility and with a good long-term prognosis.

Indications for ovarian tissue cryobanking

Certain malignancies of young adults and children, such as Hodgkin's lymphoma or Wilms' tumor or sarcoma in its early stages, are suitable for ovarian tissue banking because of the extremely low risk of ovarian metastases and good prognosis. However, disseminated or systemic malignancies, such as leukemia or advanced sarcoma, may be better excluded unless reliable screening methods become available or until follicle culture techniques are perfected.

Breast cancer is the most common cancer in women and about 5% of all invasive breast cancers occur under the age of 40 years[65,66]. The demand for fertility conservation for young women with breast cancer is high, as aggressive treatment with chemotherapy and radiation therapy can result in ovarian failure. The high estrogen milieu of pregnancy or ovulation induction with gonadotropins might stimulate cancer cell growth in estrogen-dependent breast cancer, although 80% of breast cancer in young women is estrogen receptor-negative[67]. In ovaries from therapeutic oophorectomy for advanced breast cancer, the incidence of microscopic metastases is about one in four[68], which is far from a negligible risk.

Cervical cancer in women of reproductive age is not common. However, ovarian tissue cryobanking can be useful for young women before treatment with high-dose pelvic irradiation, as ovarian involvement is extremely rare and prognosis after treatment is relatively good especially in stage I or II. Theoretically, pregnancy can be achieved by surrogacy, even if the uterus is removed surgically or damaged by radiation.

Ovarian tissue banking will be most useful for patients who need to undergo bone marrow transplantation and peripheral blood stem cell transplantation. The use of hematopoietic cell transplantation is no longer limited to leukemia and lymphoma, but has been extended to solid malignant tumors, such as breast cancer[69], and non-malignant conditions, such as lupus, rheumatoid arthritis, aplastic anemia and sickle cell disease[70]. Unfortunately, preparatory regimens using high doses of alkylating agents and/or irradiation are highly gonadotoxic and often result in premature ovarian failure. When 708 postpubertal women treated with bone marrow transplantation were followed for 12 years, 110 recovered ovarian function and 32 became pregnant[71]. Furthermore, only one out of 73 patients recovered ovarian function and no pregnancy occurred when the busulfan and cyclophosphamide regimen was used for preparing for bone marrow transplantation. Clearly, alkylating agents are highly gonadotoxic (see Chapter 2).

When the ovary cannot be saved due to a large, benign ovarian cyst or to endometriosis, healthy portions of ovarian cortex might be rescued and cryopreserved for possible future use. Although controversial, there are several other indications for ovarian tissue cryobanking that include prophylactic oophorectomy for familial ovarian cancer, ovarian ablation with breast cancer, and familial and genetic causes of premature ovarian failure, such as Turner's syndrome.

STRATEGIES FOR MATURATION OF FOLLICLES FROM FROZEN-STORED OVARIAN TISSUE

More research will be required before optimal use can be made of frozen-stored ovarian tissue for fertility, but, at least in theory, there are three strategies available: auto-transplantation, xenotransplantation and in vitro maturation (Figure 7). Auto-transplantation is already being practiced on a tentative clinical basis, but xenotransplantation has been used purely for experimental purposes. The most desirable strategy is to develop a culture system to support the growth and maturation of immature oocytes in vitro, because embryos could then be transferred free of disease to the patient. The culture techniques and media presently available are inadequate to sustain the long period of follicular development required (see Chapter 14).

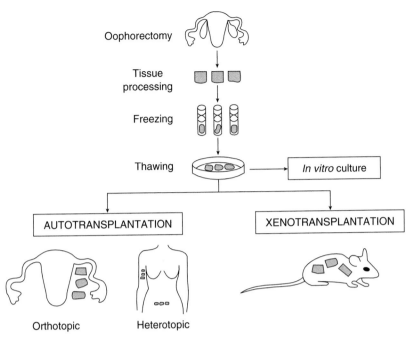

Figure 7 Strategies for development of immature oocytes in cryopreserved ovarian tissue. Reproduced from reference 12, with permission

Auto-transplantation

Frozen–thawed ovarian tissue can be autografted either orthotopically or heterotopically. The attraction of orthotopic transplantation is the restoration of normal reproductive function and natural conception. However, the relatively short lifespan of frozen–thawed ovarian grafts is of concern. Where few follicles remain and early graft exhaustion is expected, it may be more reasonable to use a heterotopic site with a rich vascular bed. Ovarian tissue has been transplanted to a number of heterotopic sites, including the subcutaneous tissue of the left axilla[72], where the graft can resume hormonal function and follicular growth (see Chapter 13).

There have been reports of successful auto-transplantation of human ovarian tissue, the first case being in a 29-year-old woman to relieve menopausal symptoms[22]. The second orthotopic transplant resulted in the return of endocrine function for 2 months in a 36-year-old woman cured of Hodgkin's lymphoma[24]. Two other cases were reported with heterotopic

transplants of fresh or thawed human ovarian tissue. Oktay and associates[23] performed ovarian auto-transplantation to the forearm on two women to restore hormonal function and follicular growth. Callejo and colleagues[25] also reported the re-establishment of ovarian hormonal secretion, albeit of a short duration, after heterotopic transplantation of fresh or frozen–thawed ovarian tissue in four women aged 46–49 years. Furthermore, Kim and co-workers[73] obtained evidence of spontaneous ovulation in human ovarian grafts after cryopreservation and heterotopic auto-transplantation into the space between the rectus sheath and the rectus muscle.

Xenotransplantation

Is xenotransplantation an alternative to auto-transplantation? It has been already demonstrated that grafting of ovarian tissue from the cat, sheep, African elephant, monkey and human to immuno-deficient mice can support follicular development up to the antral stage[74-79]. Also, generation of live young from xenografted rodent ovaries has been achieved[80]. The ovulatory capacity of human follicles in xenografts was indicated by the formation of morphologically normal corpora lutea and elevated serum progesterone in host animals[26]. Since follicles have never grown larger than 5–6 mm in diameter, the oocytes are unlikely to be fully competent, which presents another obstacle to clinical application of xenotransplantation.

In vitro maturation

Growth and maturation of germ cells from the primordial follicle stage is a long and complex process which has only been achieved in culture in a mouse model[81,82]. Whilst it is feasible in principle for human follicles, culture technology is still at a rudimentary phase and great care will be required to ensure not only that gametes become fertile in vitro but also that the correct epigenetic marking occurs. More details can be found elsewhere (Chapter 14).

TESTICULAR TISSUE BANKING

The transplantation of testicular tissue has been practiced for almost a century. It started with murky origins in 'rejuvenation science' and a dubious belief that somatic aging was primarily due to waning testicular hormone levels. This false theory encouraged entrepreneurial surgeons and quacks to transplant testicular tissue from young donor males or even from animals to reverse senescence in old men[83]. This quasi-science was discredited in the 1930s and 1940s by the advance of transplantation immunity and gerontology. Interest in testicular tissue transplantation faded with the absence of applications and so, in consequence, did frozen testis banking. But in the past decade – in parallel with the new hopes for ovarian transplantation and cryopreservation – there has been renewed interest in storing testicular tissue for fertility preservation. What was the basis for this development, and why was frozen semen banking not sufficient?

Semen banking is a mature and valuable technology, but it is not always reliable. There is much variability between men in the tolerance of spermatozoa to freezing and thawing injury. Second, it is not uncommon for a cancer patient requiring fertility preservation before sterilizing chemotherapy to fail to produce a satisfactory and timely specimen[84]. Fortunately, up to half of men who are azoospermic can eventually achieve genetic parenthood through testicular sperm extraction and ICSI of their partner's oocytes[85]. For these reasons, and for the sake of prepubertal boys undergoing sterilizing treatment, two other options are being investigated: the extraction of spermatogonial stem cells for cryopreservation and transplantation (see Chapter 10); and testicular tissue banking. It is too early to predict which strategy will eventually turn out to be most successful and, therefore, research is on dual tracks. Some centers that are already offering banking for ovarian tissue are likely to do the same for testicular tissue.

The chief hope vested in male stem cell banking is in restoring natural fertility by recolonizing the testicular tubules with proliferating germ cells. There is no option for xenogeneic transplantation (except in experimental biology) because, although primate spermatogonia survive in murine testicular tubules, they do not restore spermatogenesis[86]. If stem cell auto-transplantation is proven to be clinically successful, other options may not be needed. But, while doubts remain it is desirable to investigate tissue banking and transplantation as an alternative. Besides it has real prospects of success, although carrying the drawback of requiring assisted reproduction and requiring the female partner to undergo burdensome medical procedures to conceive.

The modern era of testicular frozen banking and transplantation originated in the 1950s in London, UK. The group was led by Alan Parkes and his wife, Ruth Deanesly, and included Christopher Polge, James Lovelock and Audrey Smith. They were investigating the tolerance of various cells and tissues to temperatures below freezing point. In 1954, they reported results for rat testes which had been cooled slowly to −79°C in glycerol, thawed rapidly and grafted into animals after removing the CPA[87]. We now know that glycerol is not an ideal CPA for this tissue, but the group nonetheless achieved a striking result. Grafts from immature testes survived freezing and thawing and initiated spermatogenesis in the host. In those days, however, it was not possible to test the fertility of the sperm using IVF techniques.

The first reinvestigation of this technique was reported nearly 50 years later[88], being prompted by remarkable progress made in the treatment of pediatric cancer. The results of Deanesly were confirmed using immature and adult inbred mice. Later, it was found that spermatogenesis and near-normal serum testosterone levels were restored by transplanting small pieces of mouse, hamster and neonatal marmoset monkey testes either autologously or by xenografting[6]. Another study from groups in Philadelphia and Münster (Germany) used the *nude* mouse as an incubator for subcutaneous xenografts from mice, pig and goat testes[7]. This indicated that testicular tissue from any species can probably resume or initiate function in an immuno-deficient host animal. Subsequently, Schlatt and co-workers[89] produced live-born young after recovering sperm from fresh, neonatal mouse grafts in *nude* mice using donor oocytes. Since there were modest numbers of mature sperm present, ICSI was required for efficient fertilization.

Testicular tissue banking and transplantation is attractive because of its simplicity and similarity to established ovarian techniques. It involves small fragments of testes (~ 1 mm^3) prepared in HEPES-buffered or Leibovitz L-15 medium by trimming with a scalpel. These slices are suitable for cryopreservation using the same slow cooling–rapid thawing protocol as used for ovaries (see above). The tissue is equilibrated for 20 min in a CPA mixture on ice containing DMSO, sucrose and serum protein and cooled in cryovials using an automated freezer. The optimal CPA mixture has not yet been identified, although we now favor EG, because of its low toxicity and high permeability, and a monosaccharide, such as fructose, which is less viscous than sucrose for the same molar concentration. After cooling to liquid nitrogen temperatures (with ice nucleation induced at −7°C) and rapid thawing, the tissue is washed by step dilutions of CPA (1.5 → 1.0 → 0.5 → 0 mol/l). Vitrification has not been tested to date. In principle, ultra-rapid freezing using very high concentrations of CPA may not seem very promising, although recent successes with ovarian tissue may be encouraging[90].

The grafting process is straightforward and usually performed subcutaneously to the belly or back where the temperatures are similar to those in the scrotum. In only one study has the scrotum been used for transplantation, and this involved cells reaggregated after complete enzymatic disaggregation of testicular tissue (tubules reformed and a few contained meiotic germ cells)[88]. The procedures are carried out under general anesthesia and, in the case of *nude* or SCID mice, under strict conditions of asepsis. Subcutaneous grafts must be anchored to the body wall to avoid displacement, and adhesion and angiogenesis are promoted if the site is scarified.

Graft viability can be assessed *in vitro* by oxygen consumption or *in vivo* after grafting. Histology is not a very effective tool for revealing acute cellular damage. Transmission electron microscopy is more valuable for revealing subtle membrane and mitochondrial damage, although it is more laborious and usually only minute samples can be studied[91]. The gold standard for assessing the technique is fertility, but this requires IVF. Spermatozoa can be recovered from syngeneic or xenogeneic transplants using mild collagenase digestion, with mincing or tearing tissue between needle points. Grafts from immature animals require 2–3 months to produce mature sperm, depending on the species. In the future, culture technology may enable the evaluation of frozen-banked tissue without the need for grafting. The preservation of whole organs for transplantation using vascular anastomosis and vasovasostomy is still in the early stages of development but may eventually become feasible[16].

PROSPECT

Surprise is sometimes expressed at the rapid development of gonadal tissue cryopreservation and transplantation and its tentative application for patient care. The cryopreservation techniques, however, rest on principles and protocols that are well-established for other cells and tissues. The greater challenge is to realize the fertility potential of the frozen material, although there is still a need for improving freezing and thawing protocols, including evaluation of vitrification. Tissue transplantation is a relatively inefficient procedure and research needs to focus on ways of minimizing the loss of cells from ischemia and safeguarding patients from risks of residual cancer cells. These goals could be achieved by producing mature gametes from immature germ cells in culture, but the prospects of effectively and safely implementing such a technology are still remote. Meanwhile, transplantation of cryopreserved ovarian tissue offers some hope for patients, including children, who wish to preserve their fertility.

References

1. Sanders JE, Buckner CD, Amos D, et al. Ovarian function following marrow transplantation for aplastic anemia or leukemia. *J Clin Oncol* 1988;6:813–18

2. Faddy MJ, Gosden RG, Gougeon A, et al. Accelerated disappearance of ovarian follicles in midlife: implications for forecasting menopause. *Hum Reprod* 1992;7:1342–6

3. Sanger WG, Armitage JO, Schmidt MA. Feasibility of semen cryopreservation in patients with malignant disease. *J Am Med Assoc* 1980;244:789–90

4. Brinster RL, Zimmermann JW. Spermatogenesis following male germ-cell transplantation. *Proc Natl Acad Sci USA* 1994;91:11298–302

5. Schlatt S, Rosiepen G, Weinbauer GF, et al. Germ cell transfer into rat, bovine, monkey and human testes. *Hum Reprod* 1999;14:144–50

6. Schlatt S, Kim SS, Gosden R. Spermatogenesis and steroidogenesis in mouse, hamster and monkey testicular tissue after cryopreservation and heterotopic grafting to castrated hosts. *Reproduction* 2002;124:339–46

7. Honaramooz A, Snedaker A, Boiani M, et al. Sperm from neonatal mammalian testes grafted in mice. *Nature* 2002;418:778–81

8. Porcu E. Oocyte freezing. *Semin Reprod Med* 2001;19:221–30

9. Pickering SJ, Braude PR, Johnson MH, et al. Transient cooling to room temperature can cause irreversible disruption of the meiotic spindle in the human oocyte. *Fertil Steril* 1990;54:102–8

10. Baka SG, Toth TL, Veeks LL, et al. Evaluation of the spindle apparatus of *in vitro* matured oocytes following cryopreservation. *Hum Reprod* 1995;10:1816–20

11. Pickering SJ, Braude PR, Johnson MH. Cryoprotection of human oocytes: inappropriate exposure to DMSO reduces fertilization rates. *Hum Reprod* 1991;6:142–3

12. Kim SS, Battaglia DE, Soules MR. The future of human ovarian cryopreservation and transplantation: fertility and beyond. *Fertil Steril* 2001;75:1049–56

13. Perez GI, Knudson CM, Leykin L, et al. Apoptosis-associated signaling pathways are required for chemotherapy-mediated female germ cell destruction. *Nat Med* 1997;3:1228–32

14. Morita Y, Perez GI, Paris F, et al. Oocyte apoptosis is suppressed by disruption of the acid sphingomyelinase gene or by sphingosine-1-phosphate therapy. *Nat Med* 2000;6:1109–14

15. Morris RT. The ovarian graft. *New York Med J* 1895;62:436

16. Yin H, Wang X, Kim SS, et al. Transplantation of intact rat gonads using vascular anastomosis: effects of cryopreservation, ischaemia and genotype. *Hum Reprod* 2003;18:1165–72

17. Parkes AS, Smith AU. Regeneration of rat ovarian tissue grafted after exposure to low temperature. *Proc R Soc Lond B Biol Sci* 1953;140:455–70

18. Deanesly R. Immature rat ovaries grafted after freezing and thawing. *J Endocrinol* 1954;11:197–200

19. Parrott DM. The fertility of mice with orthotopic ovarian grafts derived from frozen tissue. *J Reprod Fertil* 1960;1:230–41

20. Gosden RG, Baird DT, Wade JC, Webb R. Restoration of fertility to oophorectomized sheep by ovarian autografts stored at −196 degrees C. *Hum Reprod* 1994;9:597–603

21. Baird DT, Webb R, Campbell BK, *et al*. Long-term ovarian function in sheep after ovariectomy and transplantation of autografts stored at −196°C. *Endocrinology* 1999;140:462–71

22. Oktay K, Karlikaya G. Ovarian function after transplantation of frozen, banked autologous ovarian tissue. *N Engl J Med* 2000;42:1919

23. Oktay K, Economos K, Kan M, *et al*. Endocrine function and oocyte retrieval after autologous transplantation of ovarian cortical strips to the forearm. *J Am Med Assoc* 2001;286:1490–3

24. Radford JA, Lieberman BA, Brison DR, *et al*. Orthotopic reimplantation of cryopreserved ovarian cortical strips after high-dose chemotherapy for Hodgkin's lymphoma. *Lancet* 2001;357:1172–5

25. Callejo J, Salvador C, Miralles A, *et al*. Long-term ovarian function evaluation after autografting by implantation with fresh and frozen–thawed human ovarian tissue. *J Clin Endocrinol Metab* 2001;86:4489–94

26. Kim SS, Soules MR, Battaglia DE. Follicular development, ovulation, and corpus luteum formation in cryopreserved human ovarian tissue after xenotransplantation. *Fertil Steril* 2002;78:77–82

27. Gook DA, Edgar DH, Borg J, *et al*. Oocyte maturation, follicle rupture and luteinization in human cryopreserved ovarian tissue following xenografting. *Hum Reprod* 2003;18:1772–81

28. Mazur P. Kinetics of water loss from cells at subzero temperatures and the likelihood of intracellular freezing. *J Gen Physiol* 1963;47:347–69

29. Cox SL, Shaw J, Jenkin G. Transplantation of cryopreserved fetal ovarian tissue to adult recipients in mice. *J Reprod Fertil* 1996;107:315–22

30. Newton H, Aubard Y, Rutherford A, *et al*. Low temperature storage and grafting of human ovarian tissue. *Hum Reprod* 1996;11:1487–91

31. Gook DA, Edgar DH, Stern C. Effect of cooling rate and dehydration regimen on the histological appearance of human ovarian cortex following cryopreservation in 1,2–propanediol. *Hum Reprod* 1999;14:2061–8

32. Nisolle M, Casanas-Roux F, Qu J, *et al*. Histologic and ultrastructural evaluation of fresh and frozen–thawed human ovarian xenografts in nude mice. *Fertil Steril* 2000;74:122–9

33. Fahy GM, MacFarlane DR, Angell CA, *et al*. Vitrification as an approach to cryopreservation. *Cryobiology* 1984;21:407–26

34. Yin H, Kim SS, Fisher J, *et al*. Investigation of optimal conditions for equilibrating ovarian tissue with ethylene glycol prior to vitrification. *Fertil Steril* 2001;76:S101

35. Stachecki JJ, Willadsen SM. Cryopreservation of mouse oocytes using a medium with low sodium content: effect of plunge temperature. *Cryobiology* 2000;40:4–12

36. Eroglu A, Toner M, Toth TL. Beneficial effect of microinjected trehalose on the cryosurvival of human oocytes. *Fertil Steril* 2002;77:152–8

37. Rubinsky B, Arav A, Devries AL. The cryoprotective effect of antifreeze glycopeptides from Antartic fishes. *Cryobiology* 1992;29:69–79

38. Van de Abbeel E, van der Elst J, van der Linden M, *et al*. High survival rate of one-cell mouse embryos cooled rapidly to −196 degrees C after exposure to a propylene glycol–dimethylsulfoxide–sucrose solution. *Cryobiology* 1997;34:1–12

39. Newton H, Fisher J, Arnold JR, *et al*. Permeation of human ovarian tissue with cryoprotective agents in preparation for cryopreservation. *Hum Reprod* 1998;13:376–80

40. Litkouhi B, Winlow W, Gosden RG. Impact of cryoprotective agent exposure on intracellular calcium in mouse oocytes at metaphase II. *Cryo Letters* 1999;20:353–62

41. Picton HM, Kim SS, Gosden RG. Cryopreservation of gonadal tissue and cells. *Br Med Bull* 2000;56:603–15

42. Newton H, Pegg DE, Barrass R, *et al*. Osmotically inactive volume, hydraulic conductivity, and permeability to dimethyl sulphoxide of human mature oocytes. *J Reprod Fertil* 1999;117:27–33

43. Dissen GA, Lara HE, Fahrenbach WH, *et al*. Immature rat ovaries become revascularized rapidly after autotransplantation and show a gonadotropin-dependent increase in angiogenic factor gene expression. *Endocrinology* 1994;134:1146–54

44. Aubard Y, Piver P, Cogni Y, *et al*. Orthotopic and heterotopic autografts of frozen–thawed ovarian cortex in sheep. *Hum Reprod* 1999;14:2149–54

45. Kim SS, Kang HK, Lee HH, *et al*. A model to assess the protective effect of antioxidants from ischemia after ovarian transplantation. *Fertil Steril* 2003;80(Suppl 3):S144

46. Nugent D, Newton H, Gallivan L, *et al*. Protective effect of vitamin E on ischaemia–reperfusion injury in ovarian grafts. *J Reprod Fertil* 1998;114:341–6

47. Pugh CW, Ratcliffe PJ. Regulation of angiogenesis by hypoxia: role of the HIF system. *Nat Med* 2003;9:677–84

48. Zygmunt M, Herr F, Keller-Schoenwetter S, *et al*. Characterization of human chorionic gonadotropin as a novel angiogenic factor. *J Clin Endocrinol Metab* 2002;87:5290–6

49. Imthurn B, Cox SL, Jenkin G, *et al.* Gona-dotrophin administration can benefit ovarian tissue grafted to the body wall: implications for human ovarian grafting. *Mol Cell Endocrinol* 2000;163:141–6

50. Schnorr J, Oehninger S, Toner J, *et al.* Functional studies of subcutaneous ovarian transplants in non-human primates: steroidogenesis, endometrial development, ovulation, menstrual patterns and gamete morphology. *Hum Reprod* 2002;17:612–19

51. Wang X, Chen H, Yin H, *et al.* Fertility after intact ovary transplantation. *Nature* 2002; 415:385

52. Bedaiwy MA, Jeremias E, Gurunluoglu R, *et al.* Restoration of ovarian function after auto-transplantation of intact frozen–thawed sheep ovaries with microvascular anastomosis. *Fertil Steril* 2003;79:594–602

53. Tedder RS, Zuckerman MA, Goldstone AH, *et al.* Hepatitis B transmission from contaminated cryopreservation tank. *Lancet* 1995;346:137–40

54. Wakayama T, Yanagimachi R. Development of normal mice from oocytes injected with freeze-dried spermatozoa. *Nat Biotechnol* 1998;16:639–41

55. Shaw JM, Bowles J, Koopman P, *et al.* Fresh and cryopreserved ovarian tissue samples from donors with lymphoma transmit the cancer to graft recipients. *Hum Reprod* 1996;11:1668–73

56. Kim SS, Radford J, Harris M, *et al.* Ovarian tissue harvested from lymphoma patients to preserve fertility may be safe for autotransplantation. *Hum Reprod* 2001;16:2056–60

57. Ross, AA. Minimal residual disease in solid tumor malignancies: a review. *J Hematother* 1998;7:9–18

58. Shpall EJ, Jones RB, Bast RJ, *et al.* 4-Hydroperoxycyclophosphamide purging of breast cancer from the mononuclear cell fraction of bone marrow in patients receiving high-dose chemotherapy and autologous marrow support: a phase I trial. *J Clin Oncol* 1991;9:85–93

59. Purdy MH, Shpall EJ. The role and methodology for purging tumor from autologous bone marrow and peripheral blood progenitor cells. *Med Oncol* 1994;11:47–51

60. Schmidt KLT, Byskov AG, Nyboe Anderson A, *et al.* Density and distribution of primordial follicles in single pieces of cortex from 21 patients and individual pieces of cortex from three entire human ovaries. *Hum Reprod* 2003;18:1158–64

61. Kim SS, Battaglia DE, Soules MR, *et al.* Quantitative assessment of tissue damage in ovarian cortical tissue prior to transplantation. *Fertil Steril* 2001;76:S81

62. Meryman HT. Cryoprotective agents. *Cryobiology* 1971;8:173–83

63. Gook DA, Edgar DH, Stern C. The effects of cryopreservation regimens on the morphology of human ovarian tissue. *Mol Cell Endocrinol* 2000;169:99–103

64. Critchley HO, Bath LE, Wallace WH. Radiation damage to the uterus – review of the effects of treatment of childhood cancer. *Hum Fertil (Camb)* 2002;5:61–6

65. SEER 9 Registry. National Cancer Institute, 2003. http://seer.cancer.gov/publicdata

66. Weir HK, Thun MJ, Hankey BF, *et al.* Annual report to the nation on the status of cancer, 1975–2000, featuring the uses of surveillance data for cancer prevention and control. *J Natl Cancer Inst* 2003;95:1276–99

67. Puckridge PJ, Saunders CM, Ives AD, *et al.* Breast cancer and pregnancy: a diagnostic and management dilemma. *ANZ J Surg* 2003;73:500–3

68. Gagnon SS, Tetu B. Ovarian metastases of breast carcinoma. *Cancer* 1989;64:892–8

69. Rodenhuis S, Bontenbal M, Beex LV, *et al.* High-dose chemotherapy with hematopoietic stem-cell rescue for high-risk breast cancer. *N Engl J Med* 2003;349:7–16

70. Walters MC, Patience M, Leisenring W, *et al.* Bone marrow transplantation for sickle cell disease. *N Engl J Med* 1996;335:369–76

71. Sanders JE, Hawley J, Levy W, *et al.* Pregnancies following high-dose cyclophosphamide with or without high-dose busulfan or total-body irradiation and bone marrow transplantation. *Blood* 1996;87:3045–52

72. Leporrier M, von Theobald P, Roffe JL, Muller G. A new technique to protect ovarian function before pelvic irradiation. Heterotopic ovarian autotransplantation. *Cancer* 1987;60:2201–4

73. Kim SS, Hwang I, Lee H, Kim DH. Ovarian function after autotransplantation of frozen–thawed human ovarian tissue: an experience of human ovarian grafting into two heterotopic sites. *Fertil Steril* 2003;80(Suppl 3):S94

74. Gosden RG, Boulton MI, Grant K, Webb R. Follicular development from ovarian xenografts in SCID mice. *J Reprod Fertil* 1994;101:619–23

75. Gunasena KT, Lakey JR, Villines PM, *et al.* Antral follicles develop in xenografted cryo-preserved African elephant (*Loxodonta africana*) ovarian tissue. *Anim Reprod Sci* 1998;53:265–75

76. Candy CJ, Wood MJ, Whittingham DG. Follicular development in cryopreserved marmoset ovarian tissue after transplantation. *Hum Reprod* 1995;10:2334–8

77. Oktay K, Newton H, Mullen T, Gosden RG. Development of human primordial follicles to antral stages in SCID/*hpg* mice stimulated with follicle stimulating hormone. *Hum Reprod* 1998;13:1133–8

78. Weissman A, Gotlieb L, Colgan T, *et al.* Preliminary experience with subcutaneous human ovarian cortex transplantation in the NOD-SCID mouse. *Biol Reprod* 1999;60: 1462–7

79. Gook DA, McCully BA, Edgar DH, McBain JC. Development of antral follicles in human cryo-preserved ovarian tissue following xenograft-ing. *Hum Reprod* 2001;16:417–22

80. Snow M, Cox SL, Jenkin G, *et al.* Generation of live young from xenografted mouse ovaries. *Science* 2002;297:2227

81. Eppig JJ, O'Brien MJ. Development *in vitro* of mouse oocytes from primordial follicles. *Biol Reprod* 1996;54:197–207

82. O'Brien MJ, Pendola J, Eppig JJ. A revised protocol for *in vitro* development of mouse oocytes from primordial follicles dramatically improves their developmental competence. *Biol Reprod* 2003;68:1682–6

83. Gosden RG. *Cheating Time: Science, Sex and Aging.* New York: WH Freeman, 1996

84. Lass A, Akagbosu F, Abusheikha N, *et al.* A programme of semen cryopreservation for patients with malignant disease in a tertiary infertility center: lessons from 8 years' experi-ence. *Hum Reprod* 1998;13:3256–61

85. Chan PT, Schlegel PN. Nonobstructive azoospermia. *Curr Opin Urol* 2000;10:617–24

86. Nagano M, McCarrey JR, Brinster RL. Primate spermatogonial stem cells colonize mouse testis. *Biol Reprod* 2001;64:1409–16

87. Deanesly R. Spermatogenesis and endocrine activity in grafts of frozen and thawed rat testis. *J Endocrinol* 1954;11:201–6

88. Gosden RG, Matthews SJ, Kim SS, *et al.* Potential fertility in mice after isografting cryo-preserved testicular tissue. *Biol Reprod* 2000; 62(Suppl 1):212

89. Schlatt S, Honaramooz A, Boianni M, *et al.* Progeny from sperm obtained after ectopic grafting of neonatal mouse testes. *Biol Reprod* 2003;68:2331–5

90. Migishima F, Suzuki-Migishima R, Song SY, *et al.* Successful cryopreservation of mouse ovaries by vitrification. *Biol Reprod* 2003;68: 881–7

91. Oktay K, Nugent D, Newton H, *et al.* Isolation and characterization of primordial follicles from fresh and cryopreserved human ovarian tissue. *Fertil Steril* 1997;67:481–6

Fertility preservation in female cancer patients: a comprehensive approach

13

M. Sönmezer and K. Oktay

INTRODUCTION

Cancer diagnosis is surely one of the most stressful events in a person's life. However, the fact that cancer treatment may result in loss of fertility and premature ovarian failure could make the news even worse for many cancer patients of reproductive age. These patients need a compassionate, rapid and comprehensive approach to help preserve their fertility against the sterilizing effects of chemotherapy.

In the year 2003, more than 650 000 women were estimated to be afflicted with invasive cancer, and 8% or 52 000 of these women were under the age of 40[1,2]. Even though the rate of cancer incidence increased by 0.3% per year from 1987 to 1999 in women, the rate of cancer deaths declined by 0.6% per year from 1992 to 1999. This improvement in long-term survival rate was achieved mainly by the development of aggressive chemotherapy and radiotherapy, as well as bone marrow transplantation (BMT). Survival from childhood cancer has improved significantly over the past 25 years, and it is estimated that by the year 2010 approximately one in 250 young adults will have survived malignancies in childhood[3]. Between 1974–1976 and 1992–1999, the relative 5-year survival rate among children for all cancer types combined improved from 56 to 77%, being as high as > 90% for Hodgkin's disease[1,4].

However, cancer treatment with cytotoxic chemotherapy, especially when it includes alkylating agents, and ionizing radiotherapy induces premature ovarian failure in the majority of these patients. This is a significant consequence of the treatment as many patients are not only rendered infertile, but also will undergo premature menopause.

Residual ovarian function after chemotherapy is closely related to the patient's age and total cumulative chemotherapy dose. Among the chemotherapeutic agents, alkylating agents have the greatest impact on gonadal function. Among the alkylating agents that are implicated in gonadal damage are cyclophosphamide, busulfan, nitrogen mustard and L-phenylalanine mustard. These agents are believed to destroy follicle reserve through an apoptotic process. Older women are more likely to develop premature ovarian failure and permanent infertility immediately after chemotherapy, as a consequence of the age-related decline in the primordial follicle reserve[5,6]. In mice, the fraction of follicles destroyed by chemotherapy increased in proportion to the dose of alkalyting drug, but mice continued to ovulate despite a 50% loss in the pool of primordial follicles[7]. Therefore immediate reproductive function may not be an accurate marker of chemotherapy-induced gonadal failure, indicating the significance of not delaying childbearing even in patients who regain their menstrual function after chemotherapy.

In men, semen cryopreservation is an established technique for preserving fertility during the course of chemotherapy or radiotherapy, whereas for women the options are limited and more complex, including experimental technologies[8]. Advances in assisted reproductive technologies (ART) have enabled many infertile couples to conceive; however, most cancer patients of reproductive age do not have the option of utilizing established ART techniques to preserve fertility. Chemotherapy is initiated within 1–2 weeks of diagnosis in almost all cancers, with the exception of breast cancer. Cryopreservation of embryos generated by ART is among several options for these patients, but since oocyte retrieval after controlled ovarian simulation typically requires several weeks it is not practical in most cases. In addition, embryo cryopreservation is not always a suitable procedure in women without a partner. Moreover, ovarian stimulation and oocyte retrieval are not ethically acceptable in children.

In breast cancer patients, there is a 6-week hiatus between surgery and chemotherapy, but since high estrogen levels induced by traditional ovarian stimulation protocols can adversely affect breast cancer, oocyte or embryo freezing is not typically offered to these patients. Novel ovulation induction protocols using tamoxifen and aromatase inhibitors are being developed to overcome this problem in breast cancer patients[9–11].

Human oocyte cryopreservation is another attractive alternative to embryo cryopreservation. Even though some groups are reporting acceptable post-thaw fertilization and cleavage rates, results have not been consistently good enough for routine clinical application[12]. The low post-thaw survival rate, zona pellucida hardening, spindle damage and premature release of cortical granules are deemed responsible for initial low pregnancy rates. Cryopreservation of the oocyte in the germinal vesicle stage has been suggested to minimize damage to the spindle; however, only a limited number of pregnancies have been reported with frozen–thawed immature oocytes[13].

Ovarian transposition is another tool for fertility preservation when only abdomino-pelvic radiation is used in the treatment of cancer (e.g. cervical carcinoma, Ewing's sarcoma of the pelvis).

A COMPREHENSIVE APPROACH TO FERTILITY PRESERVATION

Fertility preservation procedures were initially designed to protect and restore reproductive function in cancer patients receiving cytotoxic chemotherapy or radiotherapy. The current indications extend beyond cancer, since gonadotoxic chemotherapy and radiation are used for the treatment of other systemic diseases. Patients undergoing oophorectomy for benign ovarian diseases and for prophylactic reasons may also benefit from fertility preservation.

Because each cancer patient's situation is unique, no one technique alone will be suitable for all patients who wish to preserve fertility. In our center we have developed a comprehensive approach to fertility preservation, depending on the patient's age, the presence or absence of ovarian involvement, time available, and the indication for fertility preservation.

Childhood malignancies

Cancer is the second leading cause of death in children between the ages of 1 and 14 years[1]. The survival rate for childhood cancers has increased considerably over the past 25 years, mostly due to improvements in the field of chemotherapy, BMT and stem cell transplantation (SCT). For all cancer types combined, the 5-year survival rate improved from 56 to 77% between the years 1974–1976 and 1992–1999[1]. Patients with leukemia, neuroblastoma, Hodgkin's lymphoma, non-Hodgkin's lymphoma, Wilms' tumor, Ewing's sarcoma and rabdomyosarcoma face the greatest risk of developing future ovarian failure.

In the human ovarian tissue cryopreservation trial of Poirot and colleagues, the youngest patient was 2.7 years of age[14]. Because ovarian stimulation and oocyte retrieval for oocyte or embryo preservation may neither be practical nor ethical in children, ovarian cryopreservation remains the only option for fertility preservation.

Breast cancer

Breast cancer is the leading cause of death among women, with more than 210 000 women estimated to be affected by breast cancer in the year 2003 in the USA. One out of every 228 women will develop breast cancer before the age of 40, and about 15% of cases of invasive breast cancer occur in women aged < 40 years[1,2]. Many of these patients will be subjected to cytotoxic chemotherapy that would place them at risk of premature ovarian failure.

Because there is typically a 6-week hiatus between surgery and chemotherapy, breast cancer patients may have enough time to undergo ovarian stimulation for oocyte or embryo cryopreservation, using tamoxifen or aromatase inhibitors (see below). They may also be candidates for ovarian cryopreservation, as occult ovarian metastasis is extremely rare in non-metastatic (stage I–III) breast cancer.

Cervical cancer

In the year 2002, 13 000 new cases of cervical cancer were diagnosed in the USA[15]. It is a more serious health problem worldwide, with nearly 500 000 women developing the disease each year. Even though the median age of diagnosis of cervical carcinoma is 47 years in North America, half of the cases occur before the age of 35[15]. Ovarian involvement is extremely rare in squamous cell cervical carcinoma. However, ovarian metastasis is found in up to 12% of cases with cervical adenocarcinoma, which has had an increasing trend of incidence in developed countries in recent years.

If radiation therapy only is planned, ovarian transposition may be suitable in cervical cancer patients even though the success rates with this procedure tend to vary. Ovarian cryopreservation for future auto-transplantation is another option, especially if adjuvant radiosensitizing chemotherapy is planned. Alternatively, one ovary can be transposed (usually the one on the opposite site of the main tumor) and the other can be cryopreserved. Even if there is time for ovarian stimulation, it is not considered safe to perform transvaginal oocyte aspiration in these patients as this procedure can cause profuse bleeding from the friable, cancerous cervix.

Other solid organ tumors

Radiation therapy in conjunction with conventional surgery plays an important role in the management of rectal cancer. Combination of surgery with preoperative radiotherapy not only improves local tumor control, but also overall survival and cancer-specific survival[16,17]. Radiotherapy is also utilized to improve the prognosis for some solid tumors presenting in the pelvis, such as Ewing's sarcoma, osteosarcoma or tumors of the lower spinal cord[18–20]. These patients can resort to ovarian, oocyte or embryo cryopreservation. Ovarian transposition may also be performed.

Patients undergoing bone marrow and stem cell transplantation

BMT, initially used in the treatment of leukemias, is now considered for the treatment of a number of malignant and non-malignant diseases such as systemic lupus erythematosus (SLE), aplastic anemia, sickle cell anemia and rheumatoid arthritis[21–23]. BMT and SCT are also used in patients with breast cancer and lymphoma[24]. The high-dose cytotoxic chemotherapy given to destroy the pre-existing bone marrow causes significant gonadal damage in most females. Adult patients, if there is sufficient time, can resort to conventional *in vitro* fertilization (IVF) for oocyte or embryo cryopreservation. In pediatric patients and patients who cannot delay their treatment, ovarian cryopreservation is the only choice for fertility preservation.

Autoimmune/idiopathic diseases

SLE is an autoimmune dysregulation that typically affects women of childbearing age, with an overall incidence of between 40 and 250 per 100 000[25]. High-dose cyclophosphamide is commonly used in these patients to suppress the disease, and often results in premature ovarian failure[26].

In addition, alkalyting agents are used in the treatment of other autoimmune diseases such as Behcet's disease, glomerulonephritis, inflammatory bowel diseases and pemphigus vulgaris[27–32]. These patients may also become candidates for ovarian, oocyte or embryo cryopreservation.

Benign ovarian tumors

Healthy pieces of ovarian tissue can be cryopreserved in patients undergoing oophorectomy for benign conditions[33]. If there is a concern with recurrent cyst formation, subcutaneous transplantation of the ovarian tissue is the preferred procedure, because of the ease of monitoring and removal.

Prophylactic oophorectomy

Inherited mutations, mainly in the genes *BRCA-1* and *BRCA-2*, account for almost 10% of all epithelial carcinomas. A mutation in any of these genes brings about a lifetime risk of 16–60% for developing ovarian cancer[34]. Prophylactic oophorectomy is suggested in these patients as soon as childbearing is completed or after the age of 35. Cryopreservation of ovarian tissue in those patients delaying childbearing beyond 35 years of age might be considered to decrease the risk of ovarian cancer. When the patient desires to conceive, ovarian tissue can be transplanted, preferably subcutaneously so that it can be monitored easily; once pregnancy occurs, the transplant can be removed to avoid further cancer risk. These patients may also be candidates for future *in vitro* maturation.

FERTILITY PRESERVATION OPTIONS

Embryo cryopreservation

IVF and embryo cryopreservation are standard and clinically established procedures. If the patient has a partner and enough time prior to cancer treatment, these techniques can be performed to store embryos for future use. An IVF cycle takes a minimum of 2 weeks to complete from the onset of menses; however, most cancer patients would not have sufficient time for this prior to treatment. In breast cancer,

there is typically a 6-week hiatus between surgery and chemotherapy, which would be adequate to perform ovarian stimulation and IVF. However, standard ovulation drugs are contraindicated in breast cancer patients because of resultant high levels of estradiol during stimulation.

Tamoxifen, a non-steroidal triphenylethylene anti-estrogen, was originally developed as a contraceptive agent in the UK[35]. Prior to becoming a breast cancer drug, tamoxifen was utilized as an ovulation induction drug in Europe. We recently used tamoxifen to perform ovarian stimulation prior to IVF in breast cancer patients, and found that higher numbers of embryos than in natural cycle IVF were obtained without increasing the risk of cancer recurrence in these patients[9]. In this protocol, patients received tamoxifen at 60 mg/day for a minimum of 5 days beginning on cycle day 3, and an IVF cycle was performed to cryopreserve the resulting embryos. Even though there was no difference in the number of follicles > 17 mm between treatment and control groups, the total number of mature oocytes was higher in the tamoxifen group than in the natural cycle group (1.6 vs. 0.6). Higher peak estradiol levels in the tamoxifen-treated group may raise concerns regarding stimulation of breast cancer cells. However, tamoxifen blocks the effect of supraphysiological levels of estrogen on breast tissue. Mean estradiol levels are chronically elevated in breast cancer patients on long-term tamoxifen treatment, and can be higher than in those stimulated for oocyte retrieval[36,37]. Tamoxifen inhibits the growth of breast tumors by competitive antagonism of estrogen at its receptor site.

Because tamoxifen is stimulatory on the endometrium, it cannot be used for endometrial cancer in a similar fashion. For these patients, aromatase inhibitors can be used for ovarian stimulation, IVF and embryo cryopreservation prior to radical surgery[38]. Unlike tamoxifen, aromatase inhibitors do not stimulate endometrial growth. Aromatase, an enzyme of the cytochrome P-450 superfamily and the product of the *CYP19* gene, catalyzes the reaction that converts androgenic substances to estrogens[39]. Aromatase activity is present at lower levels in many organs such as subcutaneous fat, liver, normal breast tissue, muscle and brain. Letrozole (CGS 20267) is a potent, reversible, competitive aromatase inhibitor. A single daily dose of letrozole optimally suppresses estrogen levels in postmenopausal women, and is suggested to be better than tamoxifen in the treatment of postmenopausal women with advanced-stage breast cancer[40,41]. Letrozole increases levels of follicle stimulating hormone (FSH), with a subsequent formation of multiple mature follicles[42]. In one study, ovulatory volunteer women received either 2.5 mg/day letrozole or 50 mg/day clomiphene citrate (CC). Letrozole was found to be comparable to CC in terms of the number of mature follicles, endometrial thickness at midcycle, and follicular profiles of luteinizing hormone (LH) and FSH[43]. However, the mean estradiol value on the day of the LH surge was lower in the letrozole group than in the CC group (399 ± 167 pmol/l vs. 2047 ± 930 pmol/l). Currently, we are testing the safety of ovarian stimulation with aromatase inhibitors in breast and endometrial cancer patients[10,38].

Oocyte cryopreservation

IVF and embryo cryopreservation is not an option for single patients unless they choose to use donor sperm. For single patients, unfertilized oocytes can be cryopreserved instead. Oocyte cryopreservation is attractive in theory because it would not require laparoscopy, and well-established stimulation protocols could be put to use. Unfortunately, the majority of cancer patients do not have sufficient time to complete a stimulation cycle before commencement of cancer therapy. In addition, unlike cryopreservation of embryos and spermatozoa, initial success rates with frozen–thawed oocytes have been much lower than with cryopreserved embryos[44]. However, recent studies reporting an increase in post-thaw survival and fertilization rates have rekindled interest in the cryopreservation of oocytes[45–47].

Embryos generated by intracytoplasmic sperm injection (ICSI) of thawed oocytes have a greater capacity for cell division than those generated by standard IVF[48].

It has been proposed that immature oocytes are more resistant to cryodamage than mature oocytes; however, the success rate is low. For further information on this subject, please refer to Chapter 11.

Ovarian cryopreservation and transplantation

Studies on the cryopreservation and transplantation of ovarian tissue date back to the 1950s. However, because of the unavailability of effective cryoprotectants and automated cryopreservation machines, the results met with only minimal success. The only cryoprotectant available in the 1960s, glycerol, was ineffective for cryopreservation of human oocytes and ovarian tissue[49]. After the discovery of more effective cryoprotectants, such as ethylene glycol, dimethyl sulfoxide and propanediol, rodent studies were repeated and gave encouraging results. The next step in testing the feasibility of ovarian cryopreservation and transplantation was the development of human xenograft models.

Trials using human ovarian tissue as xenografts in immuno-deficient mice

The successful animal studies (see Chapter 12) encouraged further studies to xenograft human ovarian tissue in SCID (severe combined immuno-deficient) mice. These animals are suitable for harboring human tissue because they have a mutation making them deficient in both B cells and T cells, rendering them unable to reject grafts from foreign species[50,51]. Ovarian tissue pieces can be placed subcutaneously, intramuscularly or under the kidney capsule, but concerns regarding cross-species retroviral infections should be addressed.

We demonstrated antral follicle development, estradiol production and estrogenization of the uteri in hypogonadal oophorectomized SCID mice when 1 mm³ of xenografted human ovarian tissue was stimulated with FSH[52]. Similarly, other authors showed antral follicle development and ovulation after subcutaneous or intramuscular xenografting of cryopreserved human ovarian tissue into immuno-deficient mice[53,54]. In another study, frozen–thawed human ovarian tissue was used for xenografting into immuno-deficient mice[55]. After 22 weeks of grafting, even though many follicles had initiated growth, there was still a significant number of primordial follicles remaining in each graft. No follicle growth beyond the one- to two-layer stage was observed, most probably due to lack of exogenous FSH support. Van den Broecke and colleagues transplanted cryopreserved human ovarian cortical grafts from an androgen-pretreated female-to-male transsexual patient into NOD/SCID (non-obese diabetic/severe combined immuno-deficient) mice[56]. For ovarian stimulation, daily intraperitoneal injections of 5 IU of recombinant FSH were used for 14 days. At 10, 12, 14 and 17 weeks after grafting, all stimulated groups had significantly more primary and secondary follicles than the non-stimulated control group, and progression from the primordial to the growing primary and secondary stages was most significant in the 14-week interval.

Nisolle and associates demonstrated increased fibrosis in frozen–thawed grafts 24 days after xenografting, but follicle density was similar to that of unfrozen controls[57]. In another study the same group also showed that there was no difference in survival of primordial follicles between ovarian tissue cryopreserved as $1 \text{ mm} \times 1 \text{ mm} \times 6 \text{ mm}$ pieces and that cryopreserved as $1 \text{ mm} \times 1 \text{ mm} \times 1 \text{ mm}$ pieces[58]. In summary, xenografting of human ovarian tissue provided the basis for clinical trials as well as generating another possible means to utilize banked ovarian tissue.

Development of techniques for transplanting human ovarian tissue

Ovarian tissue can be grafted to either an orthotopic location (near the infundibulopelvic ligament) or a heterotopic location (subcutaneous, subserosal, etc.).

Orthotopic ovarian transplantation

We performed the first case of laparoscopic orthotopic transplantation with frozen ovarian tissue (Figure 1)[59,60]. Ovarian tissue had been cryopreserved in 1.5 mol/l propanediol using the slow-freeze protocol. We first sutured ovarian cortical pieces to an absorbable scaffold, which was then laparoscopically implanted into the pelvic ovarian fossa. With the expectation of improving vascularization, aspirin 80 mg/day orally and FSH 150 IU/day intramuscularly were given for a week after the operation. Fifteen weeks after grafting, the patient ovulated once in response to stimulation with gonadotropins but showed signs of low ovarian reserve.

Radford and associates reported the grafting of cryopreserved ovarian tissue in a 36-year-old who had had tissue from her right ovary cryopreserved after the third recurrence of nodular sclerosing Hodgkin's lymphoma[61]. The patient was menopausal at the time when ovarian cortical strips were grafted onto the left ovary and another implanted at the site of the removed ovary. Seven months after transplantation, the patient reported resolution of the menopausal symptoms. Thereafter serum estradiol levels rose to 352 pmol/l, and pelvic ultrasonography showed an endometrial thickness of 10 mm. Despite high estrogen levels, progesterone levels never exceeded 2 nmol/l and no ovulation was detected. The cortex of frozen–thawed ovarian tissue, as well as biopsy samples of the retained left ovary, did not show evidence of neoplasia.

Heterotopic ovarian transplantation

For heterotopic transplantation, ovarian tissue is grafted into the subcutaneous space above the brachioradialis fascia of the forearm, or above the rectus fascia in the lower abdomen. Obviously, with this technique IVF–embryo transfer will always be necessary to conceive. Heterotopic transplantation has its advantages;

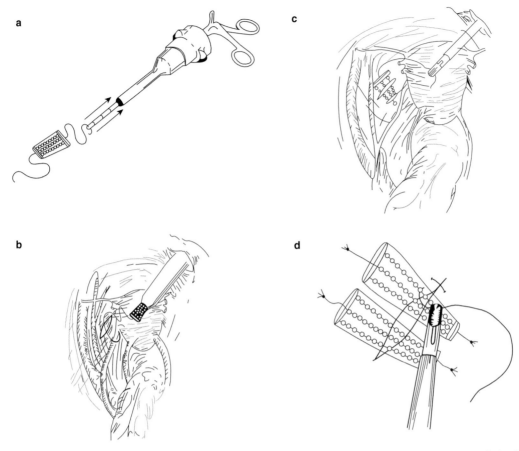

Figure 1 Procedure for laparoscopic orthotopic transplantation with frozen ovarian tissue. (a) Retrograde loading of the graft that was reconstructed by stringing the ovarian tissue between two strips of Surgicel. (b) Placement of the leading suture in the pelvic pocket and through the lower peritoneal edge. (c) Placement of the base suture through the upper peritoneal edge; by pulling on this suture, the raft is flattened against the vascular pelvic wall. (d) Closure of the peritoneum with interrupted sutures; note the placement of two grafts side by side. Reprinted from reference 60 with permission from the American Society of Reproductive Medicine

this technique does not require general anesthesia and abdominal surgery, and allows close monitoring and easy removal when necessary.

We performed subcutaneous ovarian transplantation in a 35-year-old woman with stage III squamous cervical carcinoma[33]. After grafting, she received sterilizing radiotherapy but her arm was kept out of the radiation field. Immediately after the oophorectomy, FSH and LH levels were in the postmenopausal range. Approximately 6 weeks after ovarian transplant, she reported a painless swelling at the site of the ovarian transplant. Ultrasound examination revealed one dominant and four antral follicles. After ovarian stimulation, three oocytes were retrieved, two were immature and one was in metaphase I. The metaphase I oocyte was matured *in vitro*, but ICSI did not result in fertilization. This patient had nearly 3 years of ovarian function but never ovulated spontaneously.

In a subsequent case of ovarian transplant in a 37-year-old patient whose ovary was removed for benign ovarian cyst and implanted freshly in the forearm, periodic menstruation occurred even though cycle length varied from 14 to 45 days[33]. This patient's graft also lasted for nearly 3 years.

183

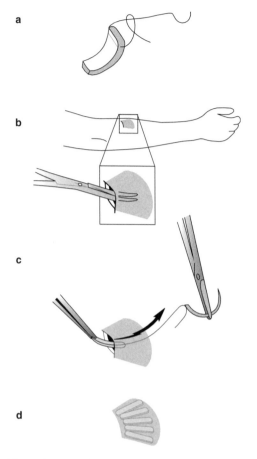

Figure 2 A surgical technique for ovarian transplantation to the forearm. (a) Preparation of the strips; (b) creating a subcutaneous pocket; (c) wedging grafts underneath the forearm skin; (d) final position of the grafts after transplantation. Reprinted from reference 62 with permission from the American Society of Reproductive Medicine

We recently described a surgical technique for transplanting ovarian cortical strips to the forearm (Figure 2)[62]. In this technique, fresh or frozen–thawed ovarian strips are placed 5–10 cm below the antecubital fossa and over the brachioradialis muscle via a small transverse incision. If the ovarian tissue has been cryopreserved first, 0.5–1.0 cm strips of 1–3 mm thickness are prepared, whereas if fresh ovarian tissue is to be grafted, the strips can be longer – 0.5–5.0 cm strips of 1–3 mm thickness will facilitate the transplantation procedure. If there are cosmetic concerns grafts can be placed more medially.

Table 1 Cancer types and the risk of ovarian metastasis

Cancers with low risk of ovarian involvement
Wilms' tumor
Ewing's sarcoma
Breast cancer (stage I–III)
Non-Hodgkin's lymphoma
Hodgkin's lymphoma
Non-genital rhabdomyosarcoma
Osteogenic sarcoma
Squamous cell carcinoma of uterine cervix

Cancers with moderate risk of ovarian involvement
Adenocarcinoma of the cervix
Colon cancer
Breast cancer (advanced stage)

Cancers with high risk of ovarian involvement
Leukemia
Neuroblastoma

It has become apparent to us from our experience with human ovarian transplantation that small ovarian pieces increase the technical difficulty of the procedure[59,60]. Therefore, the largest optimal size for the best survival of primordial follicles in tissue will have to be determined in future studies.

Risk of metastatic disease

Even though many cancers do not metastasize to ovaries, some cancers such as leukemias have a high risk for ovarian metastasis due to their systemic nature. In addition, ovarian metastasis was demonstrated in 25–50% of neuroblastoma cases[49]. Breast cancer carries a low to intermediate risk of ovarian involvement in early stages. In the absence of clinical and radiological evidence of distant metastasis, ovarian involvement is extremely rare, and most cases could be detected by a thorough clinical and radiological evaluation. Incidence of ovarian involvement is exceptionally low in Wilms' tumor, Ewing's sarcoma, lymphomas (with the exception of Burkitt's lymphoma), osteosarcomas and extragenital rhabdomyosarcomas. In squamous cell cervical cancer ovarian involvement is < 0.2%, whereas it is higher in adenocarcinoma of the cervix. The risk of ovarian involvement according to tumor type is summarized in Table 1.

There have been several animal and xenograft studies to test the risk of re-seeding cancer via ovarian transplantation. In a rodent study, most animals died of lymphoma 9–43 days after ovarian tissue from mice with a very aggressive form of lymphoma was transplanted[63]. However, this form of lymphoma is not applicable to the majority of lymphomas in humans. In another study, human frozen–thawed ovarian tissue from patients with Hodgkin's disease ($n = 13$) and non-Hodgkin's lymphoma ($n = 5$) were xenografted to NOD/LtSz-SCID mice[64]. None of the ovarian tissue transplants from lymphoma patients resulted in cancer seeding; however, in the positive control group, three mice developed lymphoma when grafted with lymph node tissue from non-Hodgkin's lymphoma patients. These results indicated that ovarian transplantation is safe in patients with non-Hodgkin's lymphoma but were not completely reassuring for those with Hodgkin's lymphoma, since, in this model, positive controls did not transmit the disease as well. However, based on clinical experience, ovarian involvement is extremely rare in Hodgkin's patients.

Regardless of the magnitude of risk of ovarian involvement, a thorough histological evaluation should be performed from multiple samples taken from ovarian tissue which is to be cryopreserved. Additionally, molecular biological techniques and immunohistochemistry can be used to screen for the presence of cancer cells in the ovary[2].

DO GONADOTROPIN RELEASING HORMONE ANALOGS REDUCE THE RISK OF OVARIAN FAILURE?

It is highly debated whether gonadal damage induced by cytotoxic chemotherapy can be prevented by co-treatment with gonadotropin releasing hormone (GnRH) agonists. Some studies have demonstrated a protective role of GnRH agonist therapy against chemotherapy-induced ovarian damage[65,66]. Ataya and co-workers demonstrated that primordial follicle loss occurring during cyclophosphamide treatment was significantly lower in rhesus monkeys that received GnRH agonist treatment, compared with untreated animals (65% vs. 29%)[67]. However, in another study, the same authors did not demonstrate any protective effect of GnRH agonist treatment against radiation-induced ovarian injury in rhesus monkeys[68].

Blumenfeld investigated the protective effect of GnRH agonists in 44 women with lymphoma, ten women with leukemia and eight women with non-malignant diseases, all of whom received chemotherapy[69]. The author compared these patients with 55 women (control group) treated with similar chemotherapy but without GnRH agonist. In almost all of the surviving patients receiving GnRH agonist/chemotherapy, spontaneous ovulation and menses occurred within 6 months; however, < 50% of the patients in the control group resumed ovarian function and regular cyclic activity. Although inhibin-A and -B decreased during GnRH agonist/chemotherapy co-treatment, it increased to normal levels in patients who resumed regular ovarian cyclicity and/or spontaneously conceived, compared with low levels in those who developed premature ovarian failure.

Meirow and colleagues showed that, despite significant follicle loss, short-term reproductive performance of cyclophosphamide-treated mice was not affected compared with controls[70]. The authors indicated that immediate reproductive performance may not be an accurate marker for assessing chemotherapy-induced ovarian injury, and suggested that damage to the ovary can be predicted more accurately by histological counting of primordial follicle number. In addition, since primordial follicles are resting and lack FSH receptors, it seems unlikely that GnRH analogs can have an effect through suppressing pituitary gonadotropin secretion[71]. In a small randomized study, Waxman and associates demonstrated that treatment with a GnRH analog was ineffective in preserving the fertility of patients receiving chemotherapy for Hodgkin's disease[72]. In that study, 30 men and 18 women were randomly allocated to receive GnRH analog prior to and for the duration of cytotoxic chemotherapy. Twenty men and eight women received GnRH analog.

Over 3 years of follow up, in the study group all males were oligospermic and four of the eight women were amenorrheic; in the control group all ten males were oligospermic and six of nine females were amenorrheic.

OVARIAN TRANSPOSITION

Repositioning of the ovaries by either laparotomy or laparoscopy has been used to preserve gonadal function[73,74]. In Hodgkin's disease, the success rate of this technique in preserving ovarian function has varied between 0% and 66%[2,75–77]. Husseinzadeh and co-workers demonstrated that ovarian function was preserved by lateral ovarian transposition at the time of laparotomy in 83% of patients receiving pelvic radiation[78], whereas in the study by Anderson's group only 17% of the women undergoing ovarian transposition before radiation therapy for cervical cancer resumed ovarian function[79]. In a recent study on 12 patients, laparoscopic oophoropexy was performed to preserve ovarian function prior to pelvic irradiation for Hodgkin's disease[80]. All patients who received minimal or no chemotherapy had evidence of ovarian function, and four of them achieved pregnancy.

Repositioning the ovaries may decrease the risk of ovarian failure, but the ovaries are still subjected to a significant amount of scattered radiation, and the surgical procedure is not without complications. Fallopian tube infarction, ovarian cyst formation and injury to the vasculature have been cited among the complications[81]. Therefore ovarian transposition may not provide a reliable means to protect ovaries against ionization radiation, nor is it useful in the case of administration of gonadotoxic chemotherapy.

FUTURE POSSIBILITIES IN FERTILITY PRESERVATION

When the risk of ovarian involvement with cancer cells is high, some other experimental options may be available in the future. It has been possible to xenograft human ovarian tissue into immuno-deficent mice and grow mature follicles in these xenografts[52,53,55]. It has also been possible to retrieve oocytes from xenografted human ovarian cortical pieces[82]. Another possibility is to isolate primordial follicles from cryopreserved ovarian tissue and grow them in vitro[83]. Even though this has been partially successful in mice, the prospect for human follicles is not clear at the present time.

DONOR EGGS AND SURROGACY

IVF with donor eggs is another alternative in cases where the patient suffers from premature menopause or low ovarian reserve as a consequence of cancer treatment[84]. The success rate with appropriate egg donors now exceeds 60% per embryo transfer. Gestational surrogacy can also be employed when patients have undergone hysterectomy or received pelvic radiation for cervical cancer. Patients with breast cancer who are considered at high risk for recurrence, or who have to be on lifelong therapy with aromatase inhibitors, may also resort to gestational surrogacy. However, the laws and regulations regarding this procedure vary significantly between countries and between each state in the USA.

CONCLUSIONS

There is a growing number of options for cancer patients facing infertility and premature ovarian failure who desire to preserve fertility prior to treatment. These options vary depending on the patient's age, the time available, the type of cancer and whether the likelihood of ovarian involvement is high. Health-care providers should have a comprehensive approach to counseling patients regarding fertility preservation procedures (Figure 3). They should also clarify with patients whether a procedure is experimental or not: with the exception of embryo cryopreservation, all of the options should currently be considered experimental. Cancer patients who may benefit from fertility preservation procedures should be referred to appropriate centers which perform the procedures under Institutional Review Board/Ethics Committee-approved protocols.

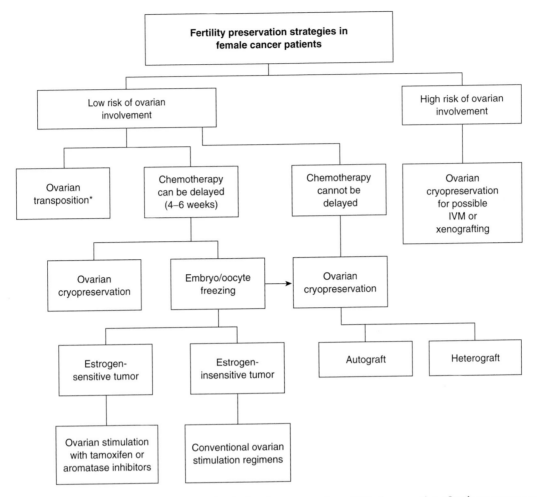

Figure 3 An algorithm for ovarian preservation in female cancer patients. With the exception of embryo cryopreservation, all strategies are experimental. *Patients receiving radiation therapy with non-gonadotoxic chemotherapy or without chemotherapy; IVM, *in vitro* maturation

References

1. Jemal A, Murray T, Samuels A, *et al.* Cancer statistics, 2003. *CA Cancer J Clin* 2003;53: 5–26

2. Oktay KH, Yih M. Preliminary experience with orthotopic and heterotopic transplantation of ovarian cortical strips. *Semin Reprod Med* 2002; 20:63–74

3. Bleyer WA. The impact of childhood cancer on the United States and the world. *CA Cancer J Clin* 1990;40:355–67

4. Bleyer WA. Cancer in older adolescents and young adults: epidemiology, diagnosis, treatment, survival, and importance of clinical trials. *Med Pediatr Oncol* 2002;38:1–10

5. Moore HC. Fertility and the impact of systemic therapy on hormonal status following treatment for breast cancer. *Curr Oncol Rep* 2000;2: 587–93

6. Howell SJ, Shalet SM. Fertility preservation and management of gonadal failure associated with

lymphoma therapy. *Curr Oncol Rep* 2002;4:
443–52

7. Meirow D, Lewis H, Nugent D, Epstein M.
Subclinical depletion of primordial follicular
reserve in mice treated with cyclophosphamide: clinical importance and proposed
accurate investigative tool. *Hum Reprod* 1999;
14:1903–7

8. Carson SA, Gentry WL, Smith AL, *et al.*
Feasibility of semen collection and cryopreservation during chemotherapy. *Hum Reprod*
1991;6:992–4

9. Oktay K, Buyuk E, Davis O, *et al.* Fertility
preservation in breast cancer patients: IVF and
embryo cryopreservation after ovarian stimulation with tamoxifen. *Hum Reprod* 2003;18:
90–5

10. Oktay K, Sonmezer M. Fertility preservation
not just ovarian cryopreservation. *Hum Reprod*
2004;19:1–4

11. Oktay K, Buyuk E, Davis OK, *et al.* A prospective comparison of tamoxifen alone and
tamoxifen–FSH combined protocol for IVF
and fertility preservation in breast cancer
patients. *ASRM* 2003;abstr. 218

12. Wininger JD, Kort HI. Cryopreservation of
immature and mature human oocytes. *Semin
Reprod Med* 2002;20:45–9

13. Tucker MJ, Wright G, Morton PC, *et al.* Birth
after cryopreservation of immature oocytes
with subsequent *in vitro* maturation. *Fertil Steril*
1998;70:578–9

14. Poirot C, Vacher-Lavenu MC, Helardot P, *et al.*
Human ovarian tissue cryopreservation: indications and feasibility. *Hum Reprod* 2002;17:
1447–52

15. Waggoner SE. Cervical cancer. *Lancet* 2003;
361:2217–25

16. Camma C, Giunta M, Fiorica F, *et al.*
Preoperative radiotherapy for resectable rectal
cancer: a meta-analysis. *J Am Med Assoc* 2000;
284:1008–15

17. Kapiteijn E, Marijnen CA, Nagtegaal ID, *et al.*
Preoperative radiotherapy combined with total
mesorectal excision for resectable rectal cancer.
N Engl J Med 2001;345:638–46

18. Rodl RW, Hoffmann C, Gosheger G, *et al.*
Ewing's sarcoma of the pelvis: combined
surgery and radiotherapy treatment. *J Surg
Oncol* 2003;83:154–60

19. Ferguson WS, Goorin AM. Current treatment
of osteosarcoma. *Cancer Invest* 2001;19:
292–315

20. Whitaker SJ, Bessell EM, Ashley SE, *et al.*
Postoperative radiotherapy in the management of spinal cord ependymoma. *J Neurosurg*
1991;74:720–8

21. Olalla JI, Ortin M, Hermida G, *et al.*
Disappearance of lupus anticoagulant after

allogeneic bone marrow transplantation. *Bone
Marrow Transplant* 1999;23:83–5

22. Tyndall A, Millikan S. Bone marrow transplantation. *Baillières Best Pract Res Clin Rheumatol*
1999;13:719–35

23. Walters MC. Bone marrow transplantation
for sickle cell disease: where do we go from
here? *J Pediatr Hematol Oncol* 1999;21:
467–74

24. Mazza P, Prudenzano A, Amurri B, *et al.*
Myeloablative therapy and bone marrow transplantation in Jehovah's Witnesses with malignancies: single center experience. *Bone Marrow
Transplant* 2003;32:433–6

25. Michet CJ Jr, McKenna CH, Elveback LR, *et al.*
Epidemiology of systemic lupus erythematosus
and other connective tissue diseases in
Rochester, Minnesota, 1950 through 1979.
Mayo Clin Proc 1985;60:105–13

26. Gladstone DE, Prestrud AA, Pradhan A, *et al.*
High-dose cyclophosphamide for severe
systemic lupus erythematosus. *Lupus* 2002;11:
405–10

27. Russell AI, Lawson WA, Haskard DO. Potential
new therapeutic options in Behcet's syndrome.
BioDrugs 2001;15:25–35

28. Schena FP. Primary glomerulonephritides with
nephrotic syndrome. Limitations of therapy in
adult patients. *J Nephrol* 1999;12(Suppl 2):
S125–30

29. Langford CA, Talar-Williams C, Barron KS,
et al. Use of a cyclophosphamide-induction
methotrexate-maintenance regimen for the
treatment of Wegener's granulomatosis:
extended follow-up and rate of relapse. *Am J
Med* 2003;114:463–9

30. Stallmach A, Wittig BM, Moser C, *et al.* Safety
and efficacy of intravenous pulse cyclophosphamide in acute steroid refractory inflammatory bowel disease. *Gut* 2003;52:377–82

31. Burt RK, Traynor A, Oyama Y, *et al.* High-
dose immune suppression and autologous
hematopoietic stem cell transplantation in
refractory Crohn disease. *Blood* 2003;101:
2064–6

32. Nousari CH, Brodsky R, Anhalt GJ. Evaluating
the role of immunoablative high-dose cyclophosphamide therapy in pemphigus vulgaris.
J Am Acad Dermatol 2003;49:148–50

33. Oktay K, Economos K, Kan M, *et al.* Endocrine
function and oocyte retrieval after autologous
transplantation of ovarian cortical strips to the
forearm. *J Am Med Assoc* 2001;286:1490–3

34. Liede A, Narod SA. Hereditary breast and
ovarian cancer in Asia: genetic epidemiology
of BRCA1 and BRCA2. *Hum Mutat* 2002;20:
413–24

35. Harper MJ, Walpole AL. Contrasting endocrine activities of cis and trans isomers in a

series of substituted triphenylethylenes. *Nature* 1966:212:87

36. Shushan A, Peretz T, Mor-Yosef S. Therapeutic approach to ovarian cysts in tamoxifen-treated women with breast cancer. *Int J Gynaecol Obstet* 1996;52:249–53

37. Klijn JG, Beex LV, Mauriac L, *et al.* Combined treatment with buserelin and tamoxifen in premenopausal metastatic breast cancer: a randomized study. *J Natl Cancer Inst* 2000;92: 903–11

38. Oktay K, Buyuk E, Rosenwaks Z, *et al.* Novel use of an aromatase inhibitor for fertility preservation via embryo cryopreservation in endometrial cancer: a case report. *ASRM* 2003;abstr. 234

39. Smith IE, Dowsett M. Aromatase inhibitors in breast cancer. *N Eng J Med* 2003;348:2431–42

40. Dowsett M, Jones A, Johnston SR, *et al. In vivo* measurement of aromatase inhibition by letrozole (CGS 20267) in postmenopausal patients with breast cancer. *Clin Cancer Res* 1995;1: 1511–15

41. Mouridsen H, Gershanovich M, Sun Y, *et al.* Phase III study of letrozole versus tamoxifen as first-line therapy of advanced breast cancer in postmenopausal women: analysis of survival and update of efficacy from the International Letrozole Breast Cancer Group. *J Clin Oncol* 2003;21:2101–9

42. Shetty G, Krishnamurthy H, Krishnamurthy HN, *et al.* Effect of estrogen deprivation on the reproductive physiology of male and female primates. *J Steroid Biochem Mol Biol* 1997;61: 157–66

43. Fisher SA, Reid RL, Van Vugt DA, *et al.* A randomized double-blind comparison of the effects of clomiphene citrate and the aromatase inhibitor letrozole on ovulatory function in normal women. *Fertil Steril* 2002;78: 280–5

44. Oktay K, Kan MT, Rosenwaks Z. Recent progress in oocyte and ovarian tissue cryopreservation and transplantation. *Curr Opin Obstet Gynecol* 2001;13:263–8

45. Yoon TK, Kim TJ, Park SE, *et al.* Live births after vitrification of oocytes in a stimulated *in vitro* fertilization–embryo transfer program. *Fertil Steril* 2003;79:1323–6

46. Boldt J, Cline D, McLaughlin D. Human oocyte cryopreservation as an adjunct to IVF–embryo transfer cycles. *Hum Reprod* 2003; 18:1250–5

47. Porcu E. Oocyte freezing. *Semin Reprod Med* 2001;19:221–30

48. Gook DA, Schiewe MC, Osborn SM, *et al.* Intracytoplasmic sperm injection and embryo development of human oocytes cryopreserved

using 1,2-propanediol. *Hum Reprod* 1995;10: 2637–41

49. Oktay K. Ovarian tissue cryopreservation and transplantation: preliminary findings and implications for cancer patients. *Hum Reprod Update* 2001;7:526–34

50. Bosma GC, Custer RP, Bosma MJ. A severe combined immunodeficiency mutation in the mouse. *Nature* 1983;301:527–30

51. Gosden RG, Boulton MI, Grant K, *et al.* Follicular development from ovarian xenografts in SCID mice. *J Reprod Fertil* 1994;101: 619–23

52. Oktay K, Newton H, Mullan J, *et al.* Development of human primordial follicles to antral stages in SCID/hpg mice stimulated with follicle stimulating hormone. *Hum Reprod* 1998; 13:1133–8

53. Weissman A, Gotlieb L, Colgan T, *et al.* Preliminary experience with subcutaneous human ovarian cortex transplantation in the NOD-SCID mouse. *Biol Reprod* 1999;60: 1462–7

54. Kim SS, Soules MR, Battaglia DE. Follicular development, ovulation, and corpus luteum formation in cryopreserved human ovarian tissue after xenotransplantation. *Fertil Steril* 2002;78:77–82

55. Oktay K, Newton H, Gosden RG. Transplantation of cryopreserved human ovarian tissue results in follicle growth initiation in SCID mice. *Fertil Steril* 2000;73:599–603

56. Van den Broecke R, Liu J, Van der Elst J, *et al.* Timing of FSH-stimulation and follicular development in cryopreserved human ovarian grafts. *Reprod Biomed Online* 2002;4:21–6

57. Nisolle M, Casanas-Roux F, Qu J, *et al.* Histologic and ultrastructural evaluation of fresh and frozen–thawed human ovarian xenografts in nude mice. *Fertil Steril* 2000;74: 122–9

58. Qu J, Godin PA, Nisolle M, *et al.* Distribution and epidermal growth factor receptor expression of primordial follicles in human ovarian tissue before and after cryopreservation. *Hum Reprod* 2000;15:302–10

59. Oktay K, Karlikaya G. Ovarian function after transplantation of frozen, banked autologous ovarian tissue. *N Engl J Med* 2000;342:1919

60. Oktay K, Aydin BA, Karlikaya G. A technique for laparoscopic transplantation of frozen–banked ovarian tissue. *Fertil Steril* 2001;75: 1212–16

61. Radford JA, Lieberman BA, Brison DR, *et al.* Orthotopic reimplantation of cryopreserved ovarian cortical strips after high-dose chemotherapy for Hodgkin's lymphoma. *Lancet* 2001;357:1172–5

62. Oktay K, Buyuk E, Rosenwaks Z, *et al.* A technique for transplantation of ovarian cortical strips to the forearm. *Fertil Steril* 2003;80: 193–8

63. Shaw JM, Bowles J, Koopman P, *et al.* Fresh and cryopreserved ovarian tissue samples from donors with lymphoma transmit the cancer to graft recipients. *Hum Reprod* 1996;11:1668–73

64. Kim SS, Radford J, Harris M, *et al.* Ovarian tissue harvested from lymphoma patients to preserve fertility may be safe for autotransplantation. *Hum Reprod* 2001;16:2056–60

65. Ataya K, Moghissi K. Chemotherapy-induced premature ovarian failure: mechanisms and prevention. *Steroids* 1989;54:607–26

66. Bokser L, Szende B, Schally AV. Protective effects of D-Trp6-luteinising hormone-releasing hormone microcapsules against cyclophosphamide-induced gonadotoxicity in female rats. *Br J Cancer* 1990;61:861–5

67. Ataya K, Rao LV, Lawrence E, *et al.* Luteinizing hormone-releasing hormone agonist inhibits cyclophosphamide-induced ovarian follicular depletion in rhesus monkeys. *Biol Reprod* 1995; 52:365–72

68. Ataya K, Pydyn E, Ramahi-Ataya A, *et al.* Is radiation-induced ovarian failure in rhesus monkeys preventable by luteinizing hormone-releasing hormone agonists? Preliminary observations. *J Clin Endocrinol Metab* 1995;80: 790–5

69. Blumenfeld Z. Ovarian rescue/protection from chemotherapeutic agents. *J Soc Gynecol Investig* 2001;8(Suppl 1):S60–4

70. Meirow D, Lewis H, Nugent D, *et al.* Subclinical depletion of primordial follicular reserve in mice treated with cyclophosphamide: clinical importance and proposed accurate investigative tool. *Hum Reprod* 1999; 14:1903–7

71. Oktay K, Briggs D, Gosden RG. Ontogeny of follicle-stimulating hormone receptor gene expression in isolated human ovarian follicles. *J Clin Endocrinol Metab* 1997;82:3748–51

72. Waxman JH, Ahmed R, Smith D, *et al.* Failure to preserve fertility in patients with Hodgkin's disease. *Cancer Chemother Pharmacol* 1987;19: 159–62

73. Morice P, Juncker L, Rey A, *et al.* Ovarian transposition for patients with cervical carcinoma treated by radiosurgical combination. *Fertil Steril* 2000;74:743–8

74. Tulandi T, Al-Took S. Laparoscopic ovarian suspension before irradiation. *Fertil Steril* 1998; 70:381–3

75. Ray GR, Trueblood HW, Enright LP, *et al.* Oophoropexy: a means of preserving ovarian function following pelvic megavoltage radiotherapy for Hodgkin's disease. *Radiology* 1970; 96:175–80

76. Thomas PR, Winstanly D, Peckham MJ, *et al.* Reproductive and endocrine function in patients with Hodgkin's disease: effects of oophoropexy and irradiation. *Br J Cancer* 1976;33:226–31

77. Hunter MC, Glees JP, Gazet JC. Oophoropexy and ovarian function in the treatment of Hodgkin's disease. *Clin Radiol* 1980;31:21–6

78. Husseinzadeh N, Nahhas WA, Velkley DE, *et al.* The preservation of ovarian function in young women undergoing pelvic radiation therapy. *Gynecol Oncol* 1984;18:373–9

79. Anderson B, LaPolla J, Turner D, *et al.* Ovarian transposition in cervical cancer. *Gynecol Oncol* 1993;49:206–14

80. Williams RS, Littell RD, Mendenhall NP. Laparoscopic oophoropexy and ovarian function in the treatment of Hodgkin disease. *Cancer* 1999;86:2138–42

81. Meirow D, Nugent D. The effects of radiotherapy and chemotherapy on female reproduction. *Hum Reprod Update* 2001;7:535–43

82. Revel A, Raanani H, Leyland N, *et al.* Human oocyte retrieval from nude mice transplanted with human ovarian cortex [abstract]. *Human Reprod* 2000;15(Abstract Book 1):13

83. Oktay K, Nugent D, Newton H, *et al.* Isolation and characterization of primordial follicles from fresh and cryopreserved human ovarian tissue. *Fertil Steril* 1997;67:481–6

84. Polak de Fried E, Notrica J, Rubinstein M, *et al.* Pregnancy after human donor oocyte cryopreservation and thawing in association with intracytoplasmic sperm injection in a patient with ovarian failure. *Fertil Steril* 1998;69:555–7

Prospects for follicle culture 14

H. M. Picton, S. E. Harris and E. L. Chambers

INTRODUCTION

The potential of the complete *in vitro* growth (IVG) and *in vitro* maturation (IVM) of mammalian oocytes was first realized some 8 years ago when Eppig and O'Brien[1] demonstrated that it was possible to produce live young from mouse oocytes grown from the primordial stages to maturity *in vitro*. More recently, Obata and colleagues[2] and O'Brien and associates[3] have repeated this work, using extended culture and micromanipulation techniques to show that the most primitive oocytes in the fetal mouse ovary can grow and differentiate into fertile mature oocytes *in vitro* with a reasonable efficiency. Despite these encouraging results, progress in IVG technology is slow and considerable effort is needed to translate the limited success of murine IVG systems into methods which will support the complete IVG of oocytes from large animals and humans.

Follicle culture has many potential applications. This technology can be used to exploit the genetic potential of commercially important domestic species. In combination with ovarian cryopreservation, IVG can be used to preserve the female germ plasm of rare or endangered species. It could also be used to generate mature oocytes for donation and research in human assisted reproduction programs. Perhaps the most important application of IVG in the context of this chapter is to develop it as a safe means of restoring the fertility of young cancer patients who are at risk of losing their fertility and who have elected to have some of their ovarian cortical tissue cryopreserved prior to the start of their cancer treatment. The advantage of using IVG of follicles as a means to restore the fertility of cancer patients is that, unlike autografting of

frozen–thawed tissue, where there may be a risk of re-introducing the malignant cells with the graft[4,5], with IVG there is no risk of re-introducing cancer cells through the embryos derived from *in vitro*-grown oocytes. However, it must be noted that the health of the oocytes and embryos derived following the complete IVG of early staged follicles has not yet been established. This chapter therefore explores the current methods used to grow primordial and preantral follicles to maturity in animals and humans and so provides insight into the prospects of follicle culture as a means to restore female fertility following ovarian cryopreservation.

FOLLICLE GROWTH *IN VIVO*

It is clear that any culture strategy designed to support the complete IVG of oocytes and follicles must mimic the developmental sequence of events seen *in vivo* in terms of follicle and oocyte growth rates, gene expression patterns and metabolic requirements. Development of follicles *in vivo* is known to be dependent on the reception of appropriate signals from the oocytes[6] and vice versa. During their extended growth phase, oocytes progressively synthesize and accumulate the payload of proteins and RNAs which are required to support both nuclear and cytoplasmic maturation of the fully grown oocytes and early post-fertilization development of the zygote[7,8]. For example, following follicle growth initiation, there is co-ordinate expression of the oocyte-specific genes *Zp-1*, *Zp-2* and *Zp-3* whose translated products form the extracellular membrane – the zona pellucida[9].

Formation of a functional zona pellucida and the formation and relocation of the cortical granules to the periphery of the mature oocyte are both essential parts of oocyte development, as the zona pellucida is directly responsible for sperm binding during fertilization and for the provision of the natural block to polyspermic fertilization. During growth, oocyte transcription and translation step up markedly and proteins, such as the cell cycle regulators which are required to both maintain meiotic arrest in growing oocytes and to reinitiate meiosis in mature oocytes, are sequentially synthesized and accumulated[8,10]. Furthermore, there are stage-specific changes in DNA methylation of the genes associated with genomic imprinting during oocyte growth[11,12].

The development of the oocyte is dependent on, and is concurrent with, that of the somatic cells of the growing follicle. The growth rates and the changes in size and morphology of follicles as they grow have been well characterized for a number of species including rodents, ruminants, primates and humans. Irrespective of species, during follicle growth the granulosa cells which surround and enclose the oocyte replicate, becoming metabolically coupled with each other through gap junctions and with the oocyte via processes passing through the developing zona pellucida that make junctional contact with the oolemma[13]. As preantral follicles grow, the thecal cell layer becomes morphologically distinguishable from the granulosa cells and the surrounding stromal tissue. The innermost layer of the theca, the theca interna, eventually assumes the appearance of typical steroid-secreting cells. Follicle antrum formation is a relatively late event in folliculogenesis, which may take several months in toto in primate and ruminant follicles in vivo[14]. During the later stages of preantral follicle growth and more importantly during antral – and preovulatory – follicle development, the granulosa and theca cells undergo differentiation and become progressively more steroidogenic in response to stimulation by the pituitary gonadotropins, follicle stimulating hormone (FSH) and luteinizing hormone (LH). Steroid production by growing follicles is therefore preceded by the induction of functional granulosa and theca cell gonadotropin receptors at the appropriate stage of follicle development[15,16].

Regardless of the type of system used to grow follicles in vitro, to be effective IVG strategies should be based at least in part on the physiological needs and the developmental time frames for oocyte growth in the body. In vivo, oocytes and their surrounding granulosa cells are closely surrounded by a complex extrafollicular milieu which includes ovarian stroma and theca cells at various stages of differentiation, branches of the systemic circulation, autonomic nervous system and scavenger cells. Many, or perhaps all, of these different cell types may influence the initiation and/or maintenance of early follicle growth through the synthesis and secretion of nutrients, hormones and/or growth factors. Overall, it would appear that the resting or growing status of follicles is regulated by the complex interaction between the growth stimulators and growth inhibitors produced by the oocyte and/or its surrounding somatic cells[17–19]. The balance between these growth factors may also regulate the susceptibility of early follicles to apoptosis[20]. It is clearly essential that the majority, if not all, of the events detailed above must be accurately replicated during follicle growth in vitro, otherwise the health, fertility and developmental potential of the mature in vitro-derived oocytes will be compromised.

THE CULTURE ENVIRONMENT

Overall, the success of follicle culture strategies appears to depend on a number of parameters including culture medium, granulosa cell association and differentiation, follicle size and follicle atresia. For example, the mutual interdependence of oocytes and granulosa cells for survival and normal development has important practical implications for IVG strategies. The granulosa–oocyte complex is a metabolically coupled unit in which the granulosa cells represent the nutrient and regulatory conduits between the oocyte and its environment throughout growth. This is regulated by phosphorylation events within the oocyte and through the glycolytic activity within the oocyte–cumulus complex during the resumption of meiosis. Importantly, both the inter-association of the somatic cells of the follicle and their differentiated status can be profoundly affected by components of the culture environment. Conversely, the physical and metabolic integrity of granulosa cell–oocyte interactions must be maintained to fully exploit the follicle's developmental potential *in vitro*.

A variety of culture systems and culture conditions have been used to support follicle growth *in vitro* for varying periods of time. The culture of follicles embedded in collagen-based matrices has proved effective in the mouse[21], as has placement of theca-free follicles upon collagen membranes[22]. Similarly, the extended incubation of intact follicles in microdrops of medium on tissue culture plastic has also proved an effective method of supporting follicle development from preantral to antral stages in the mouse[23–25], sheep[19,26], cow[27] and human[28].

The culture media used for the IVG of follicles from different species are still far from optimized. Follicle culture medium generally consists of a balanced salt solution, oxygen, bicarbonate ions, proteins, amino acids and a source of energy at a pH of 7.4, and includes defined growth factors with or without the presence of serum. The requirement for hormones, growth factors and peptides to support follicle and oocyte growth has important practical implications, as these requirements will change as follicles and oocytes develop *in vitro*. For example, inclusion of FSH in the culture medium is known to stimulate glucose utilization, estradiol production, follicle enlargement and increased granulosa cell density, and antrum formation in mouse follicles[29–31]. While the inclusion of serum is mandatory in some murine culture systems for follicular growth and survival (presumably by contributing hormones, nutrients and

growth and attachment factors such as collagen and fibronectin), in other culture systems serum may exert inhibitory effects on the phenotype of the somatic cells of the follicle. Typically, rat, ruminant and human granulosa cells cultured in the presence of serum or extracellular matrix proteins[32,33] proliferate rapidly to form epithelial monolayers and in doing so they lose the capacity to synthesize estradiol as they luteinize. In the case of long-term IVG protocols for the follicles from large animals, this remodeling may lead to the disruption of granulosa–oocyte contacts and extrusion of the oocyte, with the resultant loss of oocyte developmental potential.

In recent years, a new generation of serum-free culture media has been developed which supports the growth and normal differentiated functions of different ovarian cell types in domestic animals and humans[34–37]. Using this species-specific approach it is possible to both induce and maintain estradiol production by long-term cultures of granulosa cells, which remain exquisitely sensitive to physiological concentrations of gonadotropins and growth factors. In this system, cultured granulosa cells form distinct clumps of rounded cells that closely resemble the morphology of the cell type *in vivo*[38]. These serum-free media have proved equally effective when they are applied to IVG strategies, having been shown to maintain the extensive network of gap junctions between granulosa cells and also between the cumulus cells and the oocyte that supports follicle integrity *in vitro*. It is now possible to maintain the three-dimensional structure of ruminant[27,39] and human[28] follicles over extended periods, to induce antrum formation and oocyte growth in preantral follicles, and to induce steroidogenic function in the cultured follicles following the provision of adequate substrate[26,39].

While the growth-promoting supplements needed for follicle culture have been researched extensively in a number of species, we know relatively little about the metabolic requirements for follicle growth either *in vivo* or *in vitro* in any species. The ratio of glucose to pyruvate in the culture medium is likely to be very important for efficient energy utilization by the growing follicle. Furthermore, it is possible that the energy requirements of the oocyte and follicle cells will alter during periods of extended culture and during changing hormonal environments. Evidence to support this hypothesis is provided by a series of observations in cultured follicles. Glucose is consumed in increasing amounts by mouse follicles grown *in vitro*[30], where a high rate of glucose utilization and the glucose : lactate ratio indicated that glycolysis is an important pathway for energy production[30]. Also, human chorionic gonadotropin (hCG), in combination with FSH, elicited a large increase in the rate of glucose consumption. The reasons for this rise in glucose consumption have not been investigated but there are a number of possibilities. Glycolysis is known to be augmented in oocyte–cumulus cell complexes stimulated by FSH to recommence meiosis, due to an increase in hexokinase activity[40]. Another potential cause might relate to increased sodium pumping by granulosa cells into the antral cavity of the developing follicle(s), which would draw in fluid by osmosis, possibly facilitating ovulation. Furthermore, in the follicles of some species, for example rabbit, sodium levels are higher than in plasma/serum[41] and increase with antral follicle enlargement[42]. Sodium concentrations are also greater in growing antral follicles than in atretic follicles[42,43]. *In vivo*, ovarian glucose uptake is known to be augmented during the periovulatory period, a phenomenon known as the 'metabolic shift'[44]. It is not surprising therefore that an increase in follicle glucose consumption in response to ovulation induction was also noted by Boland and co-workers during the culture of mouse follicles[30]. Glucose is probably transported into granulosa cells by facilitated diffusion, which is responsive to endocrine and metabolic stimuli[45]. It is therefore likely that the amount and rate of glucose utilization in culture are affected by the amount of glucose available in the culture medium. Moreover, the use of combinations of hormones such as FSH and LH during IVG

may increase glucose consumption compared to FSH alone. When mouse follicles are cultured with LH in addition to FSH, steroidogenesis is greater than when follicles are cultured with FSH alone[31] as, presumably, greater energy production is required to sustain increased rates of estrogen production.

The metabolic requirements of *in vitro*-grown follicles may also be altered by suboptimal culture environments that promote cellular stress. An upregulation of lactate production has, for example, been observed in somatic cells in response to cellular stress[46]. This suggests that the culture environment and the presence/absence of the theca cell compartment and stromal cells may influence the metabolism of follicles *in vitro*[47,48]. Overall, these data highlight the need to develop a species-specific, physiological follicle culture environment.

IN VITRO GROWTH OF MAMMALIAN FOLLICLES

Primordial follicle culture

The ultimate goal for follicle culture is to be able to grow follicles from the primordial stage to maturity *in vitro* and to carry out IVM of fully grown oocytes with the production of viable embryos. Although primordial follicles are the smallest and most abundant stage of follicle development found in the mammalian ovarian cortex, the development of methods that will support the complete IVG and IVM of oocytes from these early staged follicles presents a major technical challenge for reproductive science. Despite extensive trials, the success obtained with preantral follicle cultures (detailed below) has proved difficult to repeat with isolated primordial and primary follicles, which are far more difficult to handle and culture[28,49]. A number of strategies have been tried.

Culture of isolated primordial follicles

Initial culture attempts concentrated on the IVG of isolated primordial follicles. The small size of the follicles at this stage prevents the use of manual techniques for isolation[50], and thus enzymatic methods have been routinely employed for follicle harvest. This has enabled primordial follicles to be recovered from porcine[51] and human[28,52–54] cortical tissue. Whilst a high percentage of follicles are viable following extraction (~ 71%[52]), the culture of isolated primordial follicles has proved to be relatively unsuccessful. IVG of isolated primordial follicles can be supported for up to 24 hours within a collagen gel[53], but beyond this time follicular collapse, oocyte extrusion and degeneration commonly occur. Although the presence of stromal cells around primordial follicles has been shown to improve initial culture success[55], long-term survival rates are still low. Damage to the basement membrane during the enzymatic isolation procedure and the migration of the single layer of pregranulosa cells away from the oocyte have been proposed to account for the poor in vitro success of isolated primordial follicle culture. In addition, if the growth of primordial follicles is mediated by extrafollicular growth factors then isolation will deprive them of exposure to these potential initiators, which may severely affect their ability to grow in vitro.

Culture of primordial follicles in situ

The culture of primordial follicles in situ within pieces of cortical tissue overcomes the requirement for enzymatic isolation, and also provides a complex support system that more closely resembles the ovarian environment in vivo. In early in situ IVG studies, large numbers of oocytes underwent atresia[56], and no follicular growth was observed[57]. Nevertheless, advances in our understanding of the specific requirements of cells within an in vitro environment have benefited the development of in situ culture systems, and considerable progress has been made over recent years. One of the first major breakthroughs was reported in 1996, with the demonstration that primordial follicles present within whole mouse ovaries could initiate growth in vitro and develop to multilayer stages over an 8-day period[1].

The large size of the ovaries from domestic animals and humans prevents the culture of the whole gonads, so it has been necessary to develop methods in which follicles can be grown within fragments or slices of ovarian cortex. Tissue pieces are commonly placed on a physical support, such as a porous membrane insert, in culture wells and the tissue is then covered with a meniscus of medium. In culture systems of this nature it is important that the pieces of tissue are small and thin. This ensures that the metabolic and nutritional requirements of the follicles can be adequately met by diffusion and the chance of tissue necrosis occurring in vitro is minimized. To date, pieces of fresh ovarian tissue obtained from several species have been cultured using this approach (Table 1). In all studies, initiation of primordial follicle growth was observed, and follicular development proceeded at least as far as the primary stage. Thus in situ culture is currently believed to provide the most suitable system for the initiation and maintenance of primordial follicle growth in vitro from large animals and humans.

Chorioallantoic membrane grafts

An alternative approach that incorporates the advantages of in situ cultures for primordial follicles involves placing cortical tissue fragments beneath the chorioallantoic membrane (CAM) of chick embryos[61]. The CAM is a well vascularized area that has been used widely to investigate the development of various organs[65]. Success with in ovo ovarian tissue experiments has however been limited, with few primordial follicles able to initiate growth within this environment[66]. The suitability of this methodology for use within a clinical environment is questionable, as it is likely to be beset by concerns comparable to those of xenografting with regard to the transmission of animal pathogens.

Preantral follicle culture

To date, some of the most successful follicle culture systems have been those designed to support the growth of follicles and oocyte from

Table 1 Summary of results obtained from the *in vitro* growth (IVG) of primordial follicles *in situ* in slices of fresh ovarian cortical tissue

Species	Study	Tissue piece/thickness	IVG duration	Results
Mouse	Eppig and O'Brien, 1996[1]	Whole fetal ovaries	8 days	initiation of primordial follicle growth development up to preantral (1–3 GC layers) stages
Cattle	Wandji *et al.*, 1996[58]	500 μm	0–7 days	initiation of primordial follicle growth a small number of primary follicles developed
	Braw-Tal and Yossefi, 1997[59]	1000–2000 μm	0–4 days	initiation of primordial follicle growth a small number of primary follicles developed
	Derrar *et al.*, 2000[60]	500 μm	8 days	initiation of primordial follicle growth a small number of primary follicles developed
	Fortune *et al.*, 2000[61]	500 μm	0–36 h	initiation of primordial follicle growth
Baboon	Wandji *et al.*, 1997[62]	500 μm	0–20 days	initiation of primordial follicle growth a small number of secondary follicles developed
Human	Hovatta *et al.*, 1997[63]	100–300 μm	0–21 days	primordial follicles were viable after the IVG period evidence of *in vitro* GC proliferation a small number of secondary follicles present
	Picton *et al.*, 1999[28]	80–100 μm	0–16 days	initiation of primordial follicle growth a small number of early preantral follicles developed
	Wright *et al.*, 1999[64]	1000–3000 μm	0–15 days	initiation of primordial follicle growth a small number of primary follicles developed

GC, granulosa cell

preantral stages onwards. Various methods have been developed to isolate and culture preantral follicles *in vitro*. Mechanical isolation is relatively easy for soft tissues such as fetal ovarian samples, which contain large numbers of small follicles. This method has been used successfully by a number of workers for mouse follicles[67]. The main advantage of this approach is that the theca layer remains intact and damage to the basement membrane is avoided. Many of the manually isolated follicles retain their characteristic structure when cultured individually *in vitro*, as the theca layer is important in sustaining three-dimensional development in the absence of a supporting gel and it may also promote antrum formation[68,69]. The observation that murine preantral follicles cultured without theca cells (i.e. follicles harvested by enzyme digestion) have retarded growth rates compared to their theca-enclosed counterparts (i.e. follicles harvested by mechanical isolation)[29] supports the concept that the theca cells make a significant contribution to oocyte growth and development *in vitro*, and that this effect is mediated via the granulosa cells[47,48].

In tough tissues like human, ovine or bovine ovarian cortex, it is technically difficult to mechanically isolate preantral follicles from the surrounding connective tissue. To combat this problem, researchers routinely use enzymatic methods, which are based on the use of collagenase type 1A and DNAse I, to harvest follicles[26,70,71]. This combination of enzymes softens the tissue so that the early staged follicles can be detected and mechanically detached from the surrounding stromal tissue using fine needles. While it is possible to harvest large numbers of follicles by enzymatic digestion the method is very slow, removes the theca cell layer and damages the basement membrane. Consequently, the follicles harvested by enzyme digestion methods are frequently considered to be granulosa–oocyte complexes rather than intact theca-enclosed follicles. Intact follicles can be collected from ovarian tissue for a number of species if sharp needles are used to tease apart the stroma tissue and release the follicles[19,72,73]. Alternatively, a 'sieving' method in which minced cortical tissue is pushed through a fine mesh has been employed[74]. Bovine preantral follicles have also been harvested by cutting the ovary into small pieces and the follicles loosened from the connective tissue by repeated pipetting[75].

PROSPECTS OF FOLLICLE CULTURE IN SMALL ANIMAL SPECIES

Preantral follicle culture techniques have been pioneered in rodents, with the most consistent results being achieved with mouse follicles[76]. Numerous strategies have been utilized for the culture of rodent follicles, although they are all essentially modifications of several key systems. The advantage of using rodent tissue for IVG is that their ovaries are small and contain a large number of follicles embedded within a soft stromal tissue matrix; this aids the mechanical isolation of theca-intact follicles.

Attachment cultures for intact follicles or granulosa–oocyte complexes

Damage to the basement membrane and theca cell layer(s) during enzymatic follicle isolation can result in the spontaneous migration of granulosa cells away from the oocyte once the granulosa–oocyte complexes are cultured[77]. As contact and communication between the granulosa cells and the oocyte are vital for normal oocyte growth and development, one of the main objectives of isolated granulosa–oocyte complex culture systems is to restrict the extent of this remodeling. This has been achieved by placing granulosa–oocyte cell complexes onto collagen-treated porous membranes or dishes coated with, for example, poly-L-lysine[22,78,79]. Here the outer granulosa cells attach to the collagen or lysine, which limits migration away from the oocyte, and the complexes extend a stalk of granulosa cells bearing an oocyte like the cumulus oophorus of a Graafian follicle. Perhaps because of the remodeling of the granulosa cells, this approach produces better results than suspending the complexes in collagen gels[21]. Using these systems, oocytes are able to acquire developmental competence, as demonstrated by the production of a number of live young[78].

Alternatively, intact follicles can be placed into microdrops of culture medium under oil in uncoated dishes. Here the theca cells migrate to the surface of the dish to form a monolayer, which then anchors the follicle and prevents granulosa cell migration[25]. Although follicular shape and architecture are altered using this method, all three follicular cell types remain in contact, antral-like cavities are formed and responsiveness to gonadotropin stimulation is preserved. Consequently, up to 40% of the cultured follicles produce oocytes which can be induced to undergo IVM to the metaphase II (MII) stage after 2 weeks of culture with FSH and acute exposure to stimulation with hCG (Figure 1). This technique has permitted the successful development of follicles isolated from both fresh[25] and cryopreserved[80,81] murine tissue.

Non-attached cultures of granulosa–oocyte complexes

The migration of granulosa cells in vitro can also be limited by embedding granulosa–oocyte complexes in either a collagen gel[21] or agar[82]. However, it is quite difficult to recover complexes from the gels following culture and enzymes often have to be employed to disaggregate the matrix, which may inflict additional damage on the complex[69].

Non-attached cultures of intact follicles

Perhaps the most physiological IVG model system used for the culture of murine follicles

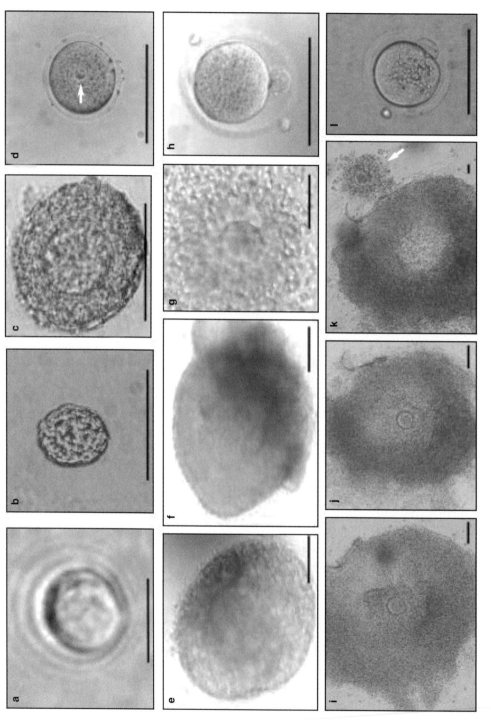

Figure 1 Isolated murine follicles and oocytes at different stages of development *in vivo* and after growth *in vitro* in an attachment culture system. Images (a)–(d) and (e)–(h) are of *in vivo*-grown follicles and oocytes: (a) primordial follicle; (b) primary follicle with 1–2 layers of granulosa cells; (c) secondary follicle with 2–3 layers of granulosa cells and one layer of theca cells; (d) immature oocyte from a secondary follicle – the germinal vesicle is visible (arrow); (e) antral follicle; (f) preovulatory follicle; (g) *in vivo*-grown cumulus–oocyte complex; (h) denuded metaphase II oocyte grown and matured *in vivo*. Images (i)–(l) are of *in vitro*-grown follicles and oocytes derived from an attachment culture system[25]: (i) *in vitro*-grown two-dimensional follicle with antral-like cavity; (j) *in vitro*-grown two-dimensional preovulatory follicle with antral-like cavity; (k) *in vitro*-grown follicle after ovulation of the cumulus–oocyte complex (arrow); (l) denuded metaphase II oocyte derived from a preantral follicle grown to maturity *in vitro*. Scale bars = 100 μm, except in (a) where bar = 20 μm. See Color Plate II

has been reported by Nayudu and Osborn[23]. These authors have shown that it is possible to grow intact mid-preantral sized mouse follicles on a porous membrane or in microdrops of medium under mineral oil. These follicles develop to the Graafian stage in about 6 days, with normal morphology and steroid production[30,83,84], and up to 80% of them ovulate in vitro in response to hCG[85] and give rise to live young[83].

PROSPECTS OF FOLLICLE CULTURE IN LARGE DOMESTIC ANIMALS AND HUMANS

Success has been more limited in experiments using follicles from large domestic animals and humans. One of the main reasons for the lack of progress is that it is technically far more difficult to recover follicles from the ovaries of these species, as detailed earlier. At the present time the culture of porcine follicles has proved to be the most successful, with a small number of meiotically competent oocytes being obtained following IVG in either collagen gels[86] or uncoated culture wells[87]. In addition, the in vitro fertilization of these IVG-derived MII-stage oocytes has led to limited blastocyst production[88].

A considerable amount of progress has also been made in methods used for the IVG of ruminant follicles. Antral cavity formation has been demonstrated in a number of studies on bovine preantral follicle culture[27,89,90], although the ability of the oocytes to undergo maturation has not been assessed. Ovine preantral follicles have been isolated from fresh tissue and grown to antral sizes over a short period, with a proportion of the oocytes being capable of progressing to MII[91]. Using the physiological serum-free culture media described earlier, granulosa–oocyte complexes and intact follicles from both fresh and cryopreserved tissue[19,26] have been successfully grown to antral sizes over 30 days in vitro. Using this approach it has also been possible to conduct a direct comparison of the growth rates of theca-free granulosa–oocyte complexes harvested by enzymatic digestion and theca-intact follicles

harvested by mechanical isolation (Figure 2). The data from the culture of sheep tissue suggest that, unlike mice, the in vitro growth and antral cavity formation rates in this species are greater in follicles lacking the theca cell layer[19]. In the theca-intact follicles, antral status was achieved in vitro by the oocyte and granulosa cell compartments breaking through the basement membrane and theca cells layers that remain tightly associated (Figure 2). This observation serves to highlight both the potential species-specific differences in the response of different sized follicles to the culture environment and the differential growth rates of rodent and ruminant follicles. The requirement for theca cell interactions in optimizing ruminant and human preantral–antral follicle culture systems may perhaps be overcome through improvement of the culture media and/or the co-culture of enzymatically isolated preantral follicles with theca cell monolayers. The optimal method for the isolation and culture of viable preantral follicles from large animal species and humans remains to be elucidated.

With regard to the IVG of human preantral granulosa–oocyte complexes and intact follicles, limited development up to antral sizes has been observed following enzymatic isolation and culture within agar[70] or collagen[53,54] gels. Mechanical isolation and IVG have also been demonstrated[92], although levels of atresia following culture were found to be high. With the same basic methods as used for the serum-free culture of sheep preantral follicles, it has been possible to induce antral cavity formation and growth of isolated human follicles over 30 days in vitro[28]. The meiotic competence and developmental capacity of human oocytes grown from preantral stages in vitro have not yet been reported. However, the systems needed to support the IVM of human oocytes in a clinical setting are relatively well established[93].

FUTURE PRIORITIES FOR FOLLICLE CULTURE

While the provision of appropriate levels of growth factors, cell survival factors, energy

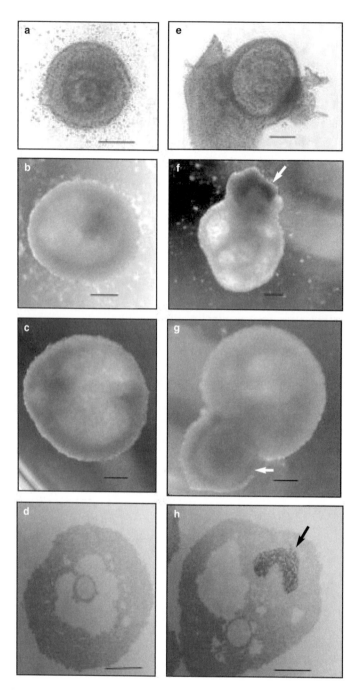

Figure 2 Growth of isolated preantral (180–220 μm diameter) sheep follicles in serum-free culture media over 30 days *in vitro*. Theca-free follicles harvested by enzyme digestion (a) develop antral cavities *in vitro* (b and c) and show no evidence of the presence of the basement membrane at the end of culture – indicated by lack of blue staining for the presence of collagen (d). In contrast, theca-enclosed follicles collected by mechanical isolation (e) show evidence of antral cavity formation by outgrowth from the dense theca and stromal cells (arrow) (f and g) that remain concentrated within one area as indicated positive staining for collagen (blue color) (h) after extended culture. Scale bars = 50 μm. Reproduced from reference 19 with permission. See Color Plate III

substrates and gases in the culture environment is clearly essential for the growth of healthy follicles *in vitro*, the length of the culture period and the use of media additives and/or supplements such as serum must be fully optimized for each species otherwise the health and developmental potential of the follicles and oocytes they contain may be compromised. In support of this hypothesis, in many species, IVM – which involves only the short-term culture of fully grown oocytes to support their nuclear and cytoplasmic maturation – followed by IVF is often associated with large offspring syndrome[94] and the aberrant expression of the imprinted gene and/or their epigenetic regulators[95]. Similarly, the mouse derived from complete IVG of a primordial follicle over approximately 3 weeks followed by fertilization *in vitro*[1] was very sickly[96], and the efficiency of embryo production and implantation in these studies was very low. While the protocols used to generate live offspring from murine primordial cultures have been substantially improved[2,3], other recent evidence from mice, sheep and cattle suggests that developmental defects can be induced in embryos following extended culture in suboptimal environments. These defects are due to the abberant expression and/or methylation of key imprinted genes[97-100]. Furthermore, additional murine culture data

suggest that whereas ovarian tissue is exposed to plasma oxygen levels of about 5% *in vivo*, growing mouse follicles *in vitro* in 5% oxygen results in an increased frequency of mature oocytes with incorrectly aligned chromosomes and many of the offspring die prematurely, compared to follicles cultured in 20% oxygen[101]. These results highlight the need for further extensive research to fully optimize the culture environment for each species whilst at the same time testing the genetic health and normality of the *in vitro*-derived oocytes.

CONCLUSION

Despite the potential benefits of growing follicles *in vitro*, many problems must still be overcome if we are ever to be able to achieve the goal of complete IVG and IVM of oocytes. Where follicle culture technology is to be used as a means to restore the fertility of young cancer patients, culture method development must progress alongside improvements in cryopreservation protocols. Furthermore, it is likely that the future success of IVG/IVM systems will only be achieved by improving our understanding of the molecular and cell biology of follicle and oocyte development. This in turn will support the development of improved, extended culture methodologies.

References

1. Eppig JJ, O'Brien MJ. Development *in vitro* of mouse oocytes from primordial follicles. *Biol Reprod* 1996;54:197–207
2. Obata Y, Kono T, Hatada I. Maturation of mouse fetal germ cells *in vitro*. *Nature* 2000; 418:497–8
3. O'Brien MJ, Pendola JK, Eppig JJ. A revised protocol for *in vitro* development of mouse oocytes from primordial follicles dramatically improved their developmental competence. *Biol Reprod* 2003;68:1682–6
4. Shaw JM, Bowles J, Koopman P, *et al*. Fresh and cryopreserved ovarian tissue samples from donors with lymphoma transmit the cancer to graft recipients. *Hum Reprod* 1996;11:1668–73
5. Kim S-S, Radford J, Harris M, *et al*. Ovarian tissue harvested from lymphoma patients to preserve fertility may be safe for autotransplantation. *Hum Reprod* 2001;16:2056–60
6. Eppig JJ, Wigglesworth K, Pendola FL. The mammalian oocyte orchestrates the rate of ovarian follicular development. *Proc Natl Acad Sci USA* 2002;99:2890–4
7. Moor RM, Dai Y, Lee C, *et al*. Oocyte maturation and embryonic failure. *Hum Reprod Update* 1998;4:223–36

8. Picton HM, Briggs D, Gosden RG. The molecular basis of oocyte growth and development. *Mol Cell Endocrinol* 1998;145:27–37

9. Green DPL. Three dimensional structure of the zona pellucida. *Rev Reprod* 1997;2:147–56

10. Fulka J Jr, First NL, Moor RM. Nuclear and cytoplasmic determinants involved in the regulation of mammalian oocyte maturation. *Mol Hum Reprod* 1998;4:41–9

11. Mertineit C, Yoder JA, Taketo T, *et al.* Sex-specific exons control DNA methyltransferase in mammalian germ cells. *Development* 1998; 125:889–97

12. Young LE, Fairburn HR. Improving the safety of embryo technologies: possible role of genomic imprinting. *Theriogenology* 2000;53:627–48

13. Anderson E, Albertini DF. Gap junctions between the oocyte and companion follicle cells in the mammalian ovary. *J Cell Biol* 1976; 71:680–6

14. Gougeon A. Regulation of ovarian follicular development in primates – facts and hypotheses. *Endocr Rev* 1996;17:121–55

15. McNatty KP, Heath DA, Lundy T, *et al.* Control of early ovarian follicular development. *J Reprod Fertil Suppl* 1999;49:123–35

16. Oktay K, Briggs D, Gosden RG. Ontogeny of follicle stimulating hormone receptor gene expression in isolated human ovarian follicles. *J Clin Endocrinol Metab* 1997;82:3748–51

17. Picton HM. Activation of follicle development: the primordial follicle. *Theriogenology* 2001;55: 1193–210

18. Trounson A, Anderiesz C, Jones G. Maturation of human oocytes *in vitro* and their developmental competence. *Reproduction* 2001;121: 51–75

19. Picton HM, Danfour MA, Harris SE, *et al.* Growth and maturation of oocytes *in vitro*. *Reprod Suppl* 2003;61:445–62

20. Braw-Tal R. The initiation of follicle growth: the oocyte or the somatic cells? *Mol Cell Endocrinol* 2002;187:11–18

21. Torrance C, Telfer E, Gosden RG. Quantitative study of the development of isolated mouse pre-antral follicles in collagen gel culture. *J Reprod Fertil* 1989;87:367–74

22. Eppig JJ, Wigglesworth K, O'Brien MJ. Comparison of embryonic developmental competence of mouse oocytes grown with and without serum. *Mol Reprod Dev* 1992;32:33–40

23. Nayudu PL, Osborn SM. Factors influencing the rate of preantral and antral growth of mouse ovarian follicles *in vitro*. *J Reprod Fertil* 1992;95:349–62

24. Boland NI, Humpherson PG, Leese HJ, *et al.* Pattern of lactate production and steroidogenesis during growth and maturation of mouse ovarian follicles *in vitro*. *Biol Reprod* 1993;48:798–806

25. Cortvrindt R, Smitz J, Van Steirteghem AC. *In vitro* maturation, fertilization and embryo development of immature oocytes from early preantral follicles from prepuberal mice in a simplified culture system. *Hum Reprod* 1996; 11:2656–66

26. Newton H, Picton H, Gosden RG. *In vitro* growth of oocyte–granulosa cell complexes isolated from cryopreserved ovine tissue. *J Reprod Fertil* 1999;115:141–50

27. Gutierrez CG, Ralph JH, Telfer E, *et al.* Growth and antrum formation of bovine preantral follicles in long-term culture *in vitro*. *Biol Reprod* 2000;62:1322–8

28. Picton HM, Mkandla A, Salha O, *et al.* Initiation of human primordial follicle growth *in vitro* in ultra-thin slices of ovarian cortex. *Hum Reprod* 1999;13:abstr. 0–020

29. Boland NI, Gosden RG. Effects of epidermal growth factor on the growth and differentiation of cultured mouse ovarian follicles. *J Reprod Fertil* 1994;101:369–74

30. Boland NI, Humpherson PG, Leese HJ, *et al.* The effect of glucose metabolism on murine follicle development and steroidogenesis *in vitro*. *Hum Reprod* 1994;9:617–23

31. Spears N, Murray AA, Allison V, *et al.* Role of gonadotrophins and steroids in the development of mouse follicles *in vitro*. *J Reprod Fertil* 1998;113:19–26

32. Amsterdam A, Rotmensch S. Structure–function relationships during granulosa cell differentiation. *Endocr Rev* 1987;8:309–37

33. Furman A, Rotmensch S, Dor J, *et al.* Culture of human granulosa cells from an *in vitro* fertilization program: effects of extracellular matrix on morphology and cyclic adenosine 3′, 5′ monophosphate production. *Fertil Steril* 1986;46:514–17

34. Campbell BK, Scaramuzzi RJ, Webb R. Induction and maintenance of oestradiol and immunoreactive inhibin production with FSH by ovine granulosa cells cultured in serum-free media. *J Reprod Fertil* 1996;106:7–16

35. Gutierrez CG, Campbell BK, Webb R. Development of a long term bovine granulosa cell culture system: induction and maintenance of estradiol production response to FSH and morphological characteristics. *Biol Reprod* 1997;56:608–16

36. Picton HM, Campbell BK, Hunter MG. Maintenance of oestradiol production and cytochrome P450 aromatase enzyme messenger ribonucleic acid expression in long-term serum-free cultures of porcine granulosa cells. *J Reprod Fertil* 1999;115:67–77

37. Wynn P, Picton HM, Krapez JA, *et al.* FSH pre-treatment promotes the numbers of human oocytes reaching metaphase II by *in vitro* maturation. *Hum Reprod* 1998;13:3132–8

38. Chang SCS, Anderson W, Lewis JC, *et al.* The porcine ovarian follicle. II. Electron microscopic study of surface features of granulosa cells at different stages of development. *Biol Reprod* 1977;16:349–57

39. Picton HM, Gosden RG. Ovarian tissue banking and *in vitro* growth and maturation of human primordial follicles. *Mol Cell Endocrinol* 2000;166:27–35

40. Downs SM, Humpherson PG, Leese HJ. Meiotic induction in cumulus cell-enclosed mouse oocytes: involvement of the pentose phosphate pathway *Biol Reprod* 1998;58:1084–94

41. Gosden RG, Hunter RHF, Telfer E, *et al.* Physiological factors underlying the formation of ovarian follicular fluid. *J Reprod Fertil* 1988;82:813–25

42. Wise T. Biochemical analysis of bovine follicular fluid: albumin, total protein, lysosomal enzymes, steroids and ascorbic acid content in relation to follicle size, rank, atresia classification and day of estrous cycle. *J Anim Sci* 1987;64:1153–69

43. Rondell PA. Follicular fluid electrolytes in ovulation. *Proc Soc Exp Biol Med* 1964;116:336–9

44. Armstrong DT, Greep RO. Effect of gonadotrophic hormones on glucose metabolism by luteinized rat ovaries. *Endocrinology* 1962;70:701–10

45. Allen WR, Nilsen-Hamilton M, Hamilton RT. Insulin and growth factors stimulate rapid posttranslational changes in glucose transport in ovarian granulosa cells. *J Cell Physiol* 1981;108:15–24

46. Elekes O, Venema K, Postema F, *et al.* Evidence that stress activates glial lactate formation *in vivo* assessed with rat hippocampus lactography. *Neurosci Lett* 1996;208:69–72

47. Kotsuji F, Kubo M, Tominaga A. Effect of interactions between granulosa and theca cells on meiotic arrest in bovine oocytes. *J Reprod Fertil* 1994;100:151–6

48. Richard FJ, Sirard MA. Effects of follicular cells on oocyte maturation. II: Theca cell inhibition of bovine oocyte maturation *in vitro*. *Biol Reprod* 1996;54:22–8

49. Hovatta O, Wright C, Krausz T, *et al.* Human primordial, primary and secondary ovarian follicles in long-term culture: effect of partial isolation. *Hum Reprod* 1999;14:2519–24

50. Gosden RG. Biology and technology of primordial follicle development. In Lauria A, Gandolfi F, Enne G, Gianaroli L, eds. *Gametes:*

Development and Function. Rome: Serono Symposia, 1998:71–83

51. Greenwald GS, Moor RM. Isolation and preliminary characterization of pig primordial follicles. *J Reprod Fertil* 1989;87:561–71

52. Oktay K, Nugent D, Newton H, *et al.* Isolation and characterization of primordial follicles from fresh and cryopreserved human ovarian tissue. *Fertil Steril* 1997;67:481–6

53. Abir R, Roizman P, Fisch B, *et al.* Pilot study of isolated early human follicles cultured in collagen gels for 24 hours. *Hum Reprod* 1999;14:1299–301

54. Abir R, Fisch B, Nitke S, *et al.* Morphological study of fully and partially isolated early human follicles. *Fertil Steril* 2001;75:141–6

55. Osborn SM, Gook DA, Stern K, *et al.* The isolation and culture of human primordial follicles from fresh ovarian tissue [abstract]. *Hum Reprod* 1997;12(Suppl 1):153

56. Blandau RJ, Warrick E, Rumery RE. *In vitro* cultivation of fetal mouse ovaries. *Fertil Steril* 1965;16:705–15

57. Baker TG, Neal P. Organ culture of cortical fragments and Graafian follicles from human ovaries. *J Anat* 1974;117:361–71

58. Wandji S-A, Srsen V, Voss AK, *et al.* Initiation *in vitro* of growth of bovine primordial follicles. *Biol Reprod* 1996;55:942–8

59. Braw-Tal R, Yossefi S. Studies *in vivo* and *in vitro* on the initiation of follicle growth in the bovine ovary. *J Reprod Fertil* 1997;109:165–71

60. Derrar N, Price CA, Sirard MA. Effect of growth factors and co-culture with ovarian medulla on the activation of primordial follicles in explants of ovarian cortex. *Theriogenology* 2000;54:587–98

61. Fortune JE, Cushman RA, Wahl CM, *et al.* The primordial to primary follicle transition. *Mol Cell Endocrinol* 2000;163:53–60

62. Wandji SA, Srsen V, Nathanielsz PW, *et al.* Initiation of growth of baboon primordial follicles *in vitro*. *Hum Reprod* 1997;12:1993–2001

63. Hovatta O, Silye R, Abir R, *et al.* Extracellular matrix improves survival of both stored and fresh human primordial and primary ovarian follicles in long-term culture. *Hum Reprod* 1997;12:1032–6

64. Wright C, Hovatta O, Margara R, *et al.* Effect of follicle stimulating hormone and serum substitution on the development and growth of early human follicles. *Hum Reprod* 1999;14:1555–62

65. Rawls ME. Transplantation of normal embryonic tissues. *Ann NY Acad Sci* 1952;55:302–12

66. Cushman RA, Wahl CM, Fortune JE. Bovine ovarian cortical pieces grafted to chick embryonic membranes: a model for studies on the

activation of primordial follicles. *Hum Reprod* 2002;17:48–54

67. Hartshorne GM. *In vitro* culture of ovarian follicles. *Rev Reprod* 1997;2:94–104
68. Qvist R, Blackwell LF, Bourne H, *et al.* Development of mouse ovarian follicles from primary to preovulatory stages *in vitro*. *J Reprod Fertil* 1990;89:169–80
69. Gosden RG, Boland NI, Spears N, *et al.* The biology and technology of follicular oocyte development *in vitro*. *Reprod Med Rev* 1993;2:129–52
70. Roy SK, Treacy BJ. Isolation and long-term culture of human pre-antral follicles. *Fertil Steril* 1993;59:783–90
71. Wandji SA, Eppig JJ, Fortune JE. FSH and growth factors affect growth and endocrine function *in vitro* of granulosa cells of bovine preantral follicle. *Theriogenology* 1996;45:817–32
72. Katska L, Alm H, Kanitz W. Isolation and culture of bovine preantral and early antral follicles. *Assoc Eur Trans Embryo News* 2002;15:10–11
73. Thomas FH, Leask R, Srsen V, *et al.* Effect of ascorbic acid on health and morphology of bovine preantral follicles during long-term culture. *Reproduction* 2001;122:487–95
74. Danfour MA. *Influence of the environment on mammalian oocyte development*. PhD thesis, University of Leeds, 2001
75. Figueiredo JR, Hulshof SC, Van den Hurk R, *et al.* Development of a new mechanical method for the isolation of intact preantral follicles from fetal, calf and adult bovine ovaries. *Theriogenology* 1993;40:789–99
76. Gosden RG, Mullan J, Picton HM, *et al.* Current perspective on primordial follicle cryopreservation and culture for reproductive medicine. *Hum Reprod Update* 2002;8:105–10
77. Nayudu PL, Fehrenbach A, Kiesel P, *et al.* Progress towards understanding follicle development *in vitro*: appearances are not deceiving. *Arch Med Res* 2001;32:587–94
78. Eppig JJ, Schroeder AC. Capacity of mouse oocytes from preantral follicles to undergo embryogenesis and development to live young after growth, maturation and fertilization *in vitro*. *Biol Reprod* 1989;41:268–76
79. Cain L, Chatterjee S, Collins TJ. *In vitro* folliculogenesis of rat preantral follicles. *Endocrinology* 1995;136:3369–77
80. Smitz JE, Cortvrindt RG. Follicle culture after ovarian cryostorage. *Maturitas* 1998;30:171–9
81. Newton H, Illingworth P. *In vitro* growth of murine preantral follicles after isolation from cryopreserved ovarian tissue. *Hum Reprod* 2001;16:423–9
82. Roy SK, Greenwald GS. Hormonal requirements for the growth and differentiation of

hamster preantral follicles in long-term culture. *J Reprod Fertil* 1989;87:103–14
83. Spears N, Boland NI, Murray AA, *et al.* Mouse oocytes derived from *in vitro* grown primary ovarian follicles are fertile. *Hum Reprod* 1994;9:527–32
84. Hartshorne GM, Sargent IL, Barlow DH. Meiotic progression of mouse oocytes throughout follicle growth and ovulation *in vitro*. *Hum Reprod* 1994;9:352–9
85. Rose UM, Hanssen RG, Kloosterboer HJ. Development and characterisation of an *in vitro* ovulation model using mouse ovarian follicles. *Biol Reprod* 1999;61:503–11
86. Hirao Y, Nagai T, Kubo M, *et al.* *In vitro* growth and maturation of pig oocytes. *J Reprod Fertil* 1994;100:333–9
87. Telfer EE, Binnie JP, McCaffery FH, *et al.* *In vitro* development of oocytes from porcine and bovine primary follicles. *Mol Cell Endocrinol* 2000;163:117–23
88. Wu J, Emery BR, Carrell DT. *In vitro* growth, maturation, fertilization and embryonic development of oocytes from porcine preantral follicles. *Biol Reprod* 2001;64:375–81
89. McCaffery FH, Leask R, Riley SC, *et al.* Culture of bovine preantral follicles in a serum-free system: markers for assessment of growth and development. *Biol Reprod* 2000;63:267–73
90. Itoh T, Kacchi M, Abe H, *et al.* Growth, antrum formation, and estradiol production of bovine preantral follicles cultured in a serum-free medium. *Biol Reprod* 2002;67:1099–105
91. Cecconi S, Barboni B, Coccia M, *et al.* *In vitro* development of sheep preantral follicles. *Biol Reprod* 1999;60:594–601
92. Abir R, Franks S, Mobberley MA, *et al.* Mechanical isolation and *in vitro* growth of preantral and small antral human follicles. *Fertil Steril* 1997;68:682–8
93. Picton HM. Oocyte maturation *in vitro*. *Curr Opin Obstet Gynecol* 2002;14:295–302
94. Leese HJ, Donnay I, Thompson JG. Human assisted conception: a cautionary tale. Lessons from domestic animals. *Hum Reprod* 1998;13(Suppl 4):184–202
95. Young LE, Sinclair KD, Wilmut I. Large offspring syndrome in cattle and sheep. *Rev Reprod* 1998;3:155–63
96. Eppig JJ, O'Brien MJ. Comparison of preimplantation developmental competence after mouse oocyte growth and development *in vitro* and *in vivo*. *Theriogenology* 1997;49:415–22
97. Doherty AS, Mann MR, Tremblay KD, *et al.* Differential effects of culture on imprinted H19 expression in the preimplantation mouse embryo. *Biol Reprod* 2000;62:1526–35

98. Khosla S, Dean W, Reik W, *et al.* Culture of preimplantation embryos and its long-term effects on gene expression and phenotype. *Hum Reprod Update* 2001;7:419–27

99. Kerjean A, Couvert P, Heams T, *et al. In vitro* follicular growth affects oocyte imprinting establishment in mice. *Eur J Hum Genet* 2003; 11:493–6

100. Young LE, Fernandes K, McEvoy TG, *et al.* Epigenetic change in IGF2R is associated with fetal overgrowth after sheep embryo culture. *Nat Genet* 2001;27:153–4

101. Hu Y, Betzendahl I, Cortvrindt R, *et al.* Effects of low O_2 and ageing on spindles and chromosomes in mouse oocytes from pre-antral follicle culture. *Hum Reprod* 2001;16:737–48

Pregnancy after pelvic irradiation 15

H. O. D. Critchley and W. H. B. Wallace

INTRODUCTION

Current therapeutic advances in the management of childhood cancer mean that the majority of children can have a realistic hope for long-term survival after treatment. Cancer in childhood is rare, within the UK approximately 1400 new cases per year, and the cumulative risk is around one in 500 by the age of 15 years. With long-term survival rates approaching 70%, it has been estimated that, by the year 2010, about one in 715 of the adult population will be a long-term survivor of childhood cancer[1,2].

The treatment of childhood cancer may involve a combination of surgery, radiotherapy, chemotherapy and bone marrow transplantation (BMT). The challenge to carers of these children is to maintain the excellent survival rates and to minimize the incidence and severity of treatment-related late effects. In the future, a successful pregnancy will depend upon a functioning hypothalamic–pituitary–ovarian axis and a uterine environment that not only is receptive to implantation but also able to accommodate normal growth of the developing fetus to term. Thus adverse effects on pregnancy potential may be mediated through the hypothalamic–pituitary–ovarian axis[3], the ovary[4,5] or the uterus[6,7]. One of the most important issues for the survivors of childhood cancer is the impact of their disease and its treatment on reproductive function and the implications for the health of their offspring. In the female, chemotherapy and radiotherapy may damage the ovary and hasten oocyte depletion, resulting in loss of hormone production, truncated fecundity and a premature menopause[8,9]. It is the recognition of the impact of cancer treatment on reproductive potential that has driven the pursuit of strategies to preserve fertility.

This chapter focuses on the effects of pelvic irradiation on pregnancy potential. Where considered important and relevant to successful achievement of a pregnancy, mention is also made of the late effects of exposure to cranial and total body irradiation (TBI).

PRIMORDIAL FOLLICLE RESERVE AND FERTILITY POTENTIAL

The human ovary contains a fixed population of primordial follicles. This pool is maximal at 5 months of gestational age, with approximately 2 million oocytes present at birth, and thereafter declines steadily throughout life[10,11]. The 'fertile window' in females is characterized by roughly 400 monthly ovulations of a mature oocyte. Follicle depletion, as a result of atresia and recruitment towards ovulation, leads to premature exhaustion of the follicle pool and menopause at a median age of 51 years. The rate of oocyte decline represents an instantaneous rate of temporal change, based upon the remaining population in the primordial follicle pool. To make it possible to predict the age of menopause in women who have been exposed to radiotherapy in a field that includes the ovaries, the extent of the radiation-induced damage to the follicle pool must be determined[12]. In an earlier study it was estimated that the dose of radiation required to destroy 50% of primordial follicles (LD_{50}) was < 4 Gy[13]. In a recent subsequent study, it has been calculated that for a given dose of radiotherapy, the surviving fraction may be determined and thus the age of menopause

207

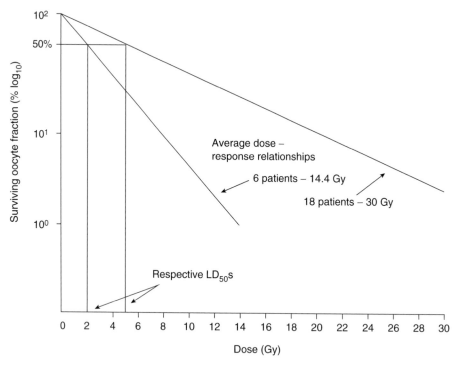

Figure 1 Dose–response relationships for the human oocyte. The mean surviving fraction of oocytes for each patient has been calculated and plotted against the dose of radiation received for (i) the six patients who received 14.4 Gy and (ii) the 18 patients who received 30 Gy. These lines represent the estimated (fractionated) dose–response relationship for the human oocyte. The LD_{50} is given by the dose required to leave a surviving fraction of 50%. Our revised LD_{50} of < 2 Gy is taken from the relationship obtained from the data for the cohort of six patients. Adapted from reference 12, with permission

predicted by the application of a mathematical model for decay[12]. Thus, based on new data and a revised mathematical model of natural oocyte decline, it is possible to determine the surviving fraction of oocytes following irradiation. The LD_{50} of the human oocyte has now been estimated to be < 2 Gy (see Figure 1).

It should thus be possible for women to be counseled about their potential reproductive lifespan and likely window of opportunity for fertility[14]. A premature loss of oocytes will result in impaired ovarian hormone production, uterine dysfunction due to inadequate estrogen exposure and an early menopause.

RADIATION-INDUCED OVARIAN DAMAGE

The degree of impairment of ovarian function is related to the radiation dose, fractionation

schedule and age at the time of cancer treatment[7,13,15]. TBI, either alone or in combination with chemotherapy, may result in impairment or loss of ovarian function. In a long-term follow-up study of 532 women at a median (range) time of 3 (1–17) years after TBI (10–15.75 Gy, single exposure or fractionated) and cyclophosphamide (200 mg/kg), ovarian failure was observed in 90% of patients. Ovarian failure was reported in 72% of patients in a separate cohort of young girls treated before puberty[16].

Exposure to abdominal and pelvic irradiation is part of the therapy for management of Wilms' tumour, pelvic rhabdomyosarcoma and Ewing's sarcoma of the pelvis or spine. Ovarian failure has been reported in 97% of young women after total abdominal irradiation (20–30 Gy) in childhood[5]. Young women exposed to flank irradiation (20–30 Gy) may have preservation of ovarian function. However, among those women who do conceive after exposure to 20–30 Gy of abdominal irradiation, there is high risk of mid-trimester miscarriage and subsequent early menopause. A retrospective study, based on data from 830 long-term female survivors in Canada[17], reported that the risk of early menopause increased significantly with an increasing dose of abdominal irradiation. The relative risk with doses < 20 Gy was 1.02, increasing to 1.37 with radiation doses of 20–35 Gy, and the relative risk was 3.27 with doses greater than 35 Gy.

Exposure to both radiotherapy and chemotherapy may damage the ovary and hasten oocyte loss. Abdominal, pelvic and total body irradiation may all lead to impairment of ovarian function[5,9,18–20]. The Five Center Study commissioned by the National Cancer Institute in North America[21,22] tracked cancer treatment survivors over 30 years, between 1945 and 1975. The study demonstrated an adjusted relative fertility in survivors of 0.85 (95% confidence interval 0.78–0.92) when compared to their siblings. An early menopause was more common among those young women who had been exposed to infradiaphragmatic irradiation and alkylating agents. The average age of menopause was 31 years and the risk of early loss of ovarian function increased with increasing age at the time of treatment[21,22].

Exposure to cranial irradiation may also impair ovarian function through effects on hypothalamic–pituitary–ovarian function. High-dose (> 24 Gy) radiotherapy to the hypothalamus and pituitary (as used for the management of brain tumors) is associated with a risk of delayed puberty. On the other hand, lower doses of cranial radiotherapy (< 24 Gy) are more often accompanied by a precocious puberty in young girls. For these reasons, girls treated with cranial irradiation should have their puberty status evaluated three to four times a year after completion of their treatment[2,23,24].

The later effects of hypothalamic–pituitary–ovarian dysfunction may be progressive with time and quite subtle. A decrease in secretion of luteinizing hormone (LH), an attenuated LH surge and shorter luteal phases have been reported among a group of women exposed to only low-dose (18–24 Gy) cranial irradiation[3]. There is an association between short luteal phases and impaired fertility and early miscarriage[25]. Data such as described above, indicate the importance of detailed follow-up for these patients if the immediate and also longer-term effects on their reproductive potential and thus pregnancy are to be evaluated.

RADIATION-INDUCED UTERINE DAMAGE

It is well recognized that both uterine development and uterine function risk compromise after pelvic irradiation, irrespective of age at the time of treatment. The degree of uterine damage is related to the total irradiation dose, the fractionation schedule employed and the site of irradiation. The risk of future compromise to growth and function of the uterus is greatest if radiation exposure takes place prepuberty. At the time of normal puberty, in response to increases in ovarian estrogen production, the uterus changes shape from a tubular to a pear-shaped organ and there is an increase in all dimensions, as well as in the thickness of the endometrium[26,27]. Uterine growth postmenarche has been demonstrated to be related to the number of years after menarche and not to the age, height or weight of the subject[26].

Both high-dose abdominal irradiation (20–30 Gy) and lower doses, as used for TBI (14.4 Gy), will result in uterine dysfunction. Uterine distensibility and blood flow are irreversibly affected by high-dose pelvic or abdominal irradiation in childhood[6]. It is likely that there are long-term effects of high-dose pelvic radiotherapy on the vasculature and development of the uterus.

There is evidence that young women exposed to TBI also suffer impaired uterine growth and blood flow[28]. In a small but important study where uterine function was evaluated in 12 women between 4 and 10.9 years after TBI and BMT for childhood leukemia and lymphoma, three subjects underwent

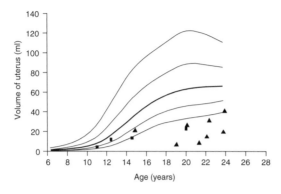

Figure 2 Volume of uterus related to age in 12 women after bone marrow transplantation and total body irradiation. Curves represent +2 SD, +1 SD, mean (bold), –1 SD and –2 SD. (▲) Patients receiving sex steroid replacement therapy; (■) no therapy. Data derived from reference 28 and redrawn with permission from Nature Publishing Group

spontaneous puberty and eight suffered a premature menopause and were administered sex steroid replacement. The remaining subject described symptoms of estrogen deficiency. Average uterine volume was reduced to 40% that of normal adult size in the women on sex steroid replacement (Figure 2). Although the women on hormone replacement experienced withdrawal bleeding (indicative of adequate estrogen priming of the endometrium), the dose of sex steroids administered was not sufficient to establish normal uterine growth and development.

It is essential that young women managed with TBI and BMT in childhood and their carers understand that if a pregnancy is achieved there is a substantial risk of early pregnancy loss and preterm birth. Thorough counseling on such issues should be a mandatory part of clinical care for these women.

There are several reports now that document adverse pregnancy outcomes among women exposed to TBI. Sanders and colleagues[16] reported data from the case records of 1326 patients treated postpuberty and 196 patients treated prepuberty either with high-dose chemotherapy alone or with TBI and BMT for a hematological malignancy or for aplastic anemia. Treatment with TBI was associated

with an increased risk of early pregnancy loss, preterm labor and delivery of a low- or very-low-birth-weight infant. There was no increased incidence of congenital abnormality. There are also reports of an excess risk of low-birth-weight infants (< 2500 g) and preterm birth among mothers who were administered abdominal irradiation for Wilms' tumor in childhood[29,30]. The infants of women exposed to such treatments do require long-term follow-up.

Relatively recently, Larsen and associates[31] described the first case histories of three women with premature menopause after TBI and BMT in childhood, who underwent ovum donation. One woman with a uterine volume in the normal range (41.8 ml) succeeded in delivering a healthy infant at 37 weeks' gestation. She had received her anticancer treatment postpuberty. A second patient, who was treated premenarche (aged 12.9 years), miscarried in the second trimester. She had a very diminished uterine volume (9.4 ml). The third patient treated postmenarche, also with an abnormal uterine volume (31.9 ml), had not conceived at the time of the publication. Pubertal status at the time of treatment with TBI may play a role in the final uterine volume attained by any patient. Furthermore, age at the time of TBI may also be a significant factor. Indeed, the observations made in the study of Larsen and co-workers[31] accord with those from the study from Bath and colleagues[7]. In the latter study uterine volume correlated with age at time of TBI; the younger the patient, the smaller the uterine volume.

It is yet to be established whether the currently prescribed doses and routes of administration of sex hormone replacement to young women with ovarian failure after pelvic irradiation provide adequate concentrations of estrogen to ensure optimal uterine growth during adolescence. This question has been addressed in a preliminary study from our group[7]. In this study, ovarian and uterine characteristics were monitored in a group of survivors treated with TBI who were administered a physiological regimen of sex steroid replacement[32]

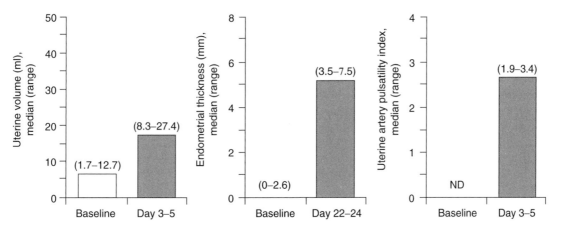

Figure 3 Administration of a physiological sex steroid replacement regimen increased uterine volume and endometrial thickness and re-established uterine artery blood flow in women ($n = 4$) with premature ovarian failure after treatment with total body irradiation for leukemia. ND, not detectable. Data derived from reference 7; redrawn from reference 50 with permission

if ovarian function was absent and also among those with endogenous sex steroid production (ovarian activity still present). Pelvic ultrasound assessed uterine blood flow, uterine size and endometrial thickness. The physiological sex steroid replacement regime (utilizing a transdermal route of estrogen delivery), which had previously been demonstrated to simulate endogenous cyclical ovarian estrogen and progesterone profiles, was administered for 3 months. At a baseline assessment of uterine volume (performed 4 weeks after discontinuation of a standard hormone replacement regimen) in the women with absent ovarian function, there was undetectable blood flow in the uterine arteries and a demonstrable reduction in uterine volume. This was in contrast to the women with endogenous ovarian function after treatment with chemotherapy or cranial irradiation, or a control group of healthy cycling women. A subsequent assessment conducted after 3 months of exposure to physiological concentrations of estrogen and progesterone demonstrated a significant increase in uterine volume from baseline (Figure 3). At baseline uterine volume was 6.5 ml; after 3 months of physiological hormone replacement, uterine volume had increased to 16.3 ml but remained significantly lower than measurements in the control

group (median 41.5 ml, range 28.1–57.9 ml). Importantly it was noted that those young girls exposed to irradiation prepuberty exhibited a far smaller increase in uterine volume than the girls exposed to irradiation postpuberty. There were also demonstrable increases in endometrial thickness and uterine blood flow after 3 months of physiological sex steroid replacement (Figure 3). Furthermore, very preliminary studies on characteristics of the endometrial tissue collected at the time of physiological sex steroid replacement revealed an appropriate functional response, as determined by immunohistochemical demonstration of endometrial sex steroid receptors[33].

Studies such as that described above do support a view that physiological sex steroid replacement may have the potential to improve uterine characteristics in some patients. The precise dose of sex steroids and administration regimens are as yet undetermined. Moreover, long-term effects are also unknown. Current knowledge about hormone replacement regimens administered to women in the usual, older menopausal age range (fifth decade) have drawn to attention the need to carefully evaluate the optimal delivery route, formulation of sex steroid and administration regimen required, to minimize adverse and optimize beneficial effects.

FERTILITY PRESERVATION AND PREGNANCY POTENTIAL

For those children and adolescents at risk of ovarian failure, the options for fertility preservation are quite limited and include ovarian translocation to reduce exposure of the ovaries to radiotherapy[34–36] and cryopreservation of ovarian cortical tissue[37–40]. Gonadotropin suppression has not been demonstrated to be protective[41–43]. The scope of this chapter prohibits further detailed discussion on these issues. Ovarian cortical tissue cryopreservation has significant ethical and legal implications and remains at present at an experimental stage only. The topic is addressed in full in Chapter 12.

Our group[44] recently reported a spontaneous conception in a teenager whose ovarian cortical tissue had been stored prior to gonadotoxic therapy for a pelvic tumor (Ewing's sarcoma on the superior pubic ramus). The patient presented postpuberty, aged 14.9 years. Her treatment involved 14 courses of chemotherapy and a radiation dose of 55 Gy to her pelvis. Owing to the high risk of post-treatment ovarian failure, informed patient and parental consent was given for laparoscopic collection of ovarian cortical strips and subsequent storage at −176°C. Her treatment was completed at age 15.8 years. Following completion of radiotherapy the patient had symptomatic and biochemical evidence of ovarian failure. She was prescribed a low-dose combined oral contraceptive pill for hormone replacement. Due to a persistent complaint of unscheduled vaginal bleeding, despite use of a variety of hormone replacement preparations, she underwent evaluation of her lower genital tract. Examination revealed an atrophic lower genital tract, with the hysteroscopic appearance of a normal uterine cavity and histological evidence of normal secretory-phase endometrium. A vaginal wall biopsy revealed evidence of radiation vaginitis, the likely source of her unscheduled vaginal spotting. The latter symptom responded to topical estrogen therapy. At times in her management when she ceased hormone replacement, her gonadotropin levels were at all times consistent with ovarian failure.

At the age of 19.7 years the patient raised the issue of fertility but continued on hormone replacement therapy. She presented at age 20.2 years with a complaint of lower abdominal pain and vaginal bleeding. An ultrasound scan revealed a totally unexpected early intrauterine pregnancy. The remainder of her pregnancy progressed without event, and both maternal and fetal health were monitored throughout the pregnancy. A cardiac assessment was indicated on account of her chemotherapeutic regimen including cardiotoxic agents, anthracyclines. Fetal growth progressed normally. Delivery was undertaken at 38 weeks' gestation by elective Cesarean section. The decision for a planned operative delivery was made on account of a wish to avoid a possible emergency Cesarean section and past history of radiotherapy and pelvic mass. Her infant, a healthy boy, weighed 2940 g (3rd–10th centile). At the time of delivery an inspection of the pelvis revealed normal ovaries and pelvic bones and no evidence of radiation damage. She had a spontaneous return of menstruation following delivery.

This particular case highlights a number of important issues for young women treated with chemotherapy and/or radiotherapy for childhood cancer. The return of ovarian function after gonadal toxic chemotherapy and biochemical evidence of absent ovarian function has been reported. Ovarian function may be preserved after radiation exposure prepuberty although spontaneous conceptions have been associated first- and second-trimester pregnancy loss, as a likely consequence of radiation damage to the uterus. Uterine function may be better preserved if radiation exposure is postpuberty. In this patient's case, had her ovarian cortical strips been replaced, then her spontaneous conception would have reasonably been attributed to a presumed re-engraftment and function of stored ovarian cortical tissue.

The second case history summarized below highlights the need to identify those women who conceive after treatment for childhood cancer as patients who may be at high risk during their pregnancy and for whom multidisciplinary care should be mandatory. The patient was aged 29 years at the time of a spontaneous conception. At the age of 2 years she underwent laminectomy to excise an abdominal, retroperitoneal neuroblastoma. She received adjuvant chemotherapy and radiotherapy. The latter total dose was 16 Gy to a field 12 cm by 9 cm in the left flank that crossed the midline, in the hope of avoiding scoliosis. Her left ovary was likely to have been in the radiation field. The right ovary and uterus would not have been in the radiation field and exposed only to a scatter dose of radiation. During childhood and adolescence she underwent several surgical procedures to manage a flaccid paralysis and urinary dysfunction. She required a permanent urinary diversion with bilateral cutaneous ureterostomies. She was monitored closely throughout her pregnancy with input from her obstetric and urological carers. Fetal growth was normal to the early third trimester (33 weeks' gestation), when she presented with preterm spontaneous rupture of the membranes. Initial conservative management had to be curtailed on account of a development of maternal pyrexia and fetal tachycardia. Augmentation of her labor with oxytocin was unsuccessful and delivery by Cesarean section undertaken. A healthy male infant was delivered (2150 g; just under the 50th centile). A multidisciplinary team (obstetric and urological) undertook her delivery. Her Cesarean section was far from straightforward owing to dense pelvic adhesions as a consequence of multiple pelvic operations and previous pelvic irradiation. Furthermore, surgical closure was difficult because of distortion of her pelvic anatomy. The operative details of this complex surgical case and further post-delivery complications and management issues have recently been reported[45]. This patient's history emphasizes the need for individualized medical care and the potential high-risk nature of pregnancy in cancer survivors.

PROGENY

Overall, there are reassuring reports that there is no increased incidence of either congenital abnormalities or childhood malignancy in children born to long-term survivors of childhood cancer[46,47]. However, these successful pregnancies mostly result from normally achieved conception. We do not know the consequences of circumventing the natural selection processes of normal sexual reproduction using assisted reproductive technologies (ART), nor the effects of ART on the complex cascade of precisely timed molecular interactions of early embryonic development. Continued surveillance of the progeny of survivors of childhood cancer remains essential[48].

Female survivors of Wilms' tumor managed with abdominal irradiation are at increased risk of several reproductive problems, including fetal loss, preterm birth and even birth defects in their offspring[20]. Flank irradiation has a particular association to the delivery of low-birth-weight infants[46]. Young women treated for acute lymphoblastic leukemia in childhood have a nearly normal reproductive pattern as young adults and do not exhibit an increased risk of congenital anomaly in their offspring[3,49].

CONCLUDING REMARKS

There has been a substantial improvement in long-term survival rates for childhood cancer. Thus current challenges include the management of disorders of gonadal function, including pubertal delay or failure, premature ovarian failure and subfertility. If female survivors of childhood cancer do achieve a pregnancy, then there is an increased risk of pregnancy loss, preterm birth and low-birth-weight infants. These pregnancies are high-risk, impose a challenge for optimal mode of delivery, and require a multidisciplinary approach to management.

ACKNOWLEDGMENTS

We are grateful to Mr Ted Pinner for help with the illustrations and to Mrs Kate Williams for her secretarial assistance.

References

1. Bleyer WA. The impact of childhood cancer on the United States and the world. *CA Cancer J Clin* 1990;40:355–67
2. Scottish Intercollegiate Guidelines Network (SIGN). Long term follow up care of survivors of childhood cancer. Guideline No. 76. Edinburgh: SIGN, 2004
3. Bath LE, Anderson RA, Critchley HO, *et al.* Hypothalamic–pituitary–ovarian dysfunction after prepubertal chemotherapy and cranial irradiation for acute leukaemia. *Hum Reprod* 2001;16:1838–44
4. Bath LE, Wallace WH, Shaw MP, *et al.* Depletion of the ovarian reserve in young women following treatment for cancer in childhood: detection by anti-Müllerian hormone, inhibin B and ovarian ultrasound. *Hum Reprod* 2003;18:2368–74
5. Wallace WH, Shalet SM, Crowne EC, *et al.* Ovarian failure following abdominal irradiation in childhood: natural history and prognosis. *Clin Oncol* 1989;1:75–9
6. Critchley HOD, Wallace WHB, Shalet SM, *et al.* Abdominal irradiation in childhood: potential for pregnancy. *Br J Obstet Gynaecol* 1992;99:392–4
7. Bath LE, Critchley HO, Chambers SE, *et al.* Ovarian and uterine characteristics after total body irradiation in childhood and adolescence: response to sex steroid replacement. *Br J Obstet Gynaecol* 1999;106:1265–72
8. Meirow D. Reproduction post chemotherapy in young cancer patients. *Mol Cell Endocrinol* 2000;169:123–31
9. Thomson AB, Critchley HOD, Kelnar CJH, Wallace WHB. Late reproductive sequelae following treatment of childhood cancer and options for fertility preservation. *Baillières Best Pract Res Clin Endocrinol Metab* 2002;16: 311–34
10. Block E. Quantitative morphological investigations of the follicular system in women. Variations at different ages. *Acta Anat (Basel)* 1952;14:108–23
11. Faddy MJ, Gosden RG, Gougeon A, *et al.* Accelerated disappearance of ovarian follicles in mid-life: implications for forecasting menopause. *Hum Reprod* 1992;7:1342–6
12. Wallace WHB, Thomson AB, Kelsey TW. The radiosensitivity of the human oocyte. *Hum Reprod* 2003;18:117–21
13. Wallace WHB, Shalet SM, Hendry JH, *et al.* Ovarian failure following abdominal irradiation in childhood: the radiosensitivity of the human oocyte. *Br J Radiol* 1989;62:995–8
14. Wallace WHB, Blacklay A, Eiser C, *et al.* Developing strategies for long-term follow up of survivors of childhood cancer. *Br Med J* 2001;323:271–4
15. Lushbaugh CC, Casarett GW. The effects of gonadal irradiation in clinical radiation in therapy; a review. *Cancer* 1976;37:1111–25
16. Sanders JE, Hawley J, Levy W, *et al.* Pregnancies following high-dose cyclophosphamide with or without high-dose busulphan or total-body irradiation and bone marrow transplantation. *Blood* 1996;87:3045–52
17. Chiarelli AM, Marrett LD, Darlington G. Early menopause and infertility in females after treatment for childhood cancer diagnosed in 1964–1988 in Ontario, Canada. *Am J Epidemiol* 1999;150:245–54
18. Sanders JE, Buckner CD, Leonard JM, *et al.* Late effects on gonadal function of cyclophosphamide, total-body irradiation, and marrow transplantation. *Transplantation* 1983;36:252–5
19. Sarafoglou K, Boulad F, Gillio A, Sklar C. Gonadal function after bone marrow transplantation for acute leukemia during childhood. *J Pediatr* 1997;130:210–16
20. Byrne J, Mulvihill JJ, Connelly RR, *et al.* Reproductive problems and birth defects in survivors of Wilms' tumor and their relatives. *Med Pediatr Oncol* 1988;16:233–40
21. Byrne J, Fears TR, Gail MH, *et al.* Early menopause in long term survivors of cancer during adolescence. *Am J Obstet Gynecol* 1992; 166:788–93
22. Byrne J. Infertility and premature menopause in childhood cancer survivors. *Med Pediatr Oncol* 1999;33:24–8
23. Davies HA, Didcock E, Didi M, *et al.* Growth, puberty and obesity after treatment for leukaemia. *Acta Paediatr Suppl* 1995;411:45–51
24. Didcock E, Davies HA, Didi M, *et al.* Pubertal growth in young adult survivors of childhood leukaemia. *J Clin Oncol* 1995;13:2503–7
25. Soules MR, McLachlan RI, Ek M, *et al.* Luteal phase deficiency: characterisation of reproductive hormones over the menstrual cycle. *J Clin Endocrinol Metab* 1989;69:804–12
26. Holm K, Laurensen EM, Brocks V, Muller J. Pubertal maturation of the internal genitalia: an ultrasound evaluation of 166 healthy girls. *Ultrasound Obstet Gynecol* 1995;6:175–81
27. Bridges NA, Cooke A, Healy MJ, *et al.* Growth of the uterus. *Arch Dis Child* 1996;75:330–1
28. Holm K, Nyson K, Brocks V, *et al.* Ultrasound B-mode changes in the uterus and ovaries and Doppler changes in the uterus after total

body irradiation and allogenic bone marrow transplantation in childhood. *Bone Marrow Transplant* 1999;23:259–63

29. Green DM, Hall B, Zevon A. Pregnancy outcome after treatment for acute lymphoblastic leukaemia during childhood or adolescence. *Cancer* 1989;64:235–44

30. Green DM. Preserving fertility in children treated for cancer [editorial]. *Br Med J* 2001; 323:1201

31. Larsen EC, Loft A, Holm K, *et al.* Oocyte donation in women cured of cancer with bone marrow transplantation including total body irradiation in adolescence. *Hum Reprod* 2000; 15:1505–8

32. Critchley HOD, Buckley CH, Anderson DC. Experience with a 'physiological' steroid replacement regimen for the establishment of a receptive endometrium in women with premature ovarian failure. *Br J Obstet Gynaecol* 1990;97:804–10

33. Critchley HOD, Bath LE, Wallace WHB. Radiation damage to the uterus – review of the effects of treatment of childhood cancer. *Hum Fertil* 2002;5:61–6

34. Clough KB, Goffinet F, Labib A, *et al.* Laparascopic unilateral ovarian transposition prior to irradiation. *Cancer* 1996;77:2638–45

35. Leporrier M, von Theobold P, Roffe J-L, Muller G. A new technique to protect ovarian function in young women undergoing pelvic irradiation. Heterotopic ovarian autotransplantation. *Cancer* 1987;60:2201–4

36. Thomas PRM, Winstanly D, Peckham MJ, *et al.* Reproductive and endocrine function in patients with Hodgkin's disease: effects of oophropexy and irradiation. *Br J Cancer* 1976; 33:226–31

37. Baird DT, Webb R, Campbell BK, *et al.* Long-term ovarian function in sheep after ovariectomy and transplantation of autografts stored at −196°C. *Endocrinology* 1999;140:462–71

38. Royal College of Obstetricians and Gynaecologists (RCOG). *Storage of Ovarian and Prepubertal Testicular Tissue: Report of a Working Party.* London: RCOG, 2000

39. Oktay K, Karlikaya G. Ovarian function after transplantation of frozen, banked, autologous ovarian tissue. *N Engl J Med* 2000;342:1919

40. Oktay K, Economos K, Kan M, *et al.* Endocrine function and oocyte retrieval after autologous transplantation of ovarian cortical strips to the forearm. *J Am Med Assoc* 2001;286:1490–3

41. Ataya K, Ramahi-Ataya A. Reproductive performance of female rats treated with cyclophosphamide and/or LHRH agonist. *Reprod Toxicol* 1993;7:229–35

42. Ataya K, Pydyn E, Ramahi-Ataya A, Orton CG. Is radiation-induced ovarian failure preventable by luteinizing hormone-releasing hormone agonist? Preliminary observations. *J Clin Endocrinol Metab* 1995;80:790–5

43. Blumenfeld Z, Avivi I, Linn S, *et al.* Prevention of irreversible chemotherapy-induced ovarian damage in young women with lymphoma by a gonadotrophin-releasing hormone agonist in parallel to chemotherapy. *Hum Reprod* 1996; 11:1620–6

44. Bath LE, Tydeman G, Critchley HOD, *et al.* Spontaneous conception in a teenager in whom ovarian cortical tissue was stored prior to gonadotoxic therapy for a pelvic tumour. Poster presented at *1st World Congress on Ovarian Cryopreservation and Ovarian Transplantation,* Brussels, June 2003

45. Patrick KIL, Wallace WHB, Critchley HOD. Late reproductive effects of cancer treatment in female survivors of childhood malignancy. *Curr Obstet Gynaecol* 2003;13:369–72

46. Hawkins MM, Smith RA. Pregnancy outcome in childhood cancer survivors: probable effects of abdominal irradiation. *Int J Cancer* 1989; 43:399–402

47. Li FP, Fine W, Jaffe N, *et al.* Offspring of patients treated for cancer in childhood. *J Natl Cancer Inst* 1979;62:1193–7

48. Grundy R, Gosden RG, Hewitt M, *et al.* Fertility preservation for children treated for cancer (1): scientific advances and research dilemmas. *Arch Dis Child* 2001;84:355–9

49. Nygaard R, Clausen N, Simes MA, *et al.* Reproduction following treatment for childhood leukemia: a population-based prospective cohort study of fertility and offspring. *Med Pediatr Oncol* 1991;19:459–66

50. Burton KA, Wallace WHB, Critchley HOD. Female reproductive potential post-treatment for childhood cancer. *Hosp Med* 2002;63:522–7

Pregnancy safety after cancer

16

S. Emery and T. Falcone

INTRODUCTION

The cure rate of childhood cancer has improved dramatically in the past few decades, meaning that more women and men are living long enough to have a family. More importantly, the outcome of pregnancy after cancer treatment is usually promising. The current survival rate for all pediatric and adolescent cancers is approximately 70%[1].

Assisted reproductive technologies (ART) have also provided some cancer patients the opportunity to preserve their fertility. Patients with ovarian failure can be offered oocyte donation. Furthermore, advances in perinatal and neonatal medicine have improved outcome in pregnancies complicated by premature birth or growth restriction, the most common adverse pregnancy complications in cancer survivors. Most evidence, albeit incomplete, suggests that the children of cancer survivors are not at increased risk for birth defects, developmental delay or childhood cancers, compared to the general population. This may be surprising given the nature of chemotherapy and radiation therapy, which is to inhibit, disrupt or otherwise alter DNA synthesis.

As the number of women delaying childbearing into their third and fourth decade increases, the additional problem of pregnancy in relatively older women is added to the issue of pregnancy in the cancer survivor. The older pregnant patient, independent of the cancer-related issues, has a higher incidence of co-morbid conditions such as diabetes and hypertension that could influence perinatal outcome.

The numerous variables that influence fetal and maternal well-being in these patients need to be considered before the patient proceeds with a pregnancy. Antenatal counseling of these patients is critical, and the risks to the mother and fetus should be discussed. The patient needs to understand that the experience of a practitioner and the literature is not vast and not all long-term outcomes are known.

THEORETICAL CONSIDERATIONS

The major questions that patients wish to discuss with their physician are:

(1) 'Can I achieve and maintain a normal pregnancy?'

(2) 'Will pregnancy cause my cancer to recur?'

(3) 'If it recurs during pregnancy, will the cancer or its treatment affect the fetus?'

(4) 'How will my treatment options be compromised by the need to protect the fetus?'

(5) 'Has my previous treatment increased the risk of birth defects in my children?'

(6) 'Are my children at risk for childhood cancers?'

Perinatal outcome

Although much of the research intended to answer these questions are reports with a small number of patients, a considerable body of evidence is mounting from which general observations can be made. To date, the largest study addressing pregnancy outcome after childhood cancer has been the Childhood Cancer Survivor Study (CCSS)[2]. The investigators studied 1915 females and 4029 pregnancies, the outcomes of interest being pregnancy loss, live births and birth weight. The strength of this study was the choice of controls: the pregnancy outcomes of the nearest age sibling were used as a control population. This study found no difference in the rate of pregnancy complications among women previously treated with chemotherapy. Women treated with pelvic irradiation tended to have more babies weighing less than 2500 g. These findings are consistent with other smaller studies demonstrating an increased risk for preterm labor, preterm delivery and low birth weight after treatment of childhood cancer with irradiation[3]. However, although statistically significant, many of these outcomes are not clinically relevant. For instance, the mean gestational age of delivery with previous irradiation was 37.23 weeks versus 38.47 weeks for non-radiated females ($p = 0.005$). The irradiated women delivered earlier, but the clinical consequences of delivery at 37 weeks versus 38 weeks are relatively insignificant. There was a disproportionate number of pregnancies delivered before 36 weeks in the irradiated group, and the risk appeared to be linear with the dose of radiation. With access to modern perinatal and neonatal services, many complications associated with such mild prematurity can be largely ameliorated. There was no increase in adverse maternal or fetal complications in the offspring of irradiated males.

Neonatal outcome

Many studies have investigated the link between the treatment of childhood cancer and the risk of congenital anomalies and childhood cancer in offspring[4,5]. There has been no consistent evidence of an increased risk of either. One large study, again using the CCSS database ($n = 1227$), looked at the pregnancy outcomes of partners of male survivors of childhood cancer[6]. Using pregnancy outcomes in the nearest sibling as a control group, these investigators found a reversal of the male-to-female ratio from 1.24 : 1.0 to

1.0 : 1.03 but no other adverse pregnancy outcomes. The National Wilms' Tumor Study Group (NWTSG)[3] found an increased incidence of congenital anomalies in offspring of previously irradiated women as well as an increased risk for malpresentation. However, the anomalies were generally mild and in no consistent pattern. For instance, one baby boy born to a previously irradiated woman had undescended testes, a self-correcting disorder. Another baby had a patent ductus arteriosus, which is amenable to simple surgery. A third, however, was born with Beckwith–Wiedemann syndrome, a microduplication syndrome possibly related to previous irradiation.

The rate of malpresentation rose with the dose of radiation from 3.2% in the non-radiated patients to 16.9% in heavily irradiated patients. However, most obstetricians do not consider malpresentation to be a significant obstacle since it can be easily diagnosed and managed. It is certainly possible that radiation of the uterus causes increased fibrosis and decreased vascularity of the myometrium, leading to decreased perfusion and less mechanical compliance[7]. This could partially explain an increased incidence of low-birth-weight babies and malpresentation. These obstacles are amenable to modern obstetric and neonatal care.

Endocrine milieu

Most management options for treating infertility secondary to previous cancer therapy[8–11] result in major, but transient, changes in the patient's endocrine milieu. Some tumors are hormonally sensitive. It is often viewed by reproductive endocrinologists that a short exposure to supraphysiological levels of sex hormones may not influence the tumor. This does not take into consideration the hormonal changes of pregnancy. The placenta produces increasing amounts of progesterone, ten- to 20-fold that of luteal phase levels, and most of the secreted progesterone (90%) enters the maternal circulation. The placenta also secretes estrone, estradiol and estriol. The highest concentration is of estriol, a weak estrogen. However, this represents at least a ten-fold increase in circulating estrogens.

Pregnancy after breast cancer

Breast cancer survivors represent a unique population. Micrometastases can theoretically be stimulated by estrogen and progesterone produced in large quantities during pregnancy. Another concern is of a new primary carcinoma stimulated by pregnancy hormones. Despite this rational consideration, most studies do not show an increased rate of recurrence in pregnancy[12,13]. These data must be interpreted with caution as the studies are with small numbers of patients and have some methodological limitations. Depending on the degree of surgical intervention and radiation exposure, breastfeeding from the affected breast may remain an option[14]. There is no evidence that lactation increases the risk of breast cancer recurrence.

PREGNANCY MANAGEMENT

Ideal pregnancy management begins preconceptionally (Table 1). Women with previous cancer who are contemplating pregnancy generally benefit from a multidisciplinary team approach. Central to the team are her oncologist and obstetrician. These will be supported by staff from other consultative services such as maternal–fetal medicine, obstetric anesthesia and neonatology. An overall assessment of the patient's candidacy for safe pregnancy should take into account effects of the previous cancer and its treatment on maternal physiology.

Specific chemotherapeutic agents used should be reviewed. Pregnancy results in significant increases in cardiac function: blood and plasma volume increase by 35–40%, stroke volume increases by 30% and total cardiac output increases by 50%. Thus, for instance, patients exposed to cardiotoxic chemotherapeutic agents such as doxorubicin (Adriamycin®) should be assessed for baseline cardiac function. If the patient has significant cardiac compromise that is compensated in

Table 1 Management protocol for patients with previous cancer

Preconception
Overall well-being assessment
Assessment of pregnancy risks
   maternal risks
   fetal risks
Consultation with relevant subspecialists
Identification of multi-specialty management team
   members
Assessment of end-organ defects from previous cancer
   or therapy
   echocardiogram
   BUN/creatinine/24 h urine total protein
   pulmonary function tests
   liver function tests
Folic acid supplementation

First and early second trimester
Transvaginal ultrasound scan for viability, gestational
   age, fetal number and location
Initiation of multi-specialty management
Baseline studies
   renal function
Reaffirmation of desire for pregnancy
   maternal risks
   fetal risks
Genetic counseling and testing
   CVS/amniocentesis
   nuchal translucency
   maternal serum screening

Second trimester
Detailed fetal anatomic survey
Serial ultrasound scans to monitor fetal growth
Follow-up laboratory tests and functional studies

Delivery
Multi-specialty management team
   maternal–fetal medicine
   obstetric anesthesia
   cardiology
   neonatology
Ultrasound scan to determine presentation
Cesarean section for obstetric indications

BUN, blood urea nitrogen; CVS, chorionic villus sampling

the non-pregnant state, pregnancy-associated physiological changes could be sufficient to cause deterioration.

Agents that cause pulmonary toxicity such as bleomycin may be associated with a pregnancy-induced deterioration in respiratory function. Minute ventilation increases by 30% as the result of increased tidal volume. There is a decrease in functional residual capacity and increased oxygen consumption that places the pregnant patient at higher risk for hypoxemia.

Similarly, baseline renal function should be assessed given the significant demands on the kidneys during pregnancy. Every attempt should be made to optimize maternal well-being before conception. Folic acid supplementation is appropriate in all women anticipating pregnancy.

Management plan

Once pregnancy is achieved, an early transvaginal ultrasound scan performed at 6–7 weeks serves to establish location, viability, gestational age and number of fetuses. If not performed in the preconceptional period, an overall assessment of well-being should be performed, including baseline function studies of potentially affected organ systems. A candid conversation about potential maternal and fetal risks must be undertaken to ensure commitment to the endeavor. If the pregnancy is unintended and/or undesired, abortion should be discussed and the appropriate referral made.

Once the pregnancy is established and baseline studies are reviewed, an overall management plan should be developed that includes continuing assessment of maternal and fetal well-being, with a focus on anticipated complications. Although available evidence does not support an increased risk of congenital anomalies in women previously treated for cancer, increased surveillance is reasonable for reassurance purposes. Additionally, given the potentially significant maternal risks in pregnancy, every effort should be made to ensure that the developing fetus is normal. Maternal serum screening or 'quad screen', that incorporates maternal age, gestational age and serum levels of α-fetoprotein, human chorionic gonadotropin, estriol and α-inhibin, is a useful screening tool for structural defects such as neural tube and ventral wall defects as well as Down syndrome and trisomy 18. It can be offered between 15 and 20 weeks of gestation[15].

ULTRASOUND

Ultrasound is a powerful tool in assessing fetal growth and development. A transabdominal or transvaginal ultrasound scan at 10–12 weeks can detect major structural developmental anomalies such as anencephaly or cystic hygroma. An increased nuchal translucency, a fluid-filled space between the fetal spine and skin, correlates with the risk for karyotypic abnormalities[16] as well as structural cardiac defects[17]. A high-resolution ultrasound scan performed at 16–20 weeks has the potential to diagnose a myriad of structural defects in the developing fetus. With increasing options for *in utero* fetal and neonatal interventions, early detection of structural anomalies can potentially improve outcome[18].

Since many of the pregnancies after childhood cancer treatment are achieved through ART, there is an increased likelihood of gestation of multiple fetuses[19]. Besides the added physiological burden to the mother, these pregnancies predispose complications such as preterm labor, hypertension and operative delivery that can substantially compound the risk status of the pregnancy[20]. Depending on the overall clinical picture, pregnancy reduction may be offered with the hope of improving pregnancy outcome for the mother and remaining baby(ies)[21]. Similarly, selective reduction of an anomalous twin that is threatening the well-being of the normal twin may be offered in order to improve overall pregnancy outcome[22].

Ultrasound is a useful tool in assessing fetal growth, amniotic fluid volume, placenta location, presentation, placental function and fetal well-being, all of which may be compromised by previous cancer and its treatment. These parameters should be assessed serially in the third trimester. Ultrasound examination every 4 weeks will identify the fetus that is growth-restricted. Assessment of the proportionality of fetal growth can give clues as to the nature of the forces inhibiting growth. For instance, women with previous pelvic irradiation tend to have smaller babies and a higher proportion of newborns weighing less than

2500 g. This is likely due to decreased uteroplacental perfusion and should lead to an asymmetric growth pattern by preferential brain perfusion at the expense of the abdomen and carcass. This pattern of growth is easily assessed by ultrasound. Similarly, decreased uteroplacental perfusion can lead to decreased fetal urine production and subsequently oligohydramnios. Because of the potential for myometrial fibrosis after pelvic irradiation, there may be an increased risk for placenta previa.

Delivery

The NWTSG found a linear increase in the risk of malpresentation with dose of irradiation. Ultrasound is efficient in determining fetal lie and presentation, and can be performed at the bedside on admission to the labor and delivery ward. Color Doppler waveform analysis can be used to assess the degree of placental resistance to forward blood flow, which correlates with adverse pregnancy outcomes[23]. Finally, the non-stress test and biophysical profile provide reassurance because of a high negative predictive value for intrauterine demise: 1.9 per 1000 and 0.8 per 1000, respectively[24].

Decisions regarding timing and route of delivery may be complex but are generally straightforward. Most women can be allowed to enter spontaneous labor at term. In these women, Cesarean delivery should be withheld for obstetric indications such as malpresentation and placenta previa. Occasionally, maternal or fetal decompensation may warrant earlier intervention. For instance, a woman with a previously irradiated pelvis may carry a growth-restricted fetus whose antenatal testing is not reassuring and requires delivery. Or, a woman with cardiac or pulmonary compromise from previous cancer treatment may no longer tolerate the physiological demands of pregnancy. In these circumstances, a multidisciplinary team approach that involves the appropriate subspecialty services such as maternal–fetal medicine, obstetric anesthesia and cardiology can convene to effect the best

outcome. Invasive hemodynamic monitoring with Swan-Ganz catheterization may be indicated in the most complex cases[25].

As stated above, newborn outcomes generally match those of the general population. The most commonly reported adverse neonatal outcomes are small for gestation and preterm birth. Although advances in perinatal and neonatal medicine over the past few decades have served to reduce the long-term sequelae of prematurity, it remains problematic to diagnose and treat. Fortunately, the degree of prematurity identified in most studies does not compare with other more common obstetric complications such as hypertension and hemorrhage[26].

Recurrence during pregnancy

Several significant psychosocial and ethical considerations present when cancer recurs or is diagnosed during pregnancy. If a cancer recurs, patients may fear that the cancer, or its management, may adversely impact fetal growth and development. Also, they may wonder if their treatment may be compromised by the physiology of pregnancy or the needs of the developing fetus. For example, increased renal plasma flow, glomerular filtration and volume of distribution could lead to suboptimal chemotherapy dosing. Ideal agents may be substituted for less effective but presumably safer regimens. Radiotherapy may be withheld due to its known detrimental effects on the developing fetus. Women may be faced with anguishing decisions of whether to terminate the pregnancy in order to maximize their management and eliminate the risk of a damaged newborn, or continue the pregnancy at the risk of compromising their care and/or the baby's well-being. Concerns over bereavement may also develop if a woman is faced with a potentially lethal recurrence. She may feel guilty for leaving the newborn, as well as other children, motherless and for burdening her husband. Finally, as our knowledge of the hereditary nature of some cancers increases, she may be concerned about the risk of passing on a predilection for cancer to her children[27].

CONCLUSIONS

Although the thought of having children after surviving cancer may seem like a daunting task fraught with difficulty, the majority of available evidence suggests that the overall pregnancy outcomes are good. Nonetheless, preconceptional assessment of probable pregnancy complications and outcomes, optimization of maternal health before pregnancy, and a multidisciplinary approach to complicated cases are advisable. It is hoped that a future national cancer registry would aid in more accurate, disease-specific assessment of risk and prediction of outcome.

References

1. Gloeckler LA, Smith MA, Gurney JG, et al. Cancer Incidence and Survival among Children and Adolescents: United States SEER Program 1975–1999. NIH Publication 99–4649. Bethesda, MD: National Cancer Institute, 1999
2. Green DM, Whitton JA, Stovall M, et al. Pregnancy outcome of female survivors of childhood cancer: a report from the Childhood Cancer Survivor Study. Am J Obstet Gynecol 2002;187:1070–80
3. Green DM, Peabody EM, Nan B, et al. Pregnancy outcome after treatment for Wilms tumor: a report from the National Wilms Tumor Study Group. J Clin Oncol 2002;20:2506–13
4. Byrne J, Rasmussen SA, Steinhorn SC, et al. Genetic disease in offspring of long-term survivors of childhood and adolescent cancer. Am J Hum Genet 1998;62:45–52
5. Green DM, Fiorello A, Zevon MA. Birth defects and childhood cancer in offspring of survivors of childhood cancer. Arch Pediatr Adolesc Med 1997;151:379–83
6. Green DM, Whitton JA, Stovall M, et al. Pregnancy outcome of partners of male survivors of childhood cancer: a report from the Childhood Cancer Survivor Study. J Clin Oncol 2003;21:716–21
7. Critchley HO, Wallace WH, Shalet SM, et al. Abdominal irradiation in childhood; the potential for pregnancy. Br J Obstet Gynaecol 1992;99:392–4
8. Pfeifer SM, Coutifaris C. Reproductive technologies 1998: options available for the cancer patient. Med Pediatr Oncol 1999;33:34–40
9. Anselmo AP, Cavalieri E, Aragona C, et al. Successful pregnancies following an egg donation program in women with previously treated Hodgkin's disease. Haematologica 2001;86:624–8
10. Kelleher S, Wishart SM, Liu PY, et al. Long-term outcomes of elective human sperm cryostorage. Hum Reprod 2001;16:2632–9
11. Falcone T, Little B. Placental steroids. In Tulchinsky D, Little B, eds. Maternal–Fetal, Endocrinology, 2nd edn. Philadelphia, PA: WB Saunders, 1994:351–65
12. Petrek JA. Pregnancy safety after breast cancer. Cancer 1994;74:528–31
13. Surbone A, Petrek JA. Childbearing issues in breast carcinoma survivors. Cancer 1997;79:1271–8
14. Higgins S, Haffty BG. Pregnancy and lactation after breast-conservative therapy for early stage breast cancer. Cancer 1994;73:2175–80
15. Haddow JE, Palomaki GE, Knight GJ, et al. Reducing the need for amniocentesis in women 35 years of age or older with serum markers for screening. N Engl J Med 1994;330:1114–18
16. Nicolaides KH, Azar G, Byrne D, et al. Fetal nuchal translucency: ultrasound screening for chromosomal defects in first trimester of pregnancy. Br Med J 1992;304:867–9
17. Hyett JA, Perdu M, Sharland GK, et al. Increased nuchal translucency at 10–14 weeks of gestation as a marker for major cardiac defects. Ultrasound Obstet Gynecol 1997;10:242–6
18. Saari-Kemppainen A, Karjalainen O, Ylostalo P, et al. Ultrasound screening and perinatal mortality: controlled trial systematic one-stage screening in pregnancy. The Helsinki Ultrasound Trial. Lancet 1990;336:387–91
19. Luke B. The changing pattern of multiple births in the United States: maternal and infant characteristics, 1973 and 1990. Obstet Gynecol 1994;84:101–6
20. American College of Obstetricians and Gynecologists (ACOG). Special Problems of Multiple Gestations. ACOG Educational Bulletin No. 253. Washington, DC: ACOG, 1989
21. Evans MI, Dommergues M, Wapner RJ, et al. Efficacy of transabdominal multifetal pregnancy reduction: collaborative experience among the world's largest centers. Obstet Gynecol 1993;82:61–6

22. Evans MI, Goldberg JD, Dommergues M, *et al.* Efficacy of second-trimester selective termination for fetal abnormalities: international collaborative experience among the world's largest centers. *Am J Obstet Gynecol* 1994;171: 90–4

23. Erskine RL, Ritchie JW. Umbilical artery blood flow characteristics in normal and growth-retarded fetuses. *Br J Obstet Gynaecol* 1985;92: 605–10

24. Manning FA, Morrison I, Harman CR, *et al.* Fetal assessment based on fetal biophysical profile scoring: experience in 19 221 referred high-risk pregnancies. II. An analysis of false-negative fetal deaths. *Am J Obstet Gynecol* 1987;157:880–4

25. Hankins GD, Wendel GD Jr, Cunningham FG, *et al.* Longitudinal evaluation of hemodynamic changes in eclampsia. *Am J Obstet Gynecol* 1984; 150:506–12

26. Chronic hypertension in pregnancy. ACOG Practice Bulletin No. 29. American College of Obstetricians and Gynecologists. *Obstet Gynecol* 2001;98:177–85

27. Schover LR. Psychosocial aspects of infertility and decisions about reproduction in young cancer survivors: a review. *Med Pediatr Oncol* 1999;33:53–9

Risks of prior cancer treatment to offspring

17

J. M. Trasler

INTRODUCTION

Cancer treatment has increased the chances of survival for children and young adults with cancers like Hodgkin's disease, leukemia and testicular cancer[1]. Surveys indicate that the majority of cancer survivors are interested in having children, especially if they did not have children at the time of diagnosis[2,3]. However, patients who have received anticancer treatment often hesitate or decline 'future fertility' because they are concerned about the potential genetic risks to their children[2,4]. Certainly, there is reason for concern since many of the drugs used in cancer treatment cause DNA damage, lead to temporary or permanent infertility, and thus could theoretically alter the genome of oocytes and sperm. Commonly used drugs include doxorubicin, cyclophosphamide, vincristine, chlorambucil, melphalan, bleomycin and 6-mercaptopurine; all of these drugs are potent germ cell mutagens and somatic cell clastogens in rodents[5,6]. From animal studies, it is clear that many chemotheraputic drugs used in human anticancer therapy cause genetic damage in germ cells, leading to fetal death, birth defects and behavioral abnormalities in the offspring[6–8].

This chapter reviews studies on the offspring of cancer survivors. Unlike environmental exposures, exposures to anticancer drugs are relatively well controlled and allow dose–response relationships to be determined. Adverse outcomes that have been studied include an increase in the rate of miscarriage or stillbirth, a change in the gender ratio of the offspring, an increased frequency of congenital anomalies and an increase in cancer in the offspring. Evidence that anticancer treatment can cause genetic damage in human germ cells is also presented. Finally, in light of the available studies, practical considerations for cancer patients and counseling issues are discussed.

MECHANISMS OF MALE- AND FEMALE-MEDIATED EFFECTS OF ANTICANCER TREATMENT

Damage resulting in an abnormality in the offspring may have a number of underlying mechanisms: non-genetic (e.g. presence of a drug in the seminal fluid), genetic (e.g. a gene mutation or chromosomal abnormality) or epigenetic (e.g. an effect on chromosomal proteins or imprinted genes)[7]. Characteristics of germ cell development and vulnerability differ in a number of ways between females and males.

Production of oocytes occurs exclusively during fetal life; the female has her maximum cohort of oocytes at birth and has exhausted her supply by menopause. The fact that oocytes are a non-renewable population makes female germ cells particularly susceptible to irreversible damage by anticancer drugs and radiation[8,9]. All postnatal oocytes are arrested in the late meiotic, diplotene phase of oogenesis, with each oocyte being diploid and containing four copies of the DNA. In the female, the meiotic division is completed only after ovulation and fertilization. The chromatin of arrested diplotene oocytes is in a diffuse state, making it vulnerable to a number of anticancer drugs[8]. Some oocytes are competent in DNA repair; theoretically they are able to correct chemotherapy-induced genetic damage. In women, effects of chemotherapy and radiation therapy appear to depend on doses and age at the time of exposure. Younger women (less than 30 years of age) who are exposed to anticancer agents are more likely to maintain reproductive function than are women receiving the same treatment regimen over the age of 30[9].

Treatment of the male with anticancer drugs prior to conception could affect the health of resulting offspring owing to a drug-induced defect in the spermatozoon (e.g. effect on DNA or chromosomal proteins) or an effect caused by the presence of the drug in seminal fluid. Special properties of the male reproductive system to take into account when considering effects on the progeny include the high mitotic activity of germ cells, the regulated/timed nature of spermatogenesis (starting with spermatogonial stem cells and resulting in spermatozoa about 64 days later; 5–7 days are then required for sperm to pass through the epididymis), and the continued proliferation of germ cells, maintained by the process of stem cell renewal/differentiation/proliferation throughout life, from puberty to death. In addition, during spermatogenesis undifferentiated cells pass through a sequence of developmental phases: mitosis (spermatogonia), meiosis (spermatocytes), differentiation (haploid-phase spermiogenesis) and maturation. From animal studies it is clear that healthy outcome in the offspring depends on the type of drug used and the germ cell type exposed[6]. Spermatogonial stem cells are predicted to face the greatest risk from chronic exposure to anticancer agents due to the potential accumulation and persistence of DNA damage. There are few agents that have been shown to cause permanent damage in spermatogonial stem cells. Differentiating spermatogonia are rapidly dividing cells and are most sensitive to killing by radiation and chemotherapy. Exposure of late germ cell types, spermatids

and spermatozoa in the epididymis, may also pose a risk to the offspring, since DNA damage induced by anticancer drugs cannot be repaired late in spermatogenesis[6,10].

INFERTILITY

Infertility is a well-known adverse reproductive effect of maternal and paternal exposure to anticancer drugs and radiation[9]. It can indicate that damage to germ cells has occurred and suggests the possibility of germ cell mutations if the agent involved is mutagenic. Ovarian dysfunction has been reported in Hodgkin's disease patients treated with alkylating agents[9,11]. Childhood cancer survivors treated with high doses of alkylating agents, especially if abdominal irradiation is included, may be at increased risk of premature menopause[12]. Many drugs are known to affect the number, motility and morphology of human sperm[13]. One of the best-known drug effects on sperm is the oligospermia and azoospermia seen in men following treatment with anticancer drugs, notably alkylating agents such as cyclophosphamide[14]. High risks for infertility in young male cancer survivors are associated with radiotherapy, especially doses of > 40 Gy to para-aortic and pelvic lymph nodes[15] and alkylating agent chemotherapy[16]. Excellent survival is now seen for some cancers such as Hodgkin's disease and treatment regimens are being optimized for efficacy as well as the prevention of long-term treatment-related side-effects. For example, Viviani and colleagues[17] compared gonadal function in 53 men with Hodgkin's disease following two effective regimens, MOPP (mechloethamine, vincristine, procarbazine and prednisone) and ABVD (doxorubicin, bleomycin, vincristine and dacarbazine). Azoospermia occurred in 28 out of 29 (97%) patients treated with MOPP, with recovery of spermatogenesis occurring in three out of 21 patients tested. In contrast, after ABVD, oligospermia was induced in 13 of 24 (54%) patients, and spermatogenesis recovered in all 13 patients.

EFFECTS OF ANTICANCER TREATMENT ON THE OFFSPRING OF CANCER SURVIVORS

Early, smaller-scale studies

A number of examples of earlier studies on the offspring of cancer survivors are described first. Most of these studies typically enroled small numbers of survivors of many types of childhood cancer, and surveillance and reporting bias were not adequately controlled. Together, these studies showed little or no increase in birth defects, cancer or genetic disease in the offspring of cancer survivors; however, methodological problems including small sample size made it difficult to draw firm conclusions.

Li and associates[18] examined outcomes in the offspring of patients treated for childhood cancer and enroled in tumor registries of the Sidney Farber Cancer Institute and the Kansas University Medical Center. There were 286 completed pregnancies reported for 146 patients (84 women, 62 men). Compared with their cousins and published data from the general population, the offspring of the cancer survivors did not have an excess of congenital anomalies or other diseases.

In 1991, Green and co-workers[19] reviewed the records of 306 men and women who had been treated for pediatric cancer and who responded to a questionnaire. There were 102 liveborn or stillborn pregnancies among 60 survivors who had had chemotherapy. Among the liveborn offspring, there was no difference in the frequency of congenital malformations in the offspring of males (7.9%) versus females (8.1%). In the same year, Hawkins[20] reported congenital malformations in 3.6% of offspring born to women exposed to potentially mutagenic therapy (abdominal/pelvic radiation or an alkylating agent) as compared to 2.1% of offspring of unexposed women. The congenital anomalies were reported by general practitioners, but were not independently confirmed by a review of medical records.

In a Canadian study, Dodds and colleagues[21] carried out a case–control study to determine whether the offspring of cancer survivors are at increased risk of congenital malformations and examined the role of anti-cancer treatment in any increase found. Parents (45 200 mothers and 41 158 fathers) of children born between 1979 and 1986 with a congenital anomaly were matched with parents (45 200 mothers and 41 158 fathers) whose children did not have a congenital anomaly. A cancer diagnosis was identified in 54 cases and 52 control mothers and in 61 cases and 65 control fathers. There were no significant associations reported between birth defects in the offspring and any type of prior cancer treatment of mothers or fathers.

In a retrospective cohort study, Kenney's group[22] examined adults (593 survivors with a mean age of 22.6 years and 409 sibling controls with a mean age of 25.2 years) who had been treated for childhood acute lymphoblastic leukemia (ALL). Among the survivors, 93 had given birth to or fathered 140 offspring while 122 sibling controls had given birth to or fathered 228 children. Although this was a small study, there was no increased risk of having offspring with birth defects amongst the childhood ALL survivors. Green and associates[23] reviewed the history of 405 former patients treated for childhood cancer. There were 148 patients reporting 280 pregnancies. The frequency of congenital anomalies was 3.3% among the liveborn offspring of the female cancer survivors and 3.3% among the liveborn offspring of the female partners of the male cancer survivors.

Owing to the nature of cancer chemotherapy regimens that take advantage of multiple drugs with different mechanisms of action to kill cancer cells, few studies on the outcomes in the offspring of individuals exposed to single agents have been carried out. Methotrexate is an example of a drug that is used as a single agent. Significantly, methotrexate is also widely distributed in tissues and has been reported in the liver up to 116 days after exposure. Therefore there is a theoretical risk of fetal exposure in babies whose mothers have taken the drug up to

4 months prior to conception. Rustin and co-workers[24] examined the outcomes of 368 pregnancies in 210 women who received single- and combined-agent chemotherapy (all patients received methotrexate) for gestational trophoblastic tumors over a 20-year period prior to pregnancy (mean time from cessation of methotrexate to pregnancy was 2.7 years). In this study the incidence of stillbirth and congenital abnormality was not significantly higher than the background rate. Green and colleagues[19] studied outcomes in 35 children born to 25 males who had received single- and multiple-dose methotrexate chemotherapy in childhood or adolescence; no significant increase in major abnormalities was found. For both females and males, Lloyd and associates[25] have suggested a minimum washout period of 6 months, to avoid adverse effects due to the persistence of methotrexate in tissues. This precaution may also be important for new chemotherapeutic drugs that are introduced into chemotherapy regimens, and pharmacological properties should be kept in mind when counseling patients.

Because of the mutagenic nature of anticancer drugs, a number of investigators have also looked for an excess of cancer in the offspring of cancer survivors. At least a few studies have not found a significantly greater risk than expected[26,27]. In 1987, Mulvihill's group[26] presented results of a multicenter retrospective cohort study of long-term survivors of childhood and adolescent cancer. Among 2308 offspring of survivors of childhood and adolescent cancer, in which 25% of patients had been treated with chemotherapy, no increased risk of cancer was seen; it should be noted that details of the chemotherapy were not given. The study had about an 80% power to detect a tripling in cancer risk, but no excess was observed. In the study by Hawkins' group[27], no malignancies were diagnosed among 382 offspring of survivors of childhood leukemia and non-Hodgkin's lymphoma followed up for a median period of 5.8 years.

Male–female differences in reproductive and offspring outcomes

Several studies have demonstrated an increased risk of fetal death and/or low birth weight among the offspring of women who have received abdominal irradiation prior to pregnancy for their cancers[18,28–30]. More recently, Chiarelli and co-workers[31] reported an increased risk of low-birth-weight offspring among women treated with abdominal/pelvic irradiation; the authors reported no increase in the risk of congenital anomalies among the offspring of females exposed to abdominal/pelvic irradiation, although malformations were ascertained by a mail questionnaire and not verified through a review of medical records. In another study, Green and colleagues[32] evaluated the effects of prior treatment with radiation therapy or chemotherapy for childhood/adolescent Wilms' tumor on live births, birth weight and birth defects. The authors received reports on 427 pregnancies, each of at least 20 weeks' duration, including 409 liveborn children; of these, 309 medical records were reviewed. Fetal malposition and preterm labor were more frequent in irradiated women, and especially so in women receiving higher radiation doses. Irradiated women were more likely to deliver babies weighing < 2500 g at birth, at less than 36 weeks' gestation. Among the offspring of irradiated women, an increased percentage had one or more congenital malformations; however, these data are considered only suggestive at present as ascertainment bias cannot be ruled out, with women whose child had one or more malformations possibly being more likely to participate. There was no suggestion that the congenital malformation rate was increased among the offspring of partners of irradiated males, as compared to unirradiated males.

Recent larger-scale studies

As outlined above, studies to date of patients treated for diverse types of cancer have not identified an increase in the frequency of congenital abnormalities, genetic disease or cancer in the offspring. However, all prior studies included too few children born to women or men treated for cancer to have sufficient statistical power to rule out an effect of cancer treatment on subsequent pregnancy outcome. It is estimated that many thousands of patients will be needed to rule out a relative risk for germ cell mutation in the range of 1.5. The results of more recent large-scale studies have been reported over the past few years or are in progress in a number of countries including the USA, the UK and Canada.

In The Five Center Study, Byrne and associates[33] conducted interviews of a large number of adult survivors of childhood and adolescent cancer treated between 1945 and 1975. Genetic disease (defined as a birth defect, a cytogenetic abnormality, a single-gene defect or altered sex ratio) occurred in 3.4% of 2198 offspring of survivors, as compared with 3.1% of 4544 offspring of sibling controls. Inclusion of controls reduced the potential for surveillance bias. With respect to older anticancer regimens, the study had 80% power to detect an increase in genetic disease as small as 40% and did not do so. Despite the large sample size, the study had a number of limitations: less than 25% of the survivors were exposed to potentially mutagenic therapy; the study was limited in its power to detect small changes in the risk of new mutations or risks due to individual agents or specific combinations of agents; and it was unable to consider dose–response relationships.

In a collaborative study from five countries (Denmark, Finland, Iceland, Norway and Sweden), Sankila and co-workers[34] used data from national cancer and birth registries to assess cancer risk in 5847 offspring of 14 652 male and female survivors of childhood or adolescent cancer. The data reflected all of the cases of cancer diagnosed in an overall population of approximately 20 million people over a 25- to 35-year period. There was no significant increased risk of non-hereditary cancer among the offspring. Based on their data, the authors suggested that the fear of cancer in their offspring should not be a reason to discourage survivors of sporadic childhood/adolescent cancer from having children, and that it is not warranted to screen for cancer in the offspring of survivors of sporadic childhood/adolescent cancer. It should be noted that an analysis of individual treatment regimens (i.e. specific drugs) was not included.

The Childhood Cancer Survivor Study (CCSS) is a multicenter study (25 centers in the USA and Canada) of more than 14 000 long-term survivors of childhood and adolescent cancer looking for evidence of induced genetic disease in offspring as well as other health effects[35]. Reports on some endpoints have been published.

Green and colleagues[36] reviewed the pregnancy outcome (rate of live births, gender ratio, abortions, miscarriages) among female participants in the CCSS; the frequency of congenital anomalies and cancer in the offspring will be reported in future articles. Among the 1915 women who reported 4029 pregnancies, there were no significant differences in pregnancy outcome by treatment. However, it should be noted that for less commonly used chemotherapy drugs (e.g. vinblastine, dacarbazine, cisplatin, carmustine, etoposide, lomustine), the statistical power to detect a modest effect was limited. The study had sufficient statistical power to detect a two-fold risk of a non-live birth for more commonly used drugs such as cyclophosphamide, doxorubicin, vincristine, actinomycin D, procarbazine, mechlorethamine and daunorubicin. The women who had received pelvic irradiation were at risk of delivering low-birth-weight infants, with significantly more of their babies likely to weigh < 2500 g at birth.

Pregnancy outcome (pregnancy loss, live births and birth weight) has also been reported for the partners of male survivors from the CCSS[37]. Of the 4106 sexually active males, 1227 had sired 2323 pregnancies of which 69% were live births, 1% stillbirths,

13% miscarriages, 13% abortions, and 5% unknown or in gestation. For the cancer survivors, a decreased male-to-female ratio (1.0 : 1.03 vs. 1.24 : 1.0) of the offspring and a lower proportion (0.77) of pregnancies resulting in a liveborn baby were reported, as compared with the offspring of the partners of the male siblings of the survivors. Sex ratio is used to examine the possibility of X-linked lethal mutations. Alterations in sex ratio have also been reported in association with occupational exposure to various substances, but the underlying mechanism is unclear and would benefit from studies in animal models[38,39]. No significant differences in pregnancy outcome by treatment were found. The rate of miscarriages was elevated for the partners of men treated with > 5000 mg/m^2 of procarbazine compared to those treated with 0–5000 mg/m^2; these findings are novel and will need further evaluation. Live-birth and miscarriage rates in partners were not affected by exposure to various doses of cyclophosphamide, another commonly used anticancer drug. The offspring of male survivors treated with non-alkylating agent chemotherapy were more likely to weigh < 2500 g. As for the CCSS female cancer survivors[36], frequencies of congenital anomalies and cancer in the offspring of male survivors will be reported in future articles.

Although results on congenital malformations and cancer from the CCSS have not been published, the results reported to date from more recent large-scale studies generally support the conclusions of earlier studies suggesting that prior treatment with anticancer drugs does not adversely affect pregnancy outcome. The CCSS findings of an altered sex ratio associated with childhood cancer or its treatment in males, as well as the procarbazine findings, will require follow-up studies. Limitations of the large studies include the fact that most of the cancer survivors were treated as children, that outdated chemotherapy regimens or drugs were used, that most of the studies included results on both mutagenic and non-mutagenic treatments, and that conceptions usually took

Table 1 Effects of anticancer treatment: evidence for concern for the offspring of cancer survivors

Anticancer drugs induce mutations in somatic cells → treatment-related second cancers

Anticancer drugs cause DNA damage and lead to infertility in men and women

Theoretical risk of alteration to the genome of human eggs and sperm

In female cancer survivors, prior pelvic irradiation is associated with lower-birth-weight babies

Association of ovarian dysfunction with anticancer treatment in women

Premature menopause has been reported in female childhood cancer survivors

Exposure to numerous anticancer drugs results in decreases in the quality and quantity of sperm

Induction of chromosomal abnormalities in human sperm up to 18 months after cancer treatment

Little evidence of selection against chromosomally abnormal sperm in humans

place many years after termination of the anticancer treatment[40].

Table 1 summarizes the effects of anticancer treatment that pose risks to the offspring of cancer survivors.

EVIDENCE OF MUTATION INDUCTION IN HUMAN SOMATIC AND GERM CELLS

Numerous animal studies indicate that preconception maternal and paternal exposures to mutagenic drugs used in human anticancer therapy can result in adverse reproductive outcomes and the transmission of genetic damage[5–9]. In man, although there is as yet no documented transmission to the offspring of heritable changes induced by anticancer drugs, as mentioned above there are limitations to the types of epidemiological studies that have been done to date. Certainly, there is evidence in humans from the observations of treatment-related second tumors in cancer survivors that mutations in somatic cells are involved in the induction of cancer[11,41]. That anticancer regimens induce mutations in somatic cells suggests that mutations can also be induced in human germ

Table 2 Animal versus human studies, and directions for the future

Animals

Rodent germ cells are susceptible to the induction of heritable mutations by ionizing radiation and drugs used in human anticancer regimens

Adverse outcomes of preconception maternal and paternal exposure to anticancer drugs include low birth weight, congenital malformations, behavioral defects, endocrine abnormalities and cross-generational effects

Humans

Large continuing investigations of human exposures to ionizing radiation and anticancer drugs have been unable to detect evidence of human heritable mutations

Future

Continued large-scale surveillance of the offspring of cancer survivors, including the study of new anticancer drugs, development of sensitive markers (e.g. mutation screens), continued study of mechanisms, prevention of adverse effects

cells. However, there are no reliable methods to relate somatic and germ cell mutations in a given individual. At least one study has suggested that anticancer therapy-induced cytogenetic damage in somatic cells may not correlate with cytogenetic damage in male germ cells[42]. Thus, there remain concerns that anticancer drugs induce heritable mutations in the germ cells of treated individuals (Table 2).

The only method currently available to assess the potential heritable risk of a given anticancer drug to human germ cells is the use of cytogenetic observations in spermatozoa; no equivalent non-invasive test is available for female germ cells. Studies on the induction of mutations by anticancer drugs in human sperm have helped to identify agents and time windows in relation to treatment that are associated with high levels of genetic damage.

Two major methods to detect cytogenetic damage in sperm are the human sperm/hamster egg technique[43] and the fluorescence *in situ* hybridization (FISH) technique. For the human sperm/hamster egg technique, capacitated human sperm are incubated with zona-free hamster eggs; following fusion there is decondensation and reconfiguration of the human sperm chromatin, allowing the examination of human sperm metaphase chromosomes for structural and numerical abnormalities. Martin and colleagues[44] demonstrated that the sperm of men treated with ionizing radiation contained a significant proportion of chromosomal aberrations up to 36 months after the termination of treatment. This study was the first demonstration of induced chromosomal aberrations in functional human sperm, showing that sperm with radiation-induced mutations were able to fertilize eggs. A number of different laboratories have reported elevated levels of structural abnormalities and aneuploidy in the sperm of treated men[42,45,46]. As with radiation, chemotherapy-induced chromosome damage has been found a number of years after the last treatment cycle, suggesting effects on spermatogonial stem cells.

More recently FISH has been used by a number of laboratories in place of the labor-intensive human sperm/hamster egg procedure. FISH allows an assessment of disomy frequencies for specific chromosomes in individual human spermatozoa and allows many thousands of sperm to be screened quickly for numerical chromosomal abnormalities. Modifications are currently being made to the FISH technique to allow it to also detect structural aberrations. Few large studies have been done to date, and negative and positive results have been reported in studies on the effects of anticancer drugs on human sperm chromosomes[47,48]. Some of the most revealing studies have examined sperm from patients before, during and at different intervals after treatment.

In a FISH study on chromosomes X, Y and 8, where pre-, during- and post-treatment sperm samples were examined, evidence of sperm aneuploidy was found in patients treated with NOVP (mitoxantrone, vincristine, vinblastine and prednisone) chemotherapy for Hodgkin's disease; however, damage decreased to pretreatment levels within 3–4 months after the end of therapy[49]. In a further study from the same group of NOVP-exposed men, this time examining chromosomes 18, 21, X and Y, about 18% of sperm carried a numerical abnormality after treatment; as in the first study, induced effects did not persist to 1–2 years after treatment[40]. Martin and associates[50] examined sperm chromosomal abnormalities (chromosomes 1, 12, X, Y) before, during and after BEP (bleomycin, etoposide and cisplatin) chemotherapy in patients with testicular cancer, and reported evidence of aneuploidy during and 12 months after treatment. In an earlier study of BEP-treated testicular cancer patients, these authors[48] did not demonstrate an increased frequency of chromosomal abnormalities 2–13 years after chemotherapy as compared to pre-chemotherapy values. De Mas and co-workers[51] have also studied the sperm of testicular cancer patients treated with BEP, showing that an increased frequency of sperm aneuploidy may persist until at least 18 months after the termination of chemotherapy.

Cytogenetic studies on sperm from treated cancer patients provide data on direct chromosomal damage in human germ cells. Although more studies are needed, evidence to date from studies of sperm chromosomes suggests an increased risk of induced chromosomal abnormalities during chemotherapy and up to 18 months after the end of treatment[40,48–51]. Together, the studies provide a rationale to advise patients against banking sperm samples during and shortly after chemotherapy. It is unclear whether the induced genetic damage is transmissible; this would require studies of the sperm of treated men with follow-up investigations of their children. Since there appears to be no selection against chromosomally abnormal sperm in humans and cytogenetically abnormal sperm can fertilize eggs, there is reason for concern, caution and further research[52,53].

CONCLUSIONS AND ISSUES FOR COUNSELING PATIENTS

Several studies have shown a significant adverse effect of prior pelvic irradiation on the birth weight of the offspring of female cancer survivors. It is important for physicians and patients to be aware of this side-effect because of the potential adverse impact low birth weight may have on health of the offspring.

For both male and female cancer survivors, to date there is no documented transmission to offspring of heritable changes induced by anti-cancer treatment. However, several studies are still ongoing and the data suggest caution. Women on chemotherapy regimens experience ovarian dysfunction[9]; however, the precise type of damage (e.g. genetic, epigenetic) that occurs in human oocytes and whether it persists after therapy are unclear. In men, evidence from human studies of decreases in the quality (including chromosomal abnormalities) and quantity of sperm after paternal exposure to anticancer drugs needs to be considered in light of the ability of cytogenetically abnormal sperm to fertilize oocytes. Numerous observations from animal studies indicate that maternal and paternal exposures to anticancer drugs result in adverse reproductive outcomes and the transmission of genetic damage to the offspring[7,8]. In animal studies, some of the outcomes resulting from preconception paternal or maternal exposures to anticancer drugs include low birth weight, congenital malformations, behavioral defects, growth retardation, endocrine abnormalities and cross-generational effects. Children are born with similar defects, and it is possible that some of these defects may be caused by preconception exposure to anticancer drugs. Cancer patients who are interested in having children should receive genetic counseling informing them of the available data. High-resolution ultrasound scanning, chorionic villus sampling and preimplantation diagnosis (aneuploidy screening) are the only screening tools that can be offered to cancer patients currently. Much progress has been made in the identification of human disease-causing mutations as well as mutation screening. For the future and to help in the counseling of patients, molecular and high-throughput DNA-based approaches could be used to search for genetic changes induced by anticancer therapy in human germ cells and the resulting offspring.

For men, the connection between alterations in fertility, including sperm abnormalities, and birth defects is unclear. The studies reporting increased chromosome aberrations in the sperm of patients who received radiotherapy or chemotherapy suggest that physicians should be cautious in predicting reproductive outcomes in these patients. Damage appears to be repaired within about 2 years after cancer treatment[10,48–51] and could be used as a rationale for recommending that male cancer patients delay conception for 2 years after all therapy ceases. The rationale for waiting at least 6 months has been used as this period of time will ensure that all spermatozoa that fertilize an egg derive from cells that were stem spermatogonia at the time of treatment and are thus predicted to carry a lower genetic risk[7,10,49].

As a preventive measure, sperm samples for cryopreservation should be collected prior to but not during cancer therapy[10]. For a number of reasons (lack of adequate counseling, lack of concern for future fertility, concern about any delay in starting anticancer treatment, effects of cancer on spermatogenesis, preadolescent cancer) some cancer survivors do not freeze their sperm prior to therapy[54]. If such patients had remained consistently azoospermic following treatment, they would have been considered infertile until recently, when intracytoplasmic sperm injection (ICSI) and related techniques became available. There are a number of reports of attempts to help patients with persistent azoospermia following chemotherapy, using testicular sperm extraction (TESE) and ICSI. So far, men with persistent azoospermia following chemotherapy represent a diverse group of patients, with different types of tumors treated with

Table 3 Counseling issues for cancer survivors

Cancer patients interested in having children should be offered genetic counseling

As a preventive measure, collect sperm for cryopreservation prior to treatment

Avoid collecting/banking eggs or sperm during or shortly after treatment

Be aware of the pharmacological properties of anticancer drugs (e.g. methotrexate)

different chemotherapy regimens. To date at least 14 live births of healthy children have been reported after TESE and ICSI in patients with persistent azoospermia after chemotherapy[55–57]. The potential genetic risks of using qualitatively abnormal testicular sperm from azoospermic cancer patients are a matter of concern and this approach deserves careful scrutiny.

Counseling issues for cancer survivors are summarized in Table 3.

In conclusion, there have been a number of studies of the late outcomes among survivors of childhood cancer. Approaches to cancer treatment change continually in the search for more effective, less toxic therapies. Radiation doses may have fallen, but newer anticancer drugs and higher doses of potentially mutagenic agents are being used. For the future, research is needed on large numbers of patients, not only on the late-occurring outcomes resulting from treatment protocols used three or more decades ago, but also for identification of risks associated with more recent treatment regimens. The need to systematically follow populations of survivors of newer anticancer treatment strategies will most likely require large multi-institutional initiatives like the CCSS.

References

1. Greenlee RT, Hill-Harman MB, Murray T, et al. Cancer statistics, 2001. *CA Cancer J Clin* 2001;51:15–36
2. Schover LR, Rybicki L, Martin BA, et al. Having children after cancer: a survey of survivors' attitudes and experiences. *Cancer* 1999;6:697–709
3. Schover LR, Brey K, Lichtin A, et al. Knowledge and experience regarding cancer, infertility, and sperm banking in younger male survivors. *J Clin Oncol* 2002;20:1880–9
4. Schover LR. Psychosocial aspects of infertility and decisions about reproduction in young

cancer patients: a review. *Med Pediatr Oncol* 1999;33:53–9

5. Shelby MD. Human germ cell mutagens. *Environ Mol Mutagen* 1994;23(Suppl 24):30–4

6. Witt KL, Bishop JB. Mutagenicity of anti-cancer drugs in mammalian germ cells. *Mutat Res* 1996;355:209–34

7. Trasler JM, Doerksen T. Teratogen update: paternal exposures–reproductive risks. *Teratology* 1999;60:161–72

8. Arnon J, Meirow D, Lewis-Roness H, *et al.* Genetic and teratogenic effects of cancer treatments on gametes and embryos. *Hum Reprod Update* 2001;7:394–403

9. Green DM. Fertility and pregnancy outcome after treatment for cancer in childhood or adolescence. *The Oncologist* 1997;2:171–9

10. Meistrich ML. Potential genetic risks of using semen collected during chemotherapy. *Hum Reprod* 1993;8:8–10

11. Robison LL, Bhatia S. Late-effects among survivors of leukaemia and lymphoma during childhood and adolescence. *Br J Haematol* 2003;122:345–59

12. Byrne J, Fears TR, Gail MH. Early menopause in long-term survivors of cancer during adolescence. *Am J Obstet Gynecol* 1992;166:788–93

13. Wyrobek AJ, Gordon LA, Burkhart JG, *et al.* An evaluation of human sperm as indicators of chemically induced alterations of spermatogenic function. *Mutat Res* 1983;115:73–148

14. Byrne J, Mulvihill JJ, Myers MH, *et al.* Effects of treatment on fertility in long-term survivors of childhood or adolescent cancer. *N Engl J Med* 1987;317:1315–21

15. Damewood MD, Grochow LB. Prospects for fertility after chemotherapy or radiation for neoplastic diseases. *Fertil Steril* 1986;45:443–59

16. Meirow D, Schenker JG. Cancer and male infertility. *Hum Reprod* 1995;10:2017–22

17. Viviani S, Santoro A, Ragni G. Gonadal toxicity after combination chemotherapy for Hodgkin's disease. Comparative results for MOPP vs ABVD. *Eur J Cancer Clin Oncol* 1985;21:601–5

18. Li FP, Gimbrere K, Gelber RD, *et al.* Outcome of pregnancy in survivors of Wilms' tumor. *J Am Med Assoc* 1987;257:216–19

19. Green DM, Zevon MA, Lowrie G, *et al.* Congenital anomalies in children of patients who received chemotherapy for cancer in childhood and adolescence. *N Engl J Med* 1991;325:141–6

20. Hawkins MM. Is there evidence of a therapy-related increase in germ cell mutation among childhood cancer survivors? *J Natl Cancer Inst* 1991;83:1642–50

21. Dodds L, Marrett LD, Tomkins DJ, *et al.* Case–control study of congenital anomalies in children of cancer patients. *Br Med J* 1993;307:164–8

22. Kenney LB, Nicholson HS, Brasseux C, *et al.* Birth defects in offspring of adult survivors of childhood acute lymphoblastic leukemia: a Children's Cancer Group/National Institutes of Health report. *Cancer* 1996;78:169–76

23. Green DM, Fiorello A, Zevon MA, *et al.* Birth defects and childhood cancer in offspring of survivors of childhood cancer. *Arch Pediatr Adolesc Med* 1997;151:379–83

24. Rustin GJ, Booth M, Dent J. Pregnancy after cytotoxic chemotherapy for gestational trophoblastic tumours. *Br Med J* 1984;288:103–6

25. Lloyd ME, Carr M, McElhatton P, *et al.* The effects of methotrexate on pregnancy, fertility and lactation. *Q J Med* 1999;92:551–63

26. Mulvihill JJ, Connelly RR, Austin DE, *et al.* Cancer in offspring of long term survivors of childhood and adolescent cancer. *Lancet* 1987;2:813–17

27. Hawkins MM, Draper GJ, Winter DL. Cancer in the offspring of survivors of childhood leukaemia and non-Hodgkin's lymphomas. *Br J Cancer* 1995;71:1335–9

28. Green DM, Fine WE, Li FP. Offspring of patients treated for unilateral Wilms' tumor in childhood. *Cancer* 1982;49:2285–8

29. Byrne J, Mulvihill JJ, Connelly RR, *et al.* Reproductive problems and birth defects in survivors of Wilms' tumor and their relatives. *Med Pediatr Oncol* 1988;16:233–40

30. Hawkins MM, Smith RA. Pregnancy outcome in childhood cancer survivors: probable effects of abdominal irradiation. *Int J Cancer* 1989;43:399–402

31. Chiarelli AM, Marrett LD, Darlington GA. Pregnancy outcomes in females after treatment for childhood cancer. *Epidemiology* 2000;11:161–6

32. Green DM, Peabody EM, Nan B, *et al.* Pregnancy outcome after treatment for Wilms' tumor: a report from the National Wilms' Tumor Study Group. *J Clin Oncol* 2002;10:2506–13

33. Byrne J, Rasmussen SA, Steinhorn SC, *et al.* Genetic disease in offspring of long-term survivors of childhood and adolescent cancer. *Am J Hum Genet* 1998;62:45–52

34. Sankila R, Olsen JH, Anderson H, *et al.* Risk of cancer among offspring of childhood-cancer survivors. *N Engl J Med* 1998;338:1339–44

35. Robison LL, Mertens AC, Boice JD, *et al.* Study design and cohort characteristics of the Childhood Cancer Survivor Study: a

multi-institutional collaborative project. *Med Pediatr Oncol* 2002;38:229–39

36. Green DM, Whitton JA, Stovall M, *et al.* Pregnancy outcome of female survivors of childhood cancer: a report from the Childhood Cancer Survivor Study. *Am J Obstet Gynecol* 2002;187:1070–80

37. Green DM, Whitton JA, Stovall M, *et al.* Pregnancy outcome of partners of male survivors of childhood cancer: a report from the Childhood Cancer Survivor Study. *J Clin Oncol* 2003;21:716–21

38. Mocarelli P, Gerthoux PM, Ferrari E, *et al.* Paternal concentrations of dioxin and sex ratio of offspring. *Lancet* 2000;355:1858–63

39. Trasler J. Paternal exposures: altered sex ratios II. *Teratology* 2001;64:3

40. Frias S, Van Hummelen P, Meistrich ML, *et al.* NOVP chemotherapy for Hodgkin's disease transiently induces sperm aneuploidies associated with the major clinical aneuploidy syndromes involving chromosomes X, Y, 18, and 21. *Cancer Res* 2003;63:44–51

41. Tucker MA, Coleman CN, Cox RS, *et al.* Risk of second cancers after treatment for Hodgkin's disease. *N Engl J Med* 1988;318:76–81

42. Genesca A, Barrios L, Miro R, *et al.* Lymphocyte and sperm chromosome studies in cancer-treated men. *Hum Genet* 1990;84:353–5

43. Rudak E, Jacobs PA, Yanagimachi R. Direct analysis of the chromosome composition of human spermatozoa. *Nature* 1978;274:911–12

44. Martin R, Hildebrand K, Yamamoto J, *et al.* An increased frequency of human sperm chromosomal abnormalities after radiotherapy. *Mutat Res* 1986;174:219–25

45. Brandriff BF, Meistrich ML, Gordon LA, *et al.* Chromosomal damage in sperm of patients surviving Hodgkin's disease following MOPP therapy with and without radiotherapy. *Hum Genet* 1994;93:295–9

46. Martin R, Rademaker A, Leonard N. Analysis of chromosomal abnormalities in human sperm after chemotherapy by karyotyping and fluorescence *in situ* hybridization (FISH). *Cancer Genet Cytogenet* 1995;80:29–32

47. Robbins WA. Cytogenetic damage measured in human sperm following cancer chemotherapy. *Mutat Res* 1996;355:235–52

48. Martin RH, Ernst S, Rademaker A, *et al.* Chromosomal abnormalities in sperm from testicular cancer patients before and after chemotherapy. *Hum Genet* 1997;99:214–18

49. Robbins WA, Meistrich ML, Moore D, *et al.* Chemotherapy induces transient sex chromosomal and autosomal aneuploidy in human sperm. *Nat Genet* 1997;16:74–8

50. Martin RH, Ernst S, Rademaker A, *et al.* Analysis of sperm chromosome complements before, during and after chemotherapy. *Cancer Genet Cytogenet* 1999;108:133–6

51. De Mas P, Daudin M, Vincent M-C, *et al.* Increased aneuploidy in spermatozoa from testicular tumour patients after chemotherapy with cisplatin, etoposide and bleomycin. *Hum Reprod* 2001;16:1204–8

52. Martin RH. Invited editorial: segregation analysis of translocations by the study of human sperm chromosome complements. *Am J Hum Genet* 1989;44:461–3

53. Martin R, Barclay L, Hildebrand K, *et al.* Cytogenetic analysis of 400 sperm from three translocation heterozygotes. *Hum Genet* 1990; 86:33–9

54. Schover LR, Brey K, Lichtin A, *et al.* Oncologists' attitudes and practices regarding banking sperm before cancer treatment. *J Clin Oncol* 2002;20:1890–7

55. Chan PT, Palermo GD, Veeck LL, *et al.* Testicular sperm extraction combined with intracytoplasmic sperm injection in the treatment of men with persistent azoospermia postchemotherapy. *Cancer* 2001;92:1632–7

56. Damani MN, Master V, Meng MV, *et al.* Postchemotherapy ejaculatory azoospermia: fatherhood with sperm from testis tissue with intracytoplasmic sperm injection. *J Clin Oncol* 2002;20:888–90

57. Meseguer M, Garrido N, Remohi J, *et al.* Testicular sperm extraction (TESE) and ICSI in patients with permanent azoospermia after chemotherapy. *Hum Reprod* 2003;6:1281–5

Psychosocial issues of fertility preservation in cancer survivors

18

K. H. Dow

INTRODUCTION

Changes in cancer treatment, involving less invasive surgery, high-dose chemotherapy and newer radiotherapy techniques, have increased the long-term survival of children, adolescents and young adults with cancer[1]. In addition, there has been a major shift in assisted reproductive technologies (ART), leading to increasing numbers of cancer survivors seeking answers to reproductive concerns such as premature ovarian failure, subfertility and infertility[2].

The purpose of this chapter is to briefly describe the background of cancer survivorship, describe the unique concerns facing childhood, adolescent and adult cancer survivors, consider the psychosocial issues facing cancer survivors, review the available evidence relating to psychosocial issues in fertility preservation after cancer, and explore potential areas for future research.

BACKGROUND ON CANCER SURVIVORSHIP

In the USA, cancer survivors total about 8.9 million people, a figure that represents 3.3% of the population[1]. Long-term cancer survival statistics are highly encouraging, with about 60% of adults and 77% of children surviving more than 5 years after diagnosis[1]. Even more optimistic are data that show that 14% of all cancer survivors were diagnosed over 20 years ago[3]. Improvement in cancer survivorship is attributed to changes in fundamental understanding about genetics, rapid translation of basic science to practice, modification of dose-limiting treatment toxicities, increases in screening and early detection activities, enhanced rehabilitation and support interventions, and changes in sociocultural factors[4].

Despite optimism and the prospects for long-term survival among childhood, adolescent and young adult cancer survivors, there is also a growing body of evidence that shows long-term and late effects such as infertility, secondary cancers, cognitive changes, cardiac and respiratory dysfunction, menopausal symptoms, and psychosocial problems[5–12]. While these young survivors express major distress over fertility preservation, these concerns are also balanced against the other potential late effects of cancer treatment. The following discussion distinguishes the different issues facing childhood and adolescent cancer survivors. Subsequently, the issues facing adult cancer survivors are discussed from the perspective of breast cancer and gynecological cancers.

CHILDHOOD AND ADOLESCENT CANCER SURVIVORS

While successfully treated and cured of their cancer as children, these survivors face the potential of long-term health risks as they grow into adulthood. Late physical effects include recurrence, secondary cancers, cardiac and pulmonary late effects, reproductive and endocrine effects, and higher mortality compared with their peers[13,14]. The recent Childhood Cancer Survivor Study (CCSS) reported that, among a cohort of over 20 000 young people who had survived childhood cancer for 5 years, there was a 10.8 times increase in mortality compared with the general population[11]. Recurrent disease leading to early death, secondary cancers, and cardiac and pulmonary toxicity were the most common and devastating late effects. A similar study conducted in Scandinavia with over 13 000 pediatric cancer survivors showed remarkably similar outcomes, with excess mortality, secondary cancers and major organ dysfunction over time[12]. These findings are important in helping to understand the background against which childhood and adolescent cancer survivors seek care for fertility preservation or infertility many years after treatment. Even though the potential for infertility is acknowledged to be among one of the most psychologically traumatic late complications of childhood cancer[15,16], decisions such as future intimacy, childbearing and child-rearing concerns may not be considered high priority when children and adolescents are initially diagnosed with cancer. Fertility concerns become a major problem when these children and adolescents grow into adulthood and are ready to start a family.

Both young men and young women can suffer infertility as a result of the effects of alkylating agents, high-dose chemotherapy and abdominal irradiation. The degree of reproductive damage is age-related, with younger prepubescent patients having less reproductive damage and earlier recovery than older adolescents. While the cytotoxic effects on the reproductive system are well known in both males and females, fewer females are referred for reproductive counseling compared with males.

Male fertility-preserving options

Patients with testicular germ cell tumors (even those with advanced and metastatic testicular cancers) and Hodgkin's disease are often diagnosed in their late adolescence or early adulthood. Cancer treatment offers excellent prospects for long-term survival and, thus,

there is a greater emphasis on fertility preservation[17]. Likewise, patients with Wilms' tumor and childhood leukemias have higher cure rates, but are most often diagnosed in childhood when the primary concern is long-term survival rather than fertility. However, these survivors also express increased desire for having children when they reach young adulthood.

There are several fertility-sparing procedures available for young males. First, they can be referred for semen cryopreservation, a routine procedure that is relatively inexpensive and technically easy to accomplish. Most important to the oncology team is that the timing of semen collection and cryopreservation does not coincide with the start of cancer treatment, making this a viable and preferred procedure. Despite the advantages, semen cryopreservation is not indicated in certain males, particularly preadolescents[15]. A second situation where cryopreservation may not be ideal is when males encounter difficulty producing a usable specimen. Two alternative procedures have been suggested. The first is testicular germ cell harvesting, where germ cells can be removed prior to treatment and stored. In theory the stored tissue can be auto-transplanted or the stored cells can be matured *in vitro* until they reach a stage for fertilization using ART. The second and presently realistic alternative is testicular sperm extraction (TESE) and intracytoplasmic sperm injection (ICSI) to provide a chance of paternity in men who become azoospermic after cancer treatment[18].

Successful pregnancy outcomes have occurred with fathers who were young cancer survivors. Horne and colleagues[19] discussed two case reports of successful pregnancy after long-term semen cryopreservation before chemotherapy and radiation therapy. In the first case report, the patient banked sperm at 20 years of age and prior to chemotherapy for Hodgkin's disease. Eleven years later, the patient's thawed semen was used in *in vitro* fertilization (IVF) with ICSI and resulted in twins following the transfer of frozen–thawed embryos. In the second case report, the patient banked sperm at 17 years of age prior to chemotherapy and radiotherapy for acute myeloid leukemia. Eight years later, his frozen sperm was used for ICSI, resulting in triplets born after the transfer of frozen–thawed embryos.

Female fertility-preserving options

Young females have fewer fertility-sparing options than males for several reasons[15]. First, fertility-sparing procedures involving ART can be time consuming, requiring at least one cycle (i.e. 4 weeks). Of high importance to the oncology team is that fertility-sparing procedures may interfere with the start of cancer treatment, making them less favorable. Embryo cryopreservation and IVF are potential options prior to treatment, but, unfortunately, females are not routinely referred for reproductive counseling. In situations where abdominal irradiation is indicated, such as in the treatment of Hodgkin's disease, lateral ovarian transposition to extrapelvic sites during staging laparotomy avoids the ovaries being included in the radiation treatment field. Lateral ovarian transposition is associated with preservation of ovarian function in about 83% of patients after pelvic irradiation[15]. In addition, this procedure is more effective than transposing the ovaries behind the uterus and protecting with a lead block during radiation therapy.

Other possible fertility-preserving procedures applied for young females with cancer include gonadotropin suppression using a gonadotropin releasing hormone (GnRH) analog to prevent follicular growth and mitosis, ovarian tissue transplantation, and oocyte cryopreservation. Oocyte cryopreservation has not been a routine procedure for fertility preservation in females because it is a time-consuming process producing a limited number of oocytes. Moreover, oocyte collection from prepubertal females is not appropriate[20,21].

Embryo cryopreservation is an established procedure which may be used, but carries both advantages and disadvantages. Embryo cryopreservation requires a male partner or donor sperm, and patients may not be able to afford this procedure. More importantly, this procedure takes at least 4 weeks, and the timing may interfere with the start of chemotherapy. Despite these disadvantages, Atkinson and co-workers[22] described a successful pregnancy with embryo cryopreservation in a patient with leukemia who had undergone bone marrow transplantation.

Frozen banking of immature ovarian follicles presents new opportunities for fertility preservation in the future. Ovarian tissue banking prior to chemotherapy and radiotherapy, followed by autograft after remission or *in vitro* maturation, may restore gonadal function and fertility. Fabbri and associates[23] obtained ovarian tissue by laparoscopy and used the cryopreservation protocol of slow freezing–rapid thawing.

Pregnancy outcomes

Childhood and adolescent cancer survivors express concern that they may transmit cancer to their children and are concerned about the health of their children. Green and colleagues[24] evaluated the effect of treatment for Wilms' tumor on complications of pregnancy and pregnancy outcomes in over 1000 female participants in the National Wilms' Tumor Study Group who were younger than 21 at the time of diagnosis and survived more than 5 years. They reported on 427 pregnancies lasting at least 20 weeks, with 409 live single births. Adverse outcomes such as fetal malposition and premature labor occurred more frequently among women who had received high-dose abdominal radiation therapy. Low birth weight (< 2500 g) coupled with young gestational age (< 36 weeks) was also most often seen in children whose mothers had received abdominal irradiation. Hershlag and Shuster[25] reported that two patients with Hodgkin's disease achieved a successful pregnancy after having received high-dose chemotherapy treatment with stem cell transplantation.

Thus, it is prudent to advise young female survivors that there may be an increased risk of low-birth-weight infants, fetal malposition and premature labor if they had received abdominal irradiation as a child. In addition, Thomson and co-workers[16] cautioned that while successful pregnancy outcomes have not shown an overall increased incidence of congenital malformations or childhood malignancies in infants born to long-term cancer survivors, we do not know the long-term consequences to children of cancer survivors with the use of ART.

Psychosocial issues

We are just beginning to evaluate the long-term psychosocial issues relating to fertility among childhood and adolescent cancer survivors, with only a few reports in the literature on this subject. Roopnarinesingh and associates[26] evaluated mood disorders in men with cancer who sought semen cryopreservation. Using a small sample of 29 men, they found that nearly 45% had anxiety and 17.2% reported depression, although most cases were of mild to moderate severity. Another report conservatively estimated that sexual dysfunction, fertility distress and infertility affected about 20% of patients[27]. This figure is likely to increase in the future, with the advent of new ART techniques.

Schover and colleagues[28] conducted a survey regarding cancer survivors' attitudes and experiences about having children after cancer. The investigators found that respondents were on average 5.5 years post-treatment. About 76% of childless cancer survivors wanted children in the future, with only 6% feeling that their cancer experience diminished their wish for children. Over 80% of respondents believed that their cancer experience would make them better parents and 94% felt healthy enough to be a parent. Nearly a quarter of the patients were distressed about infertility and believed that their health-care providers did not address the risks of birth defects or the potential for cancer in their own children.

In a follow-up study, the same authors[29] conducted a survey regarding knowledge, attitude and experiences with cancer-related infertility and sperm banking. A return rate of 27% yielded 201 surveys. Over 51% of men wanted children in the future, including 77% of men who were childless at diagnosis. Despite anxiety about their long-term survival and the potential risks to children, the men believed that the experience of cancer increased the value they placed on family closeness and believed that their cancer experience would also make them better parents. About 60% of men remembered receiving information about infertility and 50% indicated that they were given information about sperm banking.

In general, there is a wide variation in reproductive practice guidelines in the oncology setting. Fewer patients are referred for reproductive counseling. Glaser and co-workers[30] evaluated the current level of best clinical practice for sperm, ovarian and prepubertal tissue collection and storage in the pediatric oncology setting. They conducted a cross-sectional survey of the Pediatric Oncology Group and, of the 110 centers surveyed, there was a response of 69 questionnaires (63%). The investigators found that no center had guidelines concerning which young people should be offered preservation of sperm, ovarian or prepubertal testicular tissue. Furthermore, they found little agreement among the centers with respect to gamete preservation. The overwhelming majority (93%) of centers offered sperm cryopreservation, with about 10% discussing oocyte cryopreservation. The centers reported that males were more likely to be offered sperm cryopreservation compared with offers of female fertility-sparing information. Patients with Hodgkin's disease, non-Hodgkin's lymphoma and sarcomas were more readily offered fertility preservation. Fertility counseling was done by the doctors, nurses, social workers, psychologists and geneticists, and not through referral to reproductive endocrinologists and genetic counseling. Thus, there are tremendous opportunities for highly specialized oncology, reproductive endocrinology and genetic counseling professionals to collaborate on improving clinical practice, to increase the number of cancer survivors referred for counseling in a timely manner.

The aforementioned study results have tremendous implications for practice. Despite our knowledge of the effects of cancer treatment on fertility, particularly among long-term cancer survivors, information about fertility options is not well disseminated. Young cancer survivors' strong desire to have children after treatment, coupled with their belief that they will become good parents, places further importance on the timely receipt of fertility options before treatment begins.

BREAST CANCER

Breast cancer survivors experience severe distress with infertility after treatment[31,32]. Advanced maternal age (> 35 years) and alkylating agents are known risk factors that contribute to infertility[33–35]. On the other hand, other chemotherapeutic agents such as doxorubicin and the taxanes may decrease the potential for amenorrhea compared with standard chemotherapy regimens[36,37]. The overwhelming evidence from retrospective, single-institution, case–control and population-based studies demonstrates few adverse effects on survival with subsequent pregnancy.

Effects of treatment on fertility

The alkylating agent, cyclophosphamide, is a standard chemotherapy drug used for breast cancer, and has the greatest effect on amenorrhea by damaging cycling ovarian follicles[35]. The degree of amenorrhea varies but is related to the total dose of cyclophosphamide, with higher doses increasing the risk of amenorrhea. On the other hand, doxorubicin-containing chemotherapy regimens may potentially decrease the risk of amenorrhea compared with the standard chemotherapy protocol of cyclophosphamide, methotrexate and fluorouracil (CMF)[33].

Taxanes may also decrease the risk of amenorrhea. Stone and associates[38] recently reported a retrospective comparison of the rates of amenorrhea in 98 premenopausal

women treated for early-stage breast cancer. Patients receiving doxorubicin and cyclophosphamide (AC) were compared to those receiving AC + paclitaxel (Taxol™). The investigators found that the incidence of chemotherapy-induced amenorrhea increased with age but did not increase with the addition of paclitaxel. Most recently, Ibrahim and co-workers[37] reported that paclitaxel-based chemotherapy regimens (four cycles of paclitaxel followed by four cycles of FAC (fluorouracil, doxorubicin and cyclophosphamide)) may improve recovery of menstrual cycles in patients compared with standard chemotherapy using FAC for 8 weeks.

Radiotherapy has an indirect effect on the ovaries through internal radiation scatter, but the effects of primary breast irradiation on the ovaries are thought to be negligible. The overall effect of radiation on ovarian function is relatively small compared with that of chemotherapy. One adverse outcome of radiation therapy is the limited breast milk that can be produced in the irradiated breast. However, women consider this a minor outcome compared with having a healthy infant.

Effects of subsequent pregnancy on survival

Women with breast cancer often express initial worry that a subsequent pregnancy may increase their risk of disease recurrence. However, data do not show an increased risk of recurrence based on subsequent pregnancy alone. In fact, since the first retrospective institutional study of the effects of pregnancy on breast cancer survival in 1955, evidence accumulated over the past 50 years through case reports, matched comparison studies and international population-based studies support the clinical evidence showing no increase in disease recurrence after pregnancy[39–44].

Four large population-based studies examined the effect of pregnancy on survival in breast cancer survivors and came to similar conclusions showing no adverse effect of pregnancy. Kroman and colleagues[41] conducted a population-based cohort study with 5725 women aged 45 years or younger in Denmark, and found 173 women having subsequent pregnancy. Women having a full-term pregnancy after treatment had a non-significant *reduced* risk of death compared with women who had no full-term pregnancy. Miscarriages or induced abortions did not influence prognosis. Sankila's group[42] conducted a population-based matched survival study among more than 2500 Finnish women aged < 40 years, 91 of whom had subsequent pregnancy. They found that the subjects in the control group had 4.8-fold higher risk of death compared to breast cancer survivors with subsequent pregnancy. The researchers postulated a potential 'healthy mother effect' to explain why women who became pregnant may be more likely to be free of disease than women who do not have subsequent pregnancy.

Von Schoultz and co-workers[43] evaluated 2119 women with breast cancer who were below 50 years of age at diagnosis; 50 had a subsequent pregnancy. They concluded that hormonal changes associated with pregnancy after breast cancer had little influence on prognosis. Velentgas and associates[44] also observed no overall association between pregnancy after breast cancer and risk of death in 53 women with pregnancy, compared with 265 case-matched healthy controls. However, the rate of miscarriage among women with breast cancer was 24% compared with 18% in the control group who never had breast cancer. The rate of pregnancies ending in miscarriage was 70% higher than expected. They attributed the difference to an altered hormone profile after treatment that is less likely to support subsequent pregnancy.

Gelber and colleagues[45] conducted a study to evaluate the impact of subsequent pregnancy on prognosis, identifying 108 patients with early breast cancer through the International Breast Cancer Study Group, for whom data were available for 94. They came to similar conclusions: that subsequent pregnancy did not adversely affect the prognosis of early-stage breast cancer. The survival may reflect what is considered a 'healthy patient'

selection bias, but survival is also consistent with an antitumor effect of the pregnancy.

Thus, the accumulated evidence shows that women with breast cancer do not have adverse clinical outcomes with subsequent pregnancy. Some investigators even postulate that healthy women with early-stage breast cancer are more likely to become pregnant and carry to term. Infants born to mothers with breast cancer do not show an increased risk for low birth weight or birth defects compared with the general population.

Fertility-preserving options

Fortunately, today there are several ART options that were not available even a few years ago. Oktay and co-workers[46] reported the successful preservation of fertility in women with breast cancer using IVF and embryo cryopreservation after ovarian stimulation with tamoxifen. Tamoxifen was used to stimulate follicle growth and induce ovulation prior to the start of breast cancer treatment. Tamoxifen is a viable alternative for inducing ovulation because of its favorable hormonal profile for oncologists. The 12 women with breast cancer received 40–60 mg tamoxifen for a week beginning on days 2–3 of their menstrual cycle and had IVF with either fresh embryo transfer or cryopreservation. The authors[46] found that tamoxifen stimulation resulted in a higher number of embryos, and offered a safe method of fertility preservation in women with breast cancer.

Fox and associates[47] induced gonadal quiescence using the GnRH agonist leuprolide during chemotherapy in 24 women with breast cancer. The median age of patients was 35 years (range 23–42 years). All patients became amenorrheic by the third cycle of chemotherapy, but menses resumed in 23 of them within 12 months after completing chemotherapy. Subsequently there were six pregnancies in five patients, three of whom required fertility treatment. Three pregnancies resulted in miscarriage, one was terminated for Down syndrome and one resulted in a live birth. The authors concluded that while leuprolide may be associated with a high rate of preserving ovarian function, the subsequent effect on fertility might still be problematic.

Psychosocial issues

Similar to the situation for childhood and adolescent cancer survivors, there are very few reports of the actual psychosocial issues affecting young breast cancer survivors in their quest to preserve fertility and normalize their lives with families and children after treatment. In one of the few reports that directly assessed fertility concerns and pregnancy outcomes in young women with breast cancer, Dow[31] reported the results of a qualitative study of 43 women having children after treatment. She used a semi-structured interview guide to identify reasons why young women decided to become pregnant, described their concerns about pregnancy, and determined helpful behaviors in making decisions to become pregnant. Participants indicated that their pregnancy was a strong stimulus to 'get well' again. Young women with subsequent pregnancy believed that having a family after treatment had the greatest impact on improving their quality of life. Children gave them a reason to start the day and provided a normal structure in their lives. Participants expressed concerns about the potential for disease recurrence, about the need to be vigilant with cancer follow-up and breast examinations, and also about not having mammography during pregnancy. The participants identified helpful behaviors as: having a realistic perspective about a normal pregnancy, learning to live with and manage uncertainty about the future, having love and support from one's spouse, and determining the difference between personal and medical decision-making. Participants also cautioned that family members expressed grave concern about their decisions to become pregnant. Family members often may not agree with personal decisions, and thus women contemplating subsequent pregnancy must prepare themselves for a somewhat less than enthusiastic family response.

FERTILITY PRESERVATION IN WOMEN WITH GYNECOLOGICAL CANCERS

There are several fertility-sparing procedures available for women with gynecological cancers that may influence their quality of life[48]. These procedures include radical trachelectomy for cervical cancer, hormonal therapy for early endometrial cancer and conservative surgical management of early-stage epithelial ovarian cancer. ART have also been helpful in women with impaired ovarian function after gynecological cancer.

Schlaerth and colleagues[49] evaluated radical trachelectomy combined with pelvic lymphadenectomy as a fertility-sparing procedure for the treatment of women with early-stage cervical cancer. In their cohort of 12 women with early stage I cervical cancer, four pregnancies occurred; there were two third-trimester deliveries and two preterm losses at 24 and 26 weeks of gestation.

Ovarian cancers are rare in young women. However, when ovarian cancers are diagnosed in young women, they tend to be low-stage low-grade malignancies with good prospects for long-term survival and fertility preservation. Ayhan and co-workers[50] advocated several conservative approaches for ovarian tumors after surgical staging, including cystectomy, unilateral salpingo-oophorectomy, and unilateral salpingo-oophorectomy plus contralateral cystectomy. The investigators reported a spontaneous pregnancy rate of about 60–88% after these fertility-sparing surgical procedures.

These procedures, while available, may not often be offered to young women presenting with gynecological cancer. Most often, patients must be adamant about expressing their fertility-preserving concerns to bring about discussions of these procedures with their oncology team. Patients often search the Internet for lay reports in the news proclaiming fertility-preserving surgery. One particular advocacy organization, Fertile Hope, has made tremendous strides in educating individuals with cancer about the options available, which must be discussed in sufficient time prior to treatment for the individual patient to make an informed decision.

COUNSELING CANCER SURVIVORS ABOUT FERTILITY PRESERVATION

For each of the numerous fertility-preserving options available, including the storage of embryos, mature oocytes, immature oocytes and ovarian tissue, semen cryopreservation and ICSI, there are corresponding advantages and disadvantages. At the same time, decisions about which cancer patients should receive these treatments and the timing of any of these reproductive options are highly individualized. Seymour[2] has indicated that there are no specific guidelines for selection of patients, but offers six areas that need to be considered before making recommendations. These areas include:

(1) The risk of infertility with the proposed treatment plan;

(2) Potential risks of delaying chemotherapy (or any other cancer treatment);

(3) Overall prognosis of the patient;

(4) Impact of future pregnancy on the risk of recurrence;

(5) Impact of any required hormonal manipulation on the tumor itself;

(6) Possibility of tumor contamination of the harvested tissue.

An understanding of the relative importance of each of these factors will help to facilitate application of the appropriate fertility method to enable possible future childbearing.

Since the risks of infertility are known, it is imperative that patients be referred for reproductive counseling prior to treatment, so that they can make an informed decision about treatment. The oncology team, in particular, should elevate the fertility concerns of their young patients to higher priority. If ART is an option prior to treatment, then these options can and should be explored. If there are cancer treatment options available that may lessen the risk of infertility, these options also need additional explanation and discussion.

For most cancers other than leukemia, there is a window of opportunity to investigate ART options. Unfortunately, this window is often overlooked in the cancer workup. In this instance, patients who can advocate for themselves and find information on the Internet, such as Fertile Hope (www.fertilehope.org), are in the best position to negotiate additional time. In the future, we can best serve patients with fertility concerns by developing partnerships between the ART and oncology communities through joint sessions or programs at national conferences and organizations.

The overall prognosis of patients with cancer continues to increase. Childhood and adolescent cancer survivors have excellent chances for long-term survival and, based on current data, have high goals for parenting and starting a family in the future. In addition, adult survivors of breast and gynecological cancers also face long-term survival. Despite an overall good prognosis, it is still prudent to have a discussion of the 'what ifs' – where recurrence may potentially occur in the future (as in the case of breast cancer) and how the individual might incorporate these disease factors in their overall family planning.

We do know that there is little support for the stimulation of recurrence of breast cancer with subsequent pregnancy. It is helpful to discuss the question as to whether a cancer history may affect offspring. Patients worry that their children may have a higher risk of developing cancer or that their pregnancy may start a recurrence of their disease. Studies do not show that children born to either male or female cancer survivors have a higher incidence of birth defects than the general population. Studies do show that women who received abdominal irradiation at a young age have a higher risk of congenital malformation, fetal malposition and low-birth-weight infants. In addition, unless there is a known inherited susceptibility, children born to cancer survivors do not have a higher risk of developing cancer themselves. Cancer survivors who discuss their plans for future childbearing and ART options with family members may encounter mixed and strong emotions from family members.

Finally, it behoves the oncology community to learn more about ART options and to collaborate with reproductive specialists to improve the care of patients with cancer and their families.

References

1. American Cancer Society (ACS). *Facts and Figures*. Atlanta: ACS 2004

2. Seymour JF. Ovarian tissue cryopreservation for cancer patients: who is appropriate? *Reprod Fertil Dev* 2001;13:81–9

3. Hewitt M, Breen N, Devesa S. Cancer prevalence and survivorship issues: analyses of the 1992 National Health Interview Survey. *J Natl Cancer Inst* 1999;91:1480–6

4. Rowland JH, Aziz N, Tesauro G, Feuer EJ. The changing face of cancer survivorship. *Semin Oncol Nurs* 2001;17:236–40

5. Ferrell BR, Dow KH. Quality of life among long-term cancer survivors. *Oncology* 1997;11:565–76

6. Ganz PA. Late effects of cancer and its treatment. *Semin Oncol Nurs* 2001;17:241–8

7. Hancock SL, Hoppe RT. Long-term complications of treatment and causes of mortality after Hodgkin's disease. *Semin Radiat Oncol* 1996;6:225–42

8. Harpham W. Long-term survivorship: late effects. In Berger A, Portenoy R, Weissman D, eds. *Principles and Practice of Supportive Oncology*. Philadelphia, PA: Lippincott-Williams & Wilkins, 1998:889–97

9. Loescher L, Clark L, Atwood J, et al. The impact of the cancer experience on long-term survivors. *Oncol Nurs Forum* 1990;17:223–9

10. Loescher LJ, Welch-McCaffrey D, Leigh SA, et al. Surviving adult cancers. Part 1: Physiologic effects. *Ann Intern Med* 1989;111:411–32

11. Mertens AC, Yasui Y, Neglia JP, et al. Late mortality experience in five-year survivors of childhood and adolescent cancer: the Childhood Cancer Survivor Study. *J Clin Oncol* 2001;19:3163–72

12. Moller TR, Garwicz S, Barlow L, et al. Decreasing late mortality among five-year survivors of cancer in childhood and adolescence: a population-based study in the Nordic countries. *J Clin Oncol* 2001;19:3173–81

13. Hudson MM, Poquette CA, Lee J, et al. Increased mortality after successful treatment for Hodgkin's disease. *J Clin Oncol* 1998;16:3592–600

14. Neglia JP, Friedman DL, Yasui Y, et al. Second malignant neoplasms in five year survivors of childhood cancer: a report from the Childhood Cancer Survivor Study (CCSS). *J Natl Cancer Inst* 2001;93:618–29

15. Linch DC, Gosden RG, Tulandi T, et al. Hodgkin's lymphoma: choice of therapy and late complications. *Hematology* 2000:205–21

16. Thomson A, Critchley HO, Kelnar CJ, Wallace WHB. Late reproductive sequelae following treatment of childhood cancer and options for fertility preservation. *Baillieres Best Pract Res Clin Endocrinol Metab* 2002;16:311–34

17. Schrader M, Muller M, Sofikitis N, et al. 'Oncotese': testicular sperm extraction in azoospermic cancer patients before chemotherapy – new guidelines? *Urology* 2003;61:421–5

18. Damani MN, Masters V, Meng MV, et al. Postchemotherapy ejaculatory azoospermia: fatherhood with sperm from testis tissue with intracytoplasmic sperm injection. *J Clin Oncol* 2002;19:930–6

19. Horne G, Atkinson A, Brison DR, et al. Achieving pregnancy against the odds: successful implantation of frozen–thawed embryos generated by ICSI using spermatozoa banked prior to chemo/radiotherapy for Hodgkin's disease and acute leukaemia. *Hum Reprod* 2001;16:107–9

20. Oktay K, Newton H, Aubard Y, et al. Cryopreservation of immature human oocytes and ovarian tissue: an emerging technology? *Fertil Steril* 1998;69:1–7

21. Opsahl MS, Fugger EF, Sherins RJ, Schulman JD. Preservation of reproductive function before therapy for cancer: new options involving sperm and ovary cryopreservation. *Cancer J Sci Am* 1997;3:189–91

22. Atkinson HG, Apperley JF, Dawson K, et al. Successful pregnancy after embryo cryopreservation after BMT for CML. *Lancet* 1994;344:199

23. Fabbri R, Venturoli S, D'Errico A, et al. Ovarian tissue banking and fertility preservation in

cancer patients: histological and immuno-histochemical evaluation. *Gynecol Oncol* 2003; 89:259–66

24. Green DM, Peabody EM, Nan B, *et al.* Pregnancy outcome after treatment for Wilms tumor: a report from the National Wilms Tumor Study Group. *J Clin Oncol* 2002;20:2506–13

25. Hershlag A, Schuster MW. Return of fertility after autologous stem cell transplantation. *Fertil Steril* 2002;77:419–21

26. Roopnarinesingh R, Keane D, Harrison R. Detecting mood disorders in men diagnosed with cancer who seek semen cryopreservation; a chance to improve service. *Ir Med J* 2003; 96:106–7

27. Kuczyk M, Machtens S, Bokeymeyer C, *et al.* Sexual function and fertility after treatment of testicular cancer. *Curr Opin Urol* 2000;10:473–7

28. Schover LR, Rybicki LA, Martin BA, *et al.* Having children after cancer: a pilot survey of survivors' attitudes and experiences. *Cancer* 1999;86:697–709

29. Schover LR, Brey K, Lichtin A, *et al.* Knowledge and experience regarding cancer, infertility, and sperm banking in younger male survivors. *J Clin Oncol* 2002;20:1880–9

30. Glaser A, Wilkey O, Greenberg M. Sperm and ova conservation: existing standards of practice in North America. *Med Pediatr Oncol* 2000;35:114–18

31. Dow KH. Having children after breast cancer. *Cancer Pract* 1994;2:407–13

32. Dow KH, Harris JR, Roy C. Pregnancy after breast-conserving surgery and radiation therapy for breast cancer [monograph]. *J Natl Cancer Inst* 1994;16:131–7

33. Cobleigh M, Bines J, Harris D, *et al.* Amenorrhea following adjuvant chemotherapy for breast cancer. *Proc Annu Meet Am Soc Clin Oncol Abstr* 1995;14:156

34. Lower E, Blau R, Gazder P, Tummala R. The risk of premature menopause induced by chemotherapy for early breast cancer. *J Womens Health Gend Based Med* 1999;8:949–54

35. Moore H. Fertility and the impact of systemic therapy on hormonal status following treatment for breast cancer. *Curr Oncol Rep* 2000;2:587–93

36. Goodwin PJ, Ennis M, Pritchard KI, *et al.* Risk of menopause during the first year after breast cancer diagnosis. *J Clin Oncol* 1999;17:2365–70

37. Ibrahim NK, Macneil S, Headley JA, *et al.* Effect of paclitaxel (P)-based chemotherapy on the ovarian failure (OF) of breast cancer patients (pts): a retrospective study. *Proc Annu Meeting Am Soc Clin Oncol Abstr* 2003

38. Stone ERS, Novielli A, *et al.* Rate of chemotherapy related amenorrhea (CRA) associated with adjuvant adriamycin and cytoxan (AC) and adriamycin and cytoxan followed by Taxol (AC + T) in early stage breast cancer. Presented at the *San Antonio Breast Cancer Conference*, December, 2000;abstr. 224

39. Dow KH, Ferrel BR, Haberman MR, Eaton L. The meaning of quality of life in cancer survivorship. *Oncol Nurs Forum* 1999;26:519–28

40. Sutton R, Buzdar A, Hortobagyi G. Pregnancy and offspring after adjuvant chemotherapy in breast cancer patients. *Cancer* 1990;65:847–50

41. Kroman N, Jensen M, Melbye M, *et al.* Should women be advised against pregnancy after breast cancer treatment? *Lancet* 1997;350: 319–22

42. Sankila R, Heinavaara S, Hakulinen T. Survival of breast cancer patients after subsequent term pregnancy: 'healthy mother effect'. *Am J Obstet Gynecol* 1994;170:818–23

43. Von Schoultz E, Johansson J, Wilking N, Rutqvist LE. Influence of prior and subsequent pregnancy on breast cancer prognosis. *J Clin Oncol* 1995;13:430–4

44. Velentgas P, Daling JR, Malone KE, *et al.* Pregnancy after breast carcinoma: outcomes and influence on mortality. *Cancer* 1999;85: 2424–32

45. Gelber S, Coates AS, Goldhirsch A, *et al.* Effect of pregnancy on overall survival after the diagnosis of early-stage breast cancer. *J Clin Oncol* 2001;19:1671–5

46. Oktay K, Buyuk E, Davis O, *et al.* Fertility preservation in breast cancer patients: IVF and embryo cryopreservation after ovarian stimulation with tamoxifen. *Hum Reprod* 2003;18: 90–5

47. Fox KR, Scialla J, Moore H. Preventing chemotherapy-related amenorrhea using leuprolide during adjuvant chemotherapy for early-stage breast cancer. *Proc Annu Meeting Am Soc Clin Oncol Abstr* 2003

48. Renaud MC, Plante M, Roy M. Combined laparoscopic and vaginal radical surgery in cervical cancer. *Gynecol Oncol* 2000;79:59–63

49. Schlaerth JB, Spirtos NM, Schlaerth AC. Radical trachelectomy and pelvic lymphadenectomy with uterine preservation in the treatment of cervical cancer. *Am J Obstet Gynecol* 2003; 188:29–34

50. Ayhan A, Celik H, Taskiran C, *et al.* Oncologic and reproductive outcome after fertility-saving surgery in ovarian cancer. *Eur J Gynaecol Oncol* 2003;24:223–32

Legal issues in fertility preservation 19

S. L. Crockin

INTRODUCTION

Fertility preservation is a complicated matter, with distinct legal issues depending on whose fertility is at stake and what techniques are available for preserving it. The various legal issues confronting adults and children, male and female, singles and couples who face the need to preserve their fertility are addressed in this chapter. This chapter also looks at the potential responsibilities and liability of providers in the context of preserving the fertility of their patients and potential offspring, and suggests ways in which future medical advances may impact on currently identified legal issues.

ADULT MALES

Preserving male fertility through sperm collection and freezing is the most commonly recognized and likely most frequently performed of all fertility preservation measures. Legal issues raised by this practice center around informed consent for obtaining and using collected semen and, most critically, the future circumstances under which the sperm may be used and the legal status of any child or children resulting from such use. Informed consent issues may also arise over posthumous extraction. It is assumed that the reader is acquainted with the standard elements of informed consent: disclosure, comprehension, voluntariness, competence and consent[1]. Legal liability may also arise over the handling of frozen sperm samples, including mislabeling, misuse or failure to safely maintain samples in a usable, frozen state. Finally, legal issues may be raised if physicians or other medical professionals do not discuss collection and banking as an option prior to offering or administering medical treatment which may impair their patients' fertility.

Informed consent

Since frozen sperm has an indefinite 'shelf-life' and published reports indicate children have been born from sperm frozen for well over a decade, legal issues surrounding frozen sperm usage involve multiple future scenarios and therefore require carefully drawn informed consent documents.

As an initial matter, medical professionals will want to recognize those medical conditions and treatments that may impair fertility and inform their patients accordingly. Failure to explain the risks of both compromised fertility and the measures available to preserve fertility prior to treatment might give rise to a legal claim for negligence or malpractice, depending on the facts and circumstances. The author is unaware of any reported cases of this nature to date. A published report from a 2002 study found that of 201 male cancer patients between the ages of 14 and 40 diagnosed with cancer within the previous 2 years, 60% were warned about infertility and 51% offered an opportunity to bank their sperm[2].

Appropriate informed consent documents will obviously cover the adult male patient's own future volitional use of his sperm. Less commonly included, but highly recommended, is language which explicitly addresses any approved use following either the patient's incapacity or death, as well as the intended relationship of the patient to any resulting child. Both present potential legal issues that professionals and patients need to be aware of and provide for.

Adult male patients will want to consider the possibility that their present or future partner, or even another family member, may wish to have a child with their sperm at a point in time when they are incapable of giving contemporaneous informed consent to the use of the sperm due to incapacity or death. If a specific medical condition has been diagnosed, such as cancer or amyotrophic lateral sclerosis, informed consents may be tailored to explicitly identify such condition and the adult male's consent for future usage. The more specific and comprehensive the consent document, the more likely that conflicts will be avoided, and partners, physicians, sperm banks or courts can avoid the need to interpret ambiguities. In the alternative, addenda to standard informed consent documents can provide needed specificity and should be considered. Language can be drafted either on behalf of the medical provider or patients can be referred out to knowledgeable legal counsel to draft proposed language. Care should be taken to include language stating that any explicit addenda are intended to supplement and, as necessary, override a more general consent form.

Posthumous reproduction

Posthumous reproduction raises additional legal complexities and the legal status of any resulting child must be resolved under state law, which varies from state to state. A recent spate of cases have presented courts with issues involving children whose biological fathers died before their conception through either artificial insemination or *in vitro* fertilization (IVF). Most of these cases have arisen in the context of qualifying a child for Social Security survivor benefits. Although a federal entitlement, qualification for survivor benefits turns on whether or not the individual seeking that entitlement is considered under the relevant state's law to be the legal child of the deceased for purposes of intestate (without a will) inheritance[3]. Courts, therefore, must interpret and apply state laws

defining the parent–child relationship to answer that question. Most of such laws were drafted prior to, and without any thought of, the possibilities of posthumous reproduction.

Over the past decade, there have been at least six cases reported in the USA involving posthumous parenting. Anecdotally, there appear to be many more. Two of the reported cases have involved the issue of whether or not to release the sperm of a deceased man to attempt a pregnancy. Four of the reported decisions by state courts or administrative bodies have decided cases involving posthumous parenting in the context of survivor benefits for born children.

The two known cases involving whether to release sperm of a deceased man to his former fiancée or girlfriend for her to attempt a pregnancy came to opposite conclusions. A California court, in an unpublished decision, awarded some banked sperm to a deceased's fiancée, ruling that his written intention was clear and that posthumous conception was not against the public policy of that state[4]. In the second case, a Louisiana court affirmed a preliminary injunction against the use of sperm where evidence was conflicting as to the decendent's intentions for posthumous use: his extended family (including his adult son, sister and mother) all objected, he and his female partner had not been actively undergoing inseminations at the time of his death, and the written 'Act of Donation' she attempted to rely upon was drawn up by her law partner rather than a disinterested professional[5].

Decisions in Louisiana, New Jersey, Arizona and Massachusetts have come down regarding the legal parentage of posthumous born children. In Massachusetts, New Jersey and Louisiana, the children were found to be the legal children of the deceased; in Arizona the court rejected parenthood. Each court's decision was based on its interpretations of its own, controlling state law.

Judith Hart, born in 1991, is believed to be the first child publicly identified as being conceived from the sperm of a deceased man. She was conceived 3 months after her father died from esophageal cancer, using sperm he had banked for that purpose. His two adult children from a prior marriage did not contest Judith's claim to be legally recognized as one of his children. Her mother was initially denied Social Security survivor benefits on her behalf but, after a 4-year battle on both administrative and judicial levels, successfully obtained an administrative reversal of that denial. Louisiana law recognized a child as one born during his or her father's lifetime or within several months after, and therefore presumably conceived prior to, his death. During the protracted administrative dealings, the Harts also brought a civil lawsuit in federal district court, alleging discrimination based on the circumstances of the child's birth[6], which was dismissed by agreement after the Social Security Administration reversed its position. In doing so, it issued a statement acknowledging that the case, "raises significant policy issues that were not contemplated when the ... Act was passed many years ago ... recent advances in modern medical practice, particularly in the field of reproductive medicine, necessitate a careful review of current laws and regulations to ensure that they are equitable in awarding Social Security payments in cases such as this."

Following the *Hart* case, a lower state court in New Jersey in 2000 and the highest state court in Massachusetts in 2002 recognized posthumously conceived children to be legal heirs under their state's laws. In contrast, a federal district court in Arizona in 2002 denied benefits to children in similar circumstances. A brief analysis of those cases follows.

The New Jersey case, *In re the Estate of William Kolacy*[7], arose after a federal administrative law judge denied survivor benefits to twins born 18 months after their biological father's death and conceived via IVF. The lower court ruling in New Jersey essentially reversed the federal court's refusal to recognize the paternity of the twins, and was brought in the hope that establishing paternity under state law would qualify the children for federal benefits. The government argued unsuccessfully that the state court lacked jurisdiction in what it deemed was a federal Social Security matter. The court ruled

instead that, "once a child has come into existence ... a fundamental policy of the law should be to enhance and enlarge the rights of each human being to the maximum extent possible, consistent with the duty not to intrude unfairly upon the interests of other persons". The court went on to state its philosophical perspective[8]: "... [t]he ability to cause children to come into existence long after the death of a parent is a recently acquired ability for human society. There are probably wise and wonderful ways in which that ability can be used. There are also undoubtedly ... ethical problems, social policy problems and legal problems ... [o]ne would hope that a prospective parent thinking about causing a child to come into existence after the death of a genetic and biological parent would think very carefully about the potential consequences ... [t]he law should certainly be cautious about encouraging parents to move precipitously in this area."

The Massachusetts Supreme Judicial Court became the first highest appellate state court to rule on this issue in *Woodward v. Commissioner of Social Security*[9]. In that case, a federal district court certified the legal question of inheritance rights to the state court, which found the law permitted a finding of paternity for twins conceived by the decedent's widow after his death. The children were born 2 years after their father's death from cancer. As the first high state court decision on this issue, that court's ruling and reasoning may provide guidance to assisted reproduction programs looking to ensure that their consent forms concerning permissible uses of gametes and embryos adequately protect their patients and their programs.

The court identified three critical requirements for inheritance eligibility under Massachusetts law:

(1) Proof that the children are in fact the genetic children of the deceased;

(2) Proof that he affirmatively consented to posthumous reproduction;

(3) Proof that he affirmatively consented to support any resulting children.

The court emphasized the 'double consent' requirement was necessary because, while a man facing medical treatment that may leave him sterile may want to preserve the possibility of having children later in life, the mere act of storing sperm does not necessarily indicate an intention to father children after death. Even with such evidence, there may also be issues of timeliness or competing interests of other heirs (including children already in being) that preclude inheritance. The court made it clear that widows or other representatives of such children seeking inheritance rights will need to go to court to establish paternity and consent and must formally notify 'every other interested party', including other potential heirs.

Illustrating the differences amongst various state laws, another set of twins born 10 months after their biological father's death were denied benefits under Arizona law in the case of *Gillett-Netting v. Commissioner of Social Security*[10].

That case involved a married couple who had begun fertility treatment prior to the husband's cancer diagnosis. Before beginning chemotherapy treatments, the husband banked sperm so the couple could continue their fertility treatments. After the husband's death, his widow ultimately conceived twins using the sperm banked for IVF after multiple, unsuccessful artificial insemination attempts. According to both his widow and her doctor, although not put in writing, Netting knew and agreed that his sperm could be used to impregnate his wife after his death.

Under Arizona's intestate succession provisions, only a child who survives the deceased parent or was in gestation at the time of death may inherit. Because the twins had not yet been conceived at the time of death, the Social Security Administration and federal court found they were not entitled to inherit under state law and thus to benefit under the Act. The court also rejected the argument, similar to that raised but not decided in the *Hart* case, that the children's constitutional, equal protection rights had been violated.

The court explicitly rejected the claim that the laws created an impermissible and 'impenetrable barrier' to benefits based on the circumstances of the twins' births. The court stated the *circumstances* of the children's birth was IVF, not posthumous conception; characterized the latter as only an issue of timing; and further found that the children never lost the support of a parent, but had never had nor been entitled to that support nor should they have anticipated receiving it.

The Arizona court acknowledged that its decision was at odds with both *Woodward* and *Kolacy*. In doing so, the court explained that, in contrast to Arizona's relatively recently enacted laws, the Massachusetts' intestacy laws did not explicitly limit succession to children 'in gestation' and were written a century before assisted reproductive technologies were available. The court also distinguished *Kolacy* as having interpreted New Jersey law.

In Britain, one widow has successfully pursued a lengthy court battle, first to get access to her deceased husband's stored sperm and then to have him legally recognized as the father of the two children she separately conceived after his death[11]. Diane Blood's efforts have ultimately resulted in a London High Court judge ruling that the 1998 European Convention on Human Rights overrides inconsistent language in the 1990 version of British Human Fertilisation and Embryology Act, the latter of which states that a man is not the father of a child created posthumously with his sperm, as well as a change in the law. In 2003, Parliament passed the Human Fertilisation and Embryology (Deceased Fathers) Act. The Act now requires that any man wishing to be recorded as the father of a child resulting from fertility treatment after his death must have given his written consent. The Human Fertilisation and Embryology Authority (HFEA) issued a sample consent form to fulfill the requirements of the 2003 Act[12].

Posthumous parenthood raises both issues of law and concerns about intentionality. While laws clearly vary from jurisdiction to jurisdiction, courts are also being forced to interpret and in some cases stretch existing laws. Inconsistent results are inevitable. Thus, patients and providers will want to be aware of, and act as consistently as possible with, applicable law in their jurisdiction. Since the law is likely to remain unsettled for some time, it is also advisable to put in writing, as clearly and unambiguously as possible, the intentions of the adult male who is preserving his sperm. Explicitly identifying the individuals who may use the sperm, and the purposes for, circumstances under which, and time frames within which they may do so, is highly advisable. This should be done in consent forms with the sperm bank and physician. An additional written document consistent with the consent forms, but created for and executed between the adult male and intended recipient(s) of the sperm, is also advisable. Legal counsel experienced in applicable inheritance laws can provide valuable advice and language for such documentation, and patients should be encouraged to consult with independent legal counsel for that purpose. Such anticipatory steps may avoid the need to seek court orders by surviving widows, fiancées and parents, all of which have been pursued with varying outcomes.

Whether an adult male intended to father a child after his death, as opposed to after his hoped-for survival following treatment, is a significant distinction, and one that has troubled courts and ethicists alike. Even with clearly stated intentions, legal recognition of paternity will depend on both applicable state laws and public policy.

Model legislation has been proposed by various entities to attempt to clarify the parent–child relationship of a posthumously conceived child. As one example, the proposed language within the 2002 Uniform Parentage Act, at Section 707[13], which is available to individual states to adopt, states: "[i]f a spouse dies before placement of eggs, sperm or embryos, the deceased spouse is not a parent of the resulting child unless the deceased spouse consented in a record that if assisted reproduction were to occur after death, the deceased spouse would be a parent of the child." This provision makes clear that consent to posthumous reproduction and posthumous intended parentage must be in writing and explicit. It does not, however, address multiple other significant concerns, including single parents, indefinite or extended time periods, or potential competing claims by other heirs.

Until and unless uniform or model legislation is widely adopted by a majority of states, courts will be need to continue interpreting the varying inheritance laws of individual states and inconsistent rulings are likely to continue in this area. Even with uniform legislation, uncertainties are likely to arise and need to be resolved.

ADULT WOMEN

Female patients seeking to preserve their fertility face additional and unique challenges. Until medical advances reliably enable them to preserve their fertility independent of a male partner, they also face increased vulnerability from a legal perspective – whether through procedures to protect their reproductive organs during treatment, or through removing and freezing either their eggs or ovarian tissue as male patients can now do with sperm.

From an informed consent perspective, female patients need to be fully informed both of the available procedures and choices, and the respective risks associated with them. The experimental nature of egg and ovarian tissue freezing, and therefore the largely unknown likelihood of success, must be clearly explained, and criticism has been voiced about physicians' failure to adequately do so[14]. Equally important, the legal unknowns should be acknowledged with respect to issues such as future access to and use of this genetic material, and the vulnerabilities surrounding the genetic material and any resulting embryos or children.

Unfortunately, at present, the procedures most likely to be successful medically are also the choices that create the most legal vulnerability for women: creating and freezing embryos. Women without a current partner will need to identify a sperm source, whether known or anonymous. Women with partners will need to create embryos that are thereafter equally available to, and under control by, that male partner. Future changes of circumstances, such as divorce for married women, may impact the availability of those embryos. Uncertainties in the law may affect the degree to which any informed consent or private agreement is enforceable. Finally, use of donor eggs to create embryos with a current partner may raise additional uncertainties. These potential scenarios are discussed within this section.

Cases involving disputes over control and disposition of frozen embryos in the context of a divorcing couple suggest an important trend for female patients. While a number of those cases have raised the issue of aging and declining fertility for the female partner, none within the USA are reported to have involved patients with other diseases resulting in an inability to create additional eggs. These cases, which have been reviewed in extensive detail in multiple contexts by this author and others[15,16], will be summarized here only for their salient points.

Although courts are not wholly consistent, they appear to be increasingly willing to review IVF program consent forms and to analyze the enforceability or lack of enforceability of certain provisions for embryo disposition based on the intended use. Thus, a couple's prior recorded agreement to dispose of the embryos in a way that does not implicate childbearing has been enforced[17]. On the other hand, prior choices to allow one spouse to use the embryos for procreation over a current objection by the other have been increasingly rejected. Thus, in cases in Massachusetts, New Jersey and Washington state, courts have been unwilling to enforce a prior agreement to allow:

(1) A wife to use embryos following the couple's 'separation' (*A.Z. v. B.Z.*)[18];

(2) A husband to donate the embryos to another couple (*J.B. v. M.B.*)[19];

(3) A wife to use embryos created with donor eggs to be implanted in the same gestational carrier who had carried the couple's first child (*Litowitz v. Litowitz*)[20].

This trend rests on the stated principle that such usage amounts to 'forced procreation', which, as the Massachusetts court put it in its *A.Z.* decision, "is not amenable to judicial enforcement". Typically, courts are extremely reluctant to interfere with procreative or non-procreative decisions and the constitutional rights underlying them. Thus, forced sterilization, contraception restrictions and abortion laws have all been struck down as violative of individual constitutional rights[21–23]. An additional consideration is that under most states' laws, public policy considerations preclude a parent from waiving parental status and obligations such as child support. Thus, any agreement between spouses enabling one to use frozen embryos and the other to be relieved of parental rights and obligations is likely unenforceable as against public policy in most jurisdictions.

On the other hand, a female patient who has attempted to preserve her fertility in the most effective way currently available to her, i.e. through the creation and freezing of embryos, may have compelling arguments to maintaining control over them. Again, clear, explicit written documentation, drafted in consultation with experienced legal counsel, is advisable. In addition to consent forms, a written agreement between the female patient and her male partner, addressing as clearly as possible their joint intentions under various future scenarios, including disagreement, should provide useful even if not enforceable.

Although British law requires the mutual consent of both embryo creators to use their embryos, two recent developments in Britain tested that standard. Two British women, who claimed their cancer or other medical treatments rendered them unable to create more embryos, lost their High Court battles against their ex-partners' decisions to destroy embryos each couple had created prior to the women's cancer treatments. Notwithstanding the HFEA standards, the women had asked the court to adopt a balancing test between the various interests, arguing the decisive factor should be that this was their last chance to have a biological child. The women argued against the fairness of their former partners' 'veto' power, analogized the situation to a pregnancy where their partners would have no say at all, and argued that because of their infertility they were being discriminated against in violation of human rights legislation. One of the women was reportedly planning an appeal[24]. Also in England, the HFEA announced a change in its code of practice, following an incident where embryos created by a married couple using donor eggs were destroyed at the request of the ex-husband alone[25].

Use of donor eggs to create a family may raise additional and unsettled issues of parenthood by intention. Assuming the current trend is to require both partners to re-consent before either can use embryos they created at an earlier time, regardless of any prior agreement, this additional factor should be of little significance. With respect to donation or discard of embryos, or custody of children, however, there have been some reported instances where the fact of donor gametes has been argued or deemed relevant. Thus, in at least two cases in the USA, intended, genetic fathers have attempted to raise the issue of donor eggs as a factor in 'tipping the scales' toward themselves in determining the custody of children created with their former spouse who could not contribute genetic material. In each of those cases, the courts rejected the fathers' claims[26,27]. In a recent California case, the husband but not the wife involved in an embryo mix-up case involving a donor egg was granted legal paternity. His wife was found to have no standing whatsoever to the resulting child born to a single woman whom the court deems the leagal mother, despite the fact that the child was the genetic sibling of the couple's child and they had intended to use the remaining embryos for another child[28]. These incidences suggest there may be additional uncertainty and vulnerability for women who attempt to preserve their ability to parent, if not their fertility, through donor eggs and frozen embryos.

Finally, posthumous motherhood remains at least a technical possibility. Unlike posthumous

fatherhood, a second woman is obviously needed to carry and birth the child. While most state laws presume a woman who carries and births a child is the mother, recent developments in gestational surrogacy or gestational carrier arrangements, where a woman carries a genetically unrelated child for a couple or single intended parent, have successfully challenged that assumption. In many states legal mechanisms now exist to place the intended, genetic mother on the child's birth certificate rather than the gestational carrier. As but a few examples, Virginia, Illinois and Connecticut have statutory provisions[29–31]; Massachusetts, Ohio and California have case law supporting such outcomes[32–34]; and some state courts have recognized maternity for the intended mother who could provide neither the egg nor the uterus, and is essentially a mother through intentionality alone (multiple unreported trial level cases by the author and others). Whether or not a deceased woman could, under some circumstances, be legally recognized as the mother of a child born from her eggs or from embryos frozen prior to her death remains to be seen. Certainly, such scenarios would raise not only serious legal but also significant ethical and informed consent issues for patients and any resulting child or children.

MINORS AS PATIENTS

Minors as patients raise unique informed consent issues in any medical context. Elements of informed consent include not only providing a patient with adequate information as to the risks and benefits of, and alternatives to, any proposed treatment, but also relate to the ability of the patient to comprehend and make informed choices. Depending on the age and mental capacity of a minor, they may or may not be able to give informed consent. A 'mature minor' is capable of giving consent; a younger child is not. When incapable of giving informed consent for themselves, child patients – like other patients considered incompetent – may have adults do so on their behalf under a legal concept of 'substituted judgment', interpretations of which vary from state to state. In theory, such judgment is intended to mean that the designated adult makes the decision he or she feels the patient, if competent, would make. When that standard is impossible to meet, as is typically the case with a very young child, the adult is charged with making the decision he or she feels is in the minor patient's 'best interest'.

Preserving a child's fertility can be both a particularly sensitive issue and one not always recognized by providers or guardians when a child is facing a serious illness. Reports of scientific advances in the field of fertility preservation for children treated with cancer suggest that while the majority can expect to be cured and remain fertile, a significant minority remain at risk for subfertility. One reported estimate is that childhood cancer survivors represent one in 900 adults aged 15 to 44 years[35]. Another reports that 15% of child cancer survivors will have compromised reproductive function from their treatment[36]. Given the increasing survival rates for many childhood cancers and other serious illnesses for which treatment may affect future fertility, providers should be cognizant of available options for fertility preservation as well as the degree to which such options are experimental or of proven efficacy.

Treatment options range from sperm retrieval to invasive procedures in order to harvest gonadal tissue[37]. The latter procedures have been described as experimental, with some medical professionals calling for "appropriate regulation and ethical scrutiny in order to prevent the exploitation of vulnerable individuals by commercially driven technology"[38]. Providers will want to proceed cautiously in terms of providing sufficient information as to available treatments and appropriate cautions as to the level of experimentation of some of those treatments, particularly in light of the increased vulnerability of child patients.

PROVIDER LIABILITY

As discussed above, provider liability may arise from possible breaches of the informed consent doctrine. Not disclosing or not offering an available treatment that has the potential of improving a patient's chances of preserving his or her fertility, or not disclosing the experimental or unproven nature of some of such treatments, may each create liability.

In addition, providers may find themselves liable for other possible breaches of duty to their patients or to affected, surviving or even potentially future family members. Each of those potential sources of liability is discussed briefly.

First, failure to maintain cryopreserved gametes or embryos may be grounds for negligence actions. Power failures, mistaken transfers or destruction, and lost or misappropriated embryos or gametes all take on additional significance and legal vulnerability if the patients who created and stored the genetic material cannot replace it. Thus, although the standards for liability will be the same as in a suit brought by any patient, the measures of damages can be expected to be much greater for patients with compromised future fertility or deceased patients. One example reported very recently involved a faulty freezer storage tank resulting in lost sperm samples of 28 cancer patients in England[39], who have now filed a lawsuit against the hospital where the samples were stored[40].

Liability may also arise in the context of surviving relatives attempting to access or block access to cryopreserved gametes or embryos. Comprehensive informed consent documents which specifically address future uses or restrictions are recommended in an effort to minimize such litigation. Medical professionals should also not be expected to know or convey the status of the law in what are widely acknowledged to be unsettled areas of the law. Consent forms should be carefully drafted not to overstate, or indeed in many cases to state, the applicable law. Just as lawyers do not perform surgery, medical professionals will not want to advise patients as to the legal status of their fertility preservation or future family building efforts. Consent documents which acknowledge the 'unsettled state of the law', and which recommend seeking independent, experienced legal counsel, are both appropriate and protective of medical providers and patients alike. Addenda or supplemental consent forms should be considered in many circumstances.

Finally, there remains the possibility of liability to a child born following treatments to preserve the fertility of their genetic parent(s). Informed consent or other defenses to actions brought by an adult patient do not preclude lawsuits brought by a resulting child who could not have been a party to any agreement, waiver or consent. Most states have substantially developed law on the subject of 'wrongful birth' and 'wrongful life', with the majority rejecting claims for the latter essentially on the theory that any life has value over no life and therefore damages cannot be calculated. On the other hand, suits for 'wrongful birth' have been recognized in some jurisdictions, with liability assessed for the cost of rearing an affected child[41,42]. Thus, if efforts to preserve fertility result in children with genetic or other impairments, medical professionals involved in those efforts may, depending on applicable state law, find themselves vulnerable to subsequent claims by or on behalf of such children.

CONCLUSION

The legal issues surrounding fertility preservation include an increased awareness of, and a dialogue about, both the availability of treatments for that purpose and the degree to which various treatments are experimental or proven. Medical professionals will want to be informed about appropriate and available treatment options, risks and benefits, and will want to inform their adult and child patients accordingly. Carefully drafted consent documents, including supplemental consents, or separate legal agreements, drawn up in consultation with experienced legal counsel, may be determinative in patients' wishes being carried out. Both patients and their physicians may benefit from their having separate, independent legal counsel advise them on novel issues, such as the future use of cryopreserved gametes or embryos and the legal status of any resulting child.

This discussion has focused on a general understanding of the legal issues involved in fertility preservation. With rapid medical advances and state law variations, definitive guidelines are not possible. It is hoped that this discussion will increase awareness of the relevant legal issues, aid medical professionals in their efforts to provide comprehensive care to their patients, and help protect the families their patients hope to create.

References

1. Meisel A, Loren HR. Towards an informed discussion of informed consent: a review and critique of the empirical studies. *Arizona Law Rev* 1983;25:265–346
2. Schover LR, Brey K, Lichtin A, *et al.* Knowledge and experience regarding cancer, infertility, and sperm banking in younger male survivors. *J Clin Oncol* 2002;20:1880–9
3. *Woodward v. Commissioner of Social Security*, 435 Mass. 536, 760 N.E. 2d 257 (2002)
4. *Hecht v. LA City Supreme Court*, 50 Cal. App. 4th 1289 (1996); review denied, Cal.R.Ct. 976(d), 977 op. withdrawn by order of court. 1997 Cal. LEXIS 131 (1997)
5. *Hall, executrix v. Fertility Institute of New Orleans*, 647 So.2d 1348, 1994 La.App.LEXIS 3294 (1994)
6. *Hart v. Charter*, No. 94-3944 (E.D. La. dismissed March 18, 1996)
7. *In re Estate of William Kolacy*, 332 NJ Super. 593, 753 A.2d 1257 (2000)
8. *In re Estate of William Kolacy*, 332 NJ Super. 593, 605, 753 A.2d 1257 (2000)
9. *Woodward v. Commissioner of Social Security*, 435 Mass. 536, 760 N.E. 2d 257 (2002)
10. *Gillett-Netting v. Commissioner of Social Security*, 231 F.Supp. 2d 961 (2002)
11. News PA. Diane Blood wins paternity rights for children. *The Times Online* February 28, 2003
12. Human Fertilisation and Embryology (Deceased Fathers) Act (2003) Chapter 24; www.hfea.gov.uk
13. Uniform Parentage Act Sect. 707 (2002)
14. Weiss R. Fertility innovation or exploitation? *Washington Post* 1998
15. Crockin SL, Noe PH, Kraus TZ. Embryo law. In Crockin SL, ed. *Adoption and Reproductive*

Technology Law in Massachusetts. Boston: MCLE, 2000:474–81

16. Elster N. ARTistic license: should assisted reproductive technologies be regulated? In Dejonge C, Barratt C, eds. *ART: Today and Beyond.* Cambridge University Press, 2002: 366–75

17. *Kass v. Kass,* 696 N.E.2d 174 (NY 1998)

18. *A.Z. v. B.Z.,* 431 Mass. 150 (2000)

19. *J.B. v. M.B.,* 170 N.J. 9; 783 A.2d 707 (2001)

20. *In re Marriage of Litowitz,* 48 P. 3d 261 (Wash. 2002)

21. *Skinner v. Oklahoma,* 316 U.S. 535 (1942)

22. *Eisenstadt v. Baird,* 405 U.S. 438 (1972)

23. *Roe v. Wade,* 410 U.S. 113 (1973)

24. Embryo battle goes to court. *BBC News Online* updated June 30, 2003; cited October 24, 2003. Available from: http://news.bbc.co.uk/1/hi/health/3026102.stm

25. Horsey K. HFEA code to prevent embryo destruction without consent. *BioNews* May 19, 2003; cited February 6, 2004. Available from: http://www.bionews.org.uk/new.lasso?storyid=1619

26. *MacDonald v. MacDonald,* 608 N.Y. S. 2d 477 (App. Div. 1994)

27. *Ezzone v. Ezzone,* No. 96-DR-000359 (Ohio Lake County Ct. C.P. 1996)

28. *Robert B. v. Susan B.,* 109 Cal. App 4th 1109 (2003); review denied, 2003 Cal. LEXIS 6671 (2003)

29. VA. Code Ann. Sect. 20–159 to 165 (1999)

30. 1999 Ill. P.A. 91–138

31. 2001 Conn. Acts 01–163 (Reg Sess.)

32. *Culliton v. Beth Israel Deaconess Medical Center,* 435 Mass. 285 (2001)

33. *Belsito v. Clark,* 644 N.E.2d 760 (1994)

34. *Johnson v. Calvert,* 851 P.2d 776 (1993)

35. Bleyer WA. The impact of childhood cancer on the US and the world. *CA Cancer J Clin* 1990;40:355–67

36. Multidisciplinary Working Group. *A Strategy for Fertility Services for Survivors of Childhood Cancer.* British Fertility Society, 2002:1–39. Available from: http://www.britishfertilitysociety.org. uk/practicepolicy/documents/fccpaper.pdf

37. Grundy R, Gosden RG, Hewitt M, *et al.* Fertility preservation for children treated for cancer (1): scientific advances and research dilemmas. *Arch Dis Child* 2001;84:355–9

38. Grundy R, Larcher V, Gosden RG, *et al.* Fertility preservation for children treated for cancer (2): ethics of consent for gamete storage and experimentation. *Arch Dis Child* 2001;84: 360–2

39. Thompson J. Faulty freezer ruins 28 cancer patients' stored sperm. *The Independent Online* July 20, 2003; cited February 6, 2004. Available from: http://news.independent.co.uk/uk/health/story.jsp?story=425895

40. British cancer patients whose stored sperm was destroyed when storage tank failed sue hospital. *Daily Reproductive Health Reports* August 13, 2003; cited February 6, 2004. Available from: http://www.kaisernetwork.org/daily_reports/rep_index.cfm?DR_ID=19342

41. *Kush v. Lloyd,* 616 So. 2d 415, 1992 Fla. LEXIS 2017 (1992)

42. *Siemieniec v. Lutheran General Hospital,* 117 Ill. 2d 230, 512 N.E. 2d 691 (Ill. 1987)

Ethical issues of fertility preservation

20

G. Bahadur

INTRODUCTION

This chapter examines the ethical and social issues which arise from the increasing importance accorded to considerations of quality of life following effective treatment for patients with severe diseases such as cancers. The issues raised by two of the most significant and sensitive areas of medicine – cancer and fertility – concern life and death, and affect both existing families and generations to come. Rapidly developing medical technologies and techniques have attracted profound legal, societal and ethical interest given the complex array of family-making options and the issues raised by the question of ownership of any *in vitro*-preserved reproductive material – issues concerning the autonomy of individuals, their rights and the nature of informed consent. The chapter argues the need for all personnel involved with cancer patients to be aware of the complex moral and ethical issues. They need to bring together the fields of cancer and fertility to enhance the quality of life and welfare of their patients. They also need to recognize the possible medico-legal implications of failing to enhance patients' ability to preserve their fertility potential.

The chapter discusses the need for information – written, verbal and by means of informed counseling – so that patients can make appropriate decisions. It examines problematic areas in the application of fertility technologies for children, carriers of the human immunodeficiency virus (HIV), non-patients and the deceased. The issue of multiple births is discussed, as well as the fact that none of the *in vitro* fertilization (IVF) or cyro-preservation procedures have ever undergone

clinical trials in humans. This chapter also considers issues of fertility preservation when essential or non-essential surgery is involved. It offers a philosophical definition of ethics and a framework for defining ethical clinical practice, and advocates a utilitarian approach to moral problems, one that attends to the moral consequences of actions. The complex way in which morality, law and ethics interact is examined. Finally, the chapter considers the various rights – of the patient, their partner, the supporting family structure and the offspring – which need to be taken into account by practitioners involved in the preservation of fertility for cancer patients.

DEVELOPMENTS IN FERTILITY PRESERVATION

Gonadal toxicity was first reported in 1948, involving testicular damage by nitrogen mustard[1]. The first report of gonadal toxicity in women was in 1956 and was associated with busulfan treatment of chronic myeloid leukemia[2]. Freezing sperm became a practical proposition only after the discovery of the cryoprotective property of glycerol[3], 55 years ago. The first infants born from frozen semen are now over 50 years old[4]. Since then, significant progress has occurred in embryo cryopreservation[5,6], human oocyte cryopreservation[7,8] and gonadal tissue cryopreservation[9-11]. Perhaps most importantly, all of these developments, along with the field of IVF, have found human application without clinical trials, giving an added urgency to the public's need to be involved in the surrounding social, ethical, moral and legal debate. The future holds even more complex issues for the public, with the specter of reconstructed gamete and cloning technologies[12,13].

These historical landmarks have enabled us to develop techniques to preserve the fertility potential of cancer patients, the emphasis of whose treatment now lies in quality survival. Fertility can be lost irreversibly as a consequence of the treatment regimen or the disease, an issue that is especially important in the case of ever-younger patients diagnosed with cancers[14–17]. Fertility preservation for male and female cancer patients has become an important feature of the management of their disease. While it is easier to understand the application of these untested technologies on patients diagnosed with severe conditions, the utilization of such techniques in the case of non-patient, healthy groups gives rise to a different set of moral and ethical questions. Often these relate to the commercialization of untested technologies, the use of public resources (e.g. the National Health Service in the UK), or the use of invasive surgery in the case of a healthy group of patients. An example of this would be the retrieval and preservation of ovarian tissue as a source of eggs to enable one's career to progress, or even as a source of steroid supplementation in later years to postpone the menopause.

MALE CANCERS AND FERTILITY PRESERVATION

Cytotoxic drugs or radiation therapy are administered in order to control or destroy cancer cells. While the overall aim of the treatment regimen is for maximal anticancer effect, damage to other body cells may occur. Cancer treatment has a considerable association with morbidity in patients, and testicular dysfunction is amongst the most common side-effects of therapy in men. With improved survival rates, quality-of-life concerns[18] and advances in reproductive technologies have led adult cancer patients to be routinely offered sperm cryopreservation[19]. Hormonal

suppression of gonadal function before chemoradiation has been attempted in the hope of protecting against gonadal damage but its efficacy is unproven and it is impractical given the long time lapse before chemotherapy can be administered. There are immediate surgical approaches in which fertility, reproductive and sexual capabilities may be conserved. Nerve-sparing operations during prostate cancer removal may affect patients' erectile function, and often call for a back-up by sperm banking despite the normally older age of the men. This is because some men have a partner of reproductive age and, even without a younger partner, the male psyche needs to be reassured of its potency. For clinics there could be medico-legal problems in not offering a sperm banking facility. Sperm banking may be considered for patients having bladder neck resection where retrograde ejaculation may present problems in later years[20]. It has also been suggested that males with poor semen quality or attending fertility clinics may suffer a higher risk of testicular cancer[21,22].

FEMALE CANCERS AND FERTILITY PRESERVATION

Unlike men, women have a finite number of germ cells at birth which diminishes with age. About 200 000 follicles are present and functioning in the ovary at puberty, which decline with age to a few hundred at the time of menopause. Chemotherapy and radiotherapy increase the rate at which the germ cells diminish, and this brings forward the onset of menopause[23]. Premature menopause is the commonest toxicity experienced among women undergoing both chemotherapy and radiotherapy, and hormone replacement therapy (HRT) should be considered where necessary[23,24].

Preservation of fertility in women with cancer encompasses many more complex issues. First, gametes cannot be obtained readily, and complex therapeutic planning may be required which evolves around the patient's menstrual cycle, with a possible treatment delay of up to a month. The use of ovarian stimulation drugs in relation to estrogen-sensitive cancers should be considered carefully. Ethical, moral and pragmatic consideration should be given to the creation and preservation of embryos from women without partners. New technologies which utilize ovarian tissue cryopreservation or oocyte freezing should be kept in perspective[7,10,25–27]. At present, the likelihood of birth after oocyte freezing is low, and ovarian tissue freezing must be considered experimental as no human pregnancy has yet been achieved.

From epidemiological data there appears to be a link between reproductive cancers and the infertile woman[28]. Compared with nulliparous women without infertility, infertile nulliparous women have a higher risk of ovarian cancer. Endometrial cancer has a strong association with nulliparity and infertility, particularly anovulatory infertility[29]. As more pregnancies are diagnosed in women with malignancy, it has been possible to successfully deliver healthy babies despite a history of disease.

Disturbance in the menstrual cycle and early menopause need to be considered in the case of women undergoing cancer treatment. While normal ovarian function is likely to resume it is difficult to predict which women may suffer premature menopause, although younger women generally fare better. However, women should be counseled about the possibility of HRT. Any woman regaining ovarian function after chemotherapy and radiotherapy should not delay childbearing, given the very real risk of premature ovarian failure. If conception is not contemplated, HRT will have little contraceptive effect and the contraceptive pill should then be taken. Where a woman has been rendered menopausal by cancer therapy, it is unlikely that ovarian function will return.

FERTILITY, REPRODUCTIVE AND SURGICAL PRESERVATION

For women, some cancers directly concern reproductive and childbearing functions, thereby causing severe distress. Treatment of many malignancies with chemotherapy or radiation may damage the ovaries and uterus. When recovering from the treatment, these patients face significant psychological difficulties, physical and mental scarring, disturbances in their menstrual cycle and the onset of menopause. In some cases, such as borderline cancers of the ovary, fertility-sparing surgery may be applied to obviate the need for surrogacy and donor eggs. Embryo preservation is available to women but this needs a stable partner and the procedure is often restricted by time constraints and other factors experienced in infertility treatment, such as poor fertilization rates. The use of ovarian tissue cryopreservation has created excitement, because it may be applicable to children.

The applications of surgery include conservative surgery for borderline tumors of the ovary[30]; laparoscopic ovarian transposition before radiotherapy[31,32]; radical trachelectomy combined with pelvic lymphadenectomy to preserve fertility for early-stage cervical carcinoma patients[33]; and radical vaginal trachelectomy[34]. Pregnancies have been reported in these patients, but equally preterm loss needs to be considered seriously. If the cancers are extended to the endometrium, then conservation of fertility may become difficult. Fertility-sparing surgery is commonplace in women with gestational trophoblastic neoplasia, leading to evacuation of the uterus, and successful deliveries have occurred[35]. Fertility preservation in women with borderline tumors of the ovary and without children should be routinely considered. Equally, the chances of recurrence of disease will be high and the contralateral ovary should be removed after childbearing[36]. The choice of fertility treatment regime in breast cancer patients needs careful consideration in view of the risks associated with high estrogen levels[26,37]. Salvage hemipelvic irradiation for groin metastatases of vulvar cancer has proved to be an effective treatment allowing preservation of hormonal and obstetric function, although partial radiation damage to the uterus may contribute to premature labor[38]. Transposition of the ovaries is common practice in young women undergoing radical hysterectomy or pelvic irradiation for cervical cancer. The aim is to preserve hormonal function and fertility potential. Unfortunately, ovarian transposition preserves ovarian function in only 50% of patients undergoing pelvic radiotherapy after radical hysterectomy[39]. Perhaps the most complex treatment and ethical issues will be faced when cancers are discovered during a pregnancy[40].

What is unique to cancer patients who seek fertility preservation is an assumption about the potential for many decades of survival. Beyond the issue of cancer patients' reproductive capabilities lie several associated factors. The loss of sexual function and performance is intricately linked with their reproductive potential[41,42], and divorce rates are significantly higher in couples affected with cancer. For single individuals, their potential fertility preservation may be a significant positive consideration towards establishing a marriage. All of these factors could shape their general well-being[43,44].

BACKGROUND TO THE ETHICS OF FERTILITY PRESERVATION

Since the days of Hippocrates, it has been incumbent upon individuals entrusted with the medical care of others to adhere to codes of ethical practice affording protection not only to those seeking help, but also to providers of care. Rapid technological advances have revolutionized the way in which society looks at reproductive behavior and relationships. Reproductive technology presents an array of problems and dilemmas for patients, clinicians, practitioners and the public. To help unravel the complexities and to enhance decision-making, we explore how the general principles of ethics can be applied to the issues faced in preserving fertility. Reproductive cryotechnologies in particular allow for the suspension of time in the preservation of sperm, eggs, embryos and gonadal tissue. As a result of freezing and IVF, several reproductive possibilities are created which

may challenge the way we understand family structure. It has created unnatural possibilities such as that of twins being born years apart, significantly higher multiple birth rates, posthumous insemination and after-gender reassignment[45,46]. The issues that arise can be complex with respect to the legal, ethical, psychological and social well-being of patients and society.

The application of reproductive techniques in specific circumstances will undoubtedly elicit public disquiet – such as in the case of posthumous use, surrogacy, unusual family structures, and gamete and gonadal tissue utilization on behalf of adolescents and minors. This necessarily gives rise to a number of moral, ethical and legal dilemmas. It shapes how reproductive technologists and clinicians are perceived in society.

Self-regulation is something society finds increasingly unacceptable given recent advances in cloning technologies and the possibilities of designer sperm and oocyte engineering. This is why increasingly, around the world, governments are modeling practices on the UK's Human Fertilisation and Embryology Authority (HFEA)[47]. There are limitations to the HFEA, however, in so far as its remit is to oversee the field involving treatment of and research on the human embryo and the cryopreservation of sperm, oocyte and embryos. Despite its powers to regulate and inspect, serious embryo misappropriation and mix-ups have been reported in the UK. Several areas are not covered by the HFEA, such as ovarian stimulation, surgery, surrogacy not involving frozen gametes and embryos, and testicular and ovarian tissue which do not contain mature gametes, especially in the case of minors. Despite the plethora of choices available to patients, healthy individuals, clinicians and technologists, over-bureaucratic procedures often mean that clinics may not be able to offer fertility preservation even in desperate cases.

In other countries there are varying degrees of regulation and acceptable practice. For instance, embryo freezing is forbidden or restricted in Austria, Germany, Denmark and

Sweden. For a married woman with cancer this option may be problematic because of the local definition of an embryo. In Germany, it is permitted to freeze a 'pre-embryo' but the meaning of the term can be difficult to define in practice, and it may not entirely serve the patient's best interest when events such as success or abnormalities are to be investigated. In the USA, Canada and Australia, differences in regulation across states and provinces can be observed[48].

In the UK, sperm cryopreservation for personal use is allowed up to the age of 55 years and for 10 years only if over 55 years. Storage of frozen oocytes beyond the normal reproductive age of the woman may raise complex ethical issues. Additionally, whereas upon death of the male partner the widow can use the sperm posthumously, provided the consent is in place, the use of frozen oocytes presents complex issues. This will necessarily involve a surrogate who would become the legal mother irrespective of the partial surrogacy status, and the sperm has to be regarded as donor sperm. Using frozen oocytes is additionally complicated by the fact that the treatment cannot be regarded as 'together with a legal partner'. After the birth of the child it is necessary to seek a parental order and adoption of the genetic offspring. In the HFEA's consideration of the welfare of the child, while the need for a father is clearly stated by statute, the implicit need for a mother appears to be entirely overlooked. These examples provide an idea of the sort of problems facing specialists involved in preserving fertility.

WHAT ARE ETHICS?

The study of ethics is a specialized branch of philosophy. We make moral and ethical decisions without being aware of them. The decisions concern whether we think an action right or wrong, good or bad, fitting or not fitting. These choices reflect our values and priorities. We live in a cosmopolitan society composed of diverse social and religious backgrounds, and in an age of ever-increasing technological advances. For the average person these can be confusing. Sometimes a clash in values, norms and standards occurs, leading to the feeling of being threatened by chaos and ethical breakdown in society. As a society progresses, many ideals of behavior are formalized in laws that support our ethical principles and seek to resolve such dilemmas. These dilemmas may broadly be categorized as:

(1) When we value individualism, independence and individual rights too highly, people's actions taken in their own interest can collide with other people's rights.

(2) When people with different values clash on how to resolve a situation, it can lead to different views as to the appropriate ethical result. Even if such people reach a compromise, they can still feel upset by the result, because they feel their values have been trampled on by someone else.

(3) When our laws are out of line with our ethical principles and ideals, such as notions of decency and fair play, this disparity can trigger everyday dilemmas. Although people may know they are legally free to act in a certain way, they may feel guilty because they feel what they have done is not right.

(4) When profit-making considerations and concerns about appearing successful conflict with principles regarding doing the right, fair or honest thing, this can lead to hard choices. Instead of doing what is ethical, one might choose to do what is more profitable, and then one may deny doing this to continue to see oneself – or appear to others – as honest and honorable.

Historically, one of the main incentives to study ethics has been the hope that the findings might be of help to those faced with difficult moral problems. Ethics are a way of understanding and examining the moral life. Increasingly, in medicine it appears that particular cases, judgments or instances of public disquiet shape the rules and principles which eventually lead to an ethical theory. Within each discipline of medicine, ethics have been developed for the most part in a limited and utilitarian manner, often leading to highly idiosyncratic interpretations.

A FRAMEWORK FOR ETHICAL PRACTICE

It is important to have a framework upon which to base an objective analysis of a problem when the rights or wrongs of a certain action are being considered. Written procedures should be formulated to ensure that fertility preservation for patients is not overlooked. This will involve clinicians, scientists, counselors and administrators adhering to a code of practice, along with a system of external regulators and inspection, such as that provided by the HFEA in the UK. Conscientious objections to specific situations have to be taken into account and individuals be given the right to withdraw from a process. If a cryopreservation technique is involved, then care of that material may continue for many decades in the case of adolescent cancer patients.

Ethical obligations are based on three moral principles that form a general obligation for us all[49,50]:

(1) *Non-maleficence* – this principle states that moral agents ought not to harm others. This is enshrined in the injunction 'non-nocere' with which all physicians are familiar.

(2) *Beneficence* – this affirms the promotion of the welfare of others, usually through the removal or prevention of harm, as befitting the application of fertility preservation techniques and the reduction of multiple births.

(3) *Respect for autonomy* – this principle states that moral agents should not interfere with the actions and choices of other autonomous individuals.

These principles can be complicated in several ways. Fertility preservation has allowed individuals to circumvent fertility loss but in so doing has created vastly unnatural possibilities such as posthumous reproduction, the use of donor sperm, eggs and embryos, the application of genetic testing by preimplantation genetic diagnosis (PGD), and the use of surrogates. To promote the welfare of a prepubertal child with cancer by preserving his gonadal tissue will require actions which are incompatible with a respect for the child's autonomy[14,51]. The newer legal perspectives, such as that offered by the Human Rights Act of 1998 (HR Act)[52], also suggest fresh ways to interpret the Human Fertilisation and Embryology Act of 1990 (HFE Act) and the facilities offered under the National Health Service in the UK.

If such fertility preservation comes to fruition at the expense of strained national resources, then it is done at the cost of the welfare of another. Such conflicts might be considered in the light of two general ethical theories, *deontological* thought and *utilitarianism*. Deontological theories focus on the rights and wrongs of an act itself. They are not concerned with the consequences that an act will have; rather, they are concerned with identifying those features of the act which mark it as morally acceptable or otherwise. Kant stressed that every person must be treated as an end in him- or herself, rather than as a means to an end. In other words, we should not use others but should respect their integrity as individuals. Critics see deontological morality as rigid. An alternative and more flexible approach might be one which is more sensitive to the human feelings involved in any moral dilemma and one which also pays more attention to the consequences which flow from our actions, assuming that the end justifies the means. One such approach was Jeremy Bentham's utilitarianism, otherwise known as *consequentialism*, regarded by many as underpinning ethical medicine today. The utilitarian measure of good is, therefore, the maximization of happiness.

A landmark UK case involved Mrs Blood (*R v. Human Fertilisation and Embryology Authority*, 1997)[53] whose husband's sperm was retrieved surgically when he was in a coma and frozen upon her request; the patient subsequently died. Mrs Blood also managed to utilize the HR Act[52] to ensure that the deceased father's name would appear on her children's birth certificates despite posthumous conception. The tension between consequential and deontological thought can clearly be seen in such an example. It is widely regarded that pragmatism is necessary. Therefore, a utilitarian approach seems almost inevitable, and, in the sensitive field of assisted reproductive technologies, these assumptions need to be kept under review.

SERVICES AND FACILITIES

Ethical principles of beneficence, non-maleficence and respect for autonomy may clash in fertility preservation. The speed at which cancer therapy or surgery may need to be undertaken means that facilities may not be offered to the patient. Even if these were offered, patients may be under the influence of other medication that may render them incapable of reaching an informed decision.

Multiple births are common for cancer patients given that, in the UK's IVF programs, at least 50% of the individual babies are born in the context of twin and triplet pregnancies. Associated with these higher-order births is the cost of neonatal care and increased health risks for the offspring. The greater cost of multiple births may burden a family already in financial difficulties where one partner is recovering from disease. It may be an idea to introduce mandatory insurance for patients and IVF clinics for the care of high-order births. In the UK, cryopreservation facilities for gametes, embryos and only specific gonadal tissue containing mature gametes require a licence[54], irrespective of whether practitioners operate in the public or private sector. If patients pay for their sperm storage, the cost of the annual maintenance fee over the years may lead to the premature discarding of samples, thereby creating conflict with the initial reasons for sperm storage. The provision of support counseling for the

many years that follow may be cost-ineffective for a clinic in the private sector; as will be the intense and prolonged dialogue that may be needed with a widow for posthumous reproduction. Adolescent patients seen in dedicated private IVF centers may not always find them a comfortable setting for their semen cryopreservation if this service is normally for infertile adults. Constructive dialogue with adolescents may not occur and questions could arise about the effectiveness of consent. Significant commercialization has occurred in ovarian, testicular tissue and oocyte freezing programs, where the technology is barely in the research phase. This may seem to suggest that practitioners are motivated by commercial considerations. Likewise, academic sectors have been criticized over their motivation for publications, which have involved putting patients through procedures that are unclear. This raises concerns about the manner and level of counseling and informed consent the patient gives, since patients' rights and scientists' desire for knowledge do not always go hand-in-hand. Regulators may investigate, for example, disproportionately low embryo freezing programs against their high use in research, and how patients' interests may suffer as a result.

Religious views, the time lapse and the individual's feelings have also shaped the practice of cryotechnology. The development of human oocyte freezing programs follows straight on the heels of the Catholic Church's unease about freezing embryos. As donor gametes and embryos cannot be used within the Islamic faith[55], the cryopreservation of gametes and embryos for own-use to circumvent medical problems would be greatly welcomed by patients. Freezing sperm from an orthodox Jewish male patient about Sabbath time may be especially complex in relation to masturbation[56]. It is helpful to be open to these differing beliefs so that pressure is not put on patients that would discourage them or invalidate their consent. Individuals' strong views on ethical principles can furthermore be a factor in imposing specific ethics, since ethics are not regulated. Ethics can change over time, and only time will tell whether novel haploidization and cloning-type techniques will become acceptable.

AUTONOMY AND CONSENT

Respect for individual autonomy runs strong in common morality. Informed consent is the central tenet in decision-making regarding fertility preservation for most patients. Three conditions need to be met to rightfully speak of informed consent: autonomy, competence and understanding. It is important to be clear about the technologies that exist, the evolving state of the field, to be able to discuss these with unlimited time constraints, to recognize the potential as well as the limitations of the procedure, and to draw the patient's attention to any costs that may be attached to the procedures. The patient needs to recognize how they stand in relation to the current legal framework. In the UK, greater rights were conferred on individuals with the introduction of the HR Act[52], which declares that public bodies should not interfere with individual rights. As an example of the way different laws operate, in the UK the sperm provided by the adolescent can only be frozen and used with his consent. However, if the patient is under 16, parental consent only is required for any surgical procedure. The specter of parents wishing to use the germ cells of their deceased offspring can be disturbing. The process of gaining consent from adolescents storing sperm needs delicate handling[51]. Unique to the case of adolescent patients storing gametes is that, in the eventual posthumous use of gametes, the partner being treated would most likely not have been known at the time of the cryopreservation procedure.

The issue of competence remains contentious in the case of children, adolescents and adults alike. Therefore the completeness of consent will always remain a moot point. Sperm, oocyte or embryo cryopreservation for patients with mental incapacity will most likely be illegal, but because of discrimination issues, commentary on this group has so far been carefully avoided.

Ticking boxes in consent forms is invalid if the patient has not understood what they are for. For this reason it is imperative that full information is given, and that the patient be given a chance for independent counseling in addition to the counseling that may already be provided. Where statutory regulation exists, it is much easier to have a uniform approach. The patient must understand the process that they are undergoing. It is deemed that consent gained under pressure or coercion is unlikely to be effective and therefore invalid. For fertility preservation that comes under regulation, the HFEA has constructed consent forms (www.hfea.gov.uk) which other countries find a useful benchmark. It is therefore incumbent on clinicians, practitioners, counselors and technologists to be versed not just with the technological advances, but also with the wider societal issues such as the changing legal and ethical horizons.

Verbal information should be backed up with written information, given that a cancer patient's attention span may not enable him or her to grasp the full facts. A cancer patient may be drowsy through the preliminary treatment with, for example, painkillers or minor exploratory surgical procedures. The complex language making up the information may need to be simplified, especially if the patient is very young. Information needs to be further managed by a process of continued, informed counseling. For those speaking other languages the decision-making process should be through a qualified interpreter. All reasonable steps need to be taken in gaining consent for a procedure as well as disclosing personal and sensitive information about the patient's fertility.

Effective consent should always be in place. Individual's views, choices or circumstances may change over time. For instance, a form may record the choices in regard to frozen gametes and embryos after death or mental incapacitation. There may be change of partner who may be named as one with whom the treatment service is to be undertaken. It may be wrong for a clinic member to coerce a patient to alter or limit his or her choice simply because that clinic may not, for example, undertake posthumous reproduction. In these circumstances clinics should endeavor to highlight that it may still be possible to perform the procedure elsewhere. The way in which clinics practice gaining consent, by racing to complete consent forms, is an invalid basis for consent.

From the viewpoint of surgical preservation of an ovary, however, the single event consent model, rather than the continuous model, may be more valid, as the action resulting from a choice may not be reversible. The question of surgical removal of healthy or unaffected reproductive tissue needs to be looked at against the backdrop of ongoing research programs, as patients' decision-making may be subtly guided. Generally speaking, freedom in the context of informed choice may only happen in the absence of undue influence on the patient, who must decide how the benefits of fertility preservation outweigh the risks, burdens and costs.

There has been a significant recent extension to fertility preservation in the increasing demand to screen for HIV, hepatitis B and C, and additional conditions. These demands impinge upon individual autonomy and rights, and a proper process should be in place to explain the risks of undertaking such tests, which could compromise such individual freedoms as, for example, the ability to gain personal insurance. In the UK these tests are now required by the HFEA before cryopreservation of reproductive material is undertaken. The offer of testing has become a coercive offer; i.e. refusal on the patient's part would result in being denied the service, thereby leading to an overall loss of autonomy. This may be morally justified when the safety of other samples stored in the same bank is considered, along with the welfare of recipients and offspring.

Perhaps one of the most significant areas in which individual autonomy and rights will be threatened is the development and application of genetic tests for serious diseases such as cancers. More controversial still will be the application of PGD of individual embryos, given the fierce and compassionate views

held across society in relation to the human embryo[57]. Notwithstanding the complex moral issues relating to the embryo, the creation and use of embryos by nuclear transfer, or cloning, could become a possibility for those patients without conventional gametes. More recently, the creation and use of embryos for tissue typing of human leukocyte antigen extended the scope for PGD to determine if an embryo was clear of disease and also tissue-compatible with an existing, affected sibling needing umbilical cord cells for transplantation[58]. The Hashmi case[59,60] in the UK sparked off a wide debate as to whether reproductive techniques were being abused, whether the creation of the child was for the sake of the existing sibling, and what it meant for the autonomy and rights of the unborn child who would be brought into the world for this purpose. The application of PGD in cancers is likely to present complex issues, given that a sizable proportion of those wishing to preserve their fertility may well have cancer. PGD for mutations in cancer-implicated genes such as breast cancer genes (*BRCA-1* and *-2*) is probably going to be even more controversial, given that the penetrance of these mutations is incomplete (the lifetime risk of a female carrier is 50–85%; her risk of developing ovarian cancer is 20–65%), and preventive interventions may effectively reduce morbidity and mortality in carriers[61,62]. Fertility preservation in the case of HIV-positive couples has remained a contentious issue despite the reported successes[63,64]. This is because of the need for a dedicated area and the necessity for advanced testing procedures to be available on the day of insemination along with proper counseling support, especially if the mother is positive and there is an associated risk of vertical HIV transmission. It is these possible applications which make the public uneasy about the ever-changing pace of reproductive technologies.

RIGHTS

This leads us to the place of rights, which remains controversial in an ethical debate. In most cases when we say that someone has a right to do something, we imply that it would be wrong to interfere with his doing it, or at least that some special grounds are needed to justify any interference[52,65,66]. Rights can also be described as claim rights (positive rights) or liberty rights (negative rights). The HR Act, Article 12, incorporates the right to form a family, thereby acknowledging the unacceptability of obstructing someone in the exercise of that right, rather than demanding positive action. A young cancer patient can decide not to do anything in terms of cryopreserving his sperm before cytotoxic treatment and this wish has to be respected. In fact the position has not changed here, since under the HFE Act it would be illegal to take a sample from a patient or donor without fully informed consent or under pressure. A case when a woman has her oocytes frozen and then wishes to exercise her rights to use the cryopreserved oocyte has to be seen as an instance of a positive right.

Future ethical debates face the prospect of a slippery slope with the choice and power individuals have increasing under the HR Act. This declares that public bodies should not interfere with privacy or family life unless they can justify this in terms of protecting public health or morals, or protecting the rights of others. It means, for instance, that the HFEA cannot simply ban anything it considers ethically unacceptable. Under the HR Act, the HFEA would have to prove its right to infringe on people's choice and articulate quite precisely why it is interfering, in terms of public health or morals.

LAW, MORALITY AND ETHICS

Law and ethics operate and interact sometimes in unison, sometimes in conflict. The judge Lord Colebridge stated, "it would not be correct to say that every moral obligation involves a legal duty; but every legal duty is founded on a moral obligation" (*R v. Instan* (1893) 1 QB at 453)[67]. The law is a more powerful instrument than ethics because its provisions are more authoritative, enshrined by political legislation, stated by courts, subjected to public scrutiny, enforceable by legal professionals and the police, open to appeals and, by the nature of the institution, open to reform. Against this, a law that is considered to lack an ethical dimension, to be at best crudely pragmatic and at worst ethically bankrupt, is impoverished in its capacity to educate and inspire those it governs to distinguish right conduct from wrong. Law frames the setting within which ethical choices may be practically exercised, but ethics frame the limits within which law is voluntarily obeyed and respected as an expression of the values of the society to which it applies. The contributions that ethics should make to law and legal process, and the appropriateness of resolving ethical conflicts by law, are matters of continuing social debate. Ethics and morality are distinguishable but are frequently treated as the same, as is normally the case in reproductive medicine[68].

Whilst ethics committees are encouraged, they are not necessarily supported by statute. This is because of the potential for conflict, and the danger that moral values could clash or be inconsistent with existing statutory position. The role and workings of ethics committees is unclear[69] and so is the make-up of their membership[70], which is probably chosen by the head clinician to fit in with the clinic's ethos. Statutory support for ethics committees would most likely cause chaos and inconsistency in the interpretation of statutory instruments.

WHAT IS UNETHICAL?

Given our different ethical perspectives it may be difficult to determine what is unethical. Still we have our own ideas about what we consider to cross the line beyond what we believe is acceptable. With fertility preservation, I propose that the patient whose fertility is threatened should have every opportunity to make an informed choice to enable him or her to preserve their fertility. Unethical practices would include unsafe procedures which may harm individuals, the unborn and society; those that cause a loss of patient autonomy; those that raise false hopes; those bringing about unhealthy commercial gain, or breaking the law; and finally, cases where individuals might exploit gray areas in the law. Cancer patients in particular may be vulnerable in the decision-making process if they are under the influence of medication, and care and time should be devoted in gaining their autonomy.

A significant concern has been the speed of commercial exploitation of gonadal tissue and oocyte cryotechnology when the procedures are barely at an experimental level. It is useful to note, for example, that the primordial follicles are unevenly distributed throughout the cortex of an ovary. Histological analyses on an ovarian fragment may therefore be non-representative and this type of limitation must be made transparent[71]. The limits of the technologies and tests should be well recognized and the patients informed. Multiple births resulting from indiscriminate use of IVF have led to a significant burden on national resources and an increase in the costs of neonatal care. Perhaps wealthy IVF clinics should be encouraged to take out insurance against such higher-order births and their costs. Healthy oocyte donors and surrogates need to be carefully counseled about undergoing stimulated IVF cycles[72]. Individuals seeking to preserve their fertility are also likely to resort to IVF techniques. A recent review suggests an association between the use of assisted reproductive techniques and increased risks of problems in the resulting children, and these developments should be relayed to prospective patients[73].

Unusual areas of reproductive technology, which contemplate or proceed with the revival of deceased cancer patients by cloning, raise serious concerns about the effect on families, in addition to those relating to safety. The constant review of women with borderline tumors is essential given the recurrence rate. Support for surrogates should be given to ensure their emotional well-being is safely satisfied. The outcome of using post-chemotherapy sperm and possibly oocytes remains of concern for future generations, given that the consequences are as yet unknown.

CONCLUSION

Advances in cancer treatment and improved prospects of survival call for greater emphasis to be laid on patients' quality of life, an aspect of which is fertility preservation. The application of these advances has been extended to children, creating problems as to patient autonomy and consent. These complexities also relate to changing laws. Whilst IVF-type procedures, cryotechnology and surgical fertility preservation make various options possible, there is a need for practitioners at all levels to support patients on a long-term basis. This is to ensure that effective consent can be upheld, and informed decisions are taken to preserve patients' fertility potential. Clinicians need to enhance the welfare of patients' offspring by, for example, lessening multiple births from the overuse of IVF techniques, which is often an option for individuals seeking to preserve their fertility. It is incumbent upon practitioners not just to understand the technical and clinical aspects of procedures, but also to develop a deep sense of social responsibility, together with an equivalent level of understanding of the legal, moral and ethical issues.

References

1. Spitz S. The histological effects of nitrogen mustards on human tumors and tissues. *Cancer* 1948;1:383–98
2. Louis L, Lemaryi LR, Best WR. Treatment of chronic granulocytic leukemia with myleran. *Arch Intern Med* 1956;97:299–308
3. Polge C, Smith AU, Parkes AS. Revival of spermatozoa after vitrification and dehydration at low temperature. *Nature* 1949;164:666
4. Bunge RG, Sherman JK. Fertilisation capacity of frozen human spermatozoa. *Nature* 1953;172:767

5. Whittingham DG, Leibo SP, Mazur P. Survival of mouse embryos frozen to −196°C and −269°C. *Science* 1972;178:411–14

6. Trounson A, Mohr L. Human pregnancy following cryopreservation, thawing and transfer of an eight-cell embryo. *Nature* 1983;305:707–9

7. Porcu E, Fabbri R, Seracchioli R, et al. Birth of six healthy children after intracytoplasmic sperm-injection of cryopreserved human oocytes. *Hum Reprod* 1998;13:124

8. Chen C. Pregnancy after human oocyte cryopreservation. *Lancet* 1986;i:884–6

9. Parkes AS, Smith AU. Regeneration of rat ovarian tissue grafted after exposure to low temperatures. *Proc R Soc Lond B Biol Sci* 1953;140:455–70

10. Bahadur G, Steele SJ. Ovarian tissue cryopreservation for patients. *Hum Reprod* 1996;11:2215–16

11. Newton H, Aubard Y, Rutherford A, et al. Low temperature storage and grafting of human ovarian tissue. *Hum Reprod* 1996;11:1487–91

12. He Z, Liu HC, Rosenwaks Z. Cryopreservation of nuclear material as a potential method of fertility preservation. *Fertil Steril* 2003;79:347–54

13. Garcia-Ximene F, Escriba MJ. Viable offspring derived from cryopreserved haploid rabbit parthenotes. *Theriogenology* 2002;57:1319–25

14. Bahadur G, Ralph D. Gonadal tissue cryopreservation in boys with paediatric cancers. *Hum Reprod* 1999;14:11–17

15. Damani MN, Mittal R, Oates RD. Testicular tissue extraction in a young male with 47, XXY Klinefelter's syndrome: potential strategy for preservation of fertility. *Fertil Steril* 2001;76:1054–6

16. Revel A, Koler M, Simon A, et al. Oocyte collection during cryopreservation of ovarian cortex. *Fertil Steril* 2003;97:1237–9

17. Schlatt S. Germ cell transplantation. *Mol Cell Endocrinol* 2002;186:163–7

18. Richards MA, Stockton D, Babb P, et al. How many deaths have been avoided through improvements in cancer survival? *Br Med J* 2000;320:895–8

19. Bahadur G. Fertility issues for cancer patients. *Mol Cell Endocrinol* 2000;169:117–22

20. Abdel-Basir Sayed M. Bladder neck resection with preservation of antegrade ejaculation: basic technique. *J Endourol* 2003;17:109–11

21. Jacobson R, Bostofte E, Engholm G, et. al. Risk of testicular cancer in men with abnormal semen characteristics: cohort study. *Br Med J* 2000;321:789–92

22. Scott SD, Lee RD, Mulhall JP. Should all infertile males undergo urologic evaluation before assisted reproductive technologies? Two cases

23. of testicular cancer presenting with infertility. *Fertil Steril* 2001;75:1226–7

23. Bines J, Oleske DM, Cobleigh MA. Ovarian function in premenopausal women treated with adjuvant chemotherapy for breast cancer. *J Clin Oncol* 1996;14:1718–29

24. Byrne J, Fears TR, Gail MH, et al. Early menopause in long-term survivors of cancer during adolescence. *Am J Obstet Gynecol* 1992;166:788–93

25. Hreinsson JG, Otala M, Fridstrom M, et al. Follicles are found in the ovaries of adolescent girls with Turners syndrome. *J Clin Endocrinol Metab* 2002;87:3618–23

26. Oktay KH, Yih M. Preliminary experience with orthotopic and heterotopic transplantation of ovarian cortical strips. *Semin Reprod Med* 2002;20:63–74

27. Wang X, Chen H, Yin H, et al. Fertility after intact ovary transplantation. *Nature* 2002;415:385

28. Nieto JJ, Rolfe KJ, MacLean AB, et al. Ovarian cancer and infertility: a genetic link? *Lancet* 1999;354:649

29. Duckitt K, Templeton, AA. Cancer in women with infertility. *Curr Opin Obstet Gynecol* 1998;10:199–203

30. Maker AP, Trope C. Fertility preservation in gynecologic cancer. *Acta Obstet Gynecol Scand* 2001;80:794–802

31. Morice P, Juncker L, Rey A, et al. Ovarian transposition for patients with cervical carcinoma treated by radiosurgical combination. *Fertil Steril* 2000;74:743–8

32. Visvanathan DK, Cutner AS, Cassoni AM, et al. A new technique of laparoscopic ovariopexy before irradiation. *Fertil Steril* 2003;79:1204–6

33. Schlaerth JB, Spirtos NM, Schlaerth AC. Radical trachelectomy and pelvic lymphadenectomy with uterine preservation in the treatment of cervical cancer. *Am J Obstet Gynecol* 2003;188:29–34

34. Burnett AF, Roman LD, O'Meara AT, et al. Radical vaginal trachelectomy and pelvic lymphadenectomy for preservation of fertility in early cervical carcinoma. *Gynecol Oncol* 2003;88:419–23

35. Case AM, Wilson S, Colgan TJ, et al. Fertility sparing surgery, with subsequent pregnancy, in persistent gestational trophoblastic neoplasia. *Hum Reprod* 2001;16:360–4

36. Donnez J, Munschke A, Berliere M, et al. Safety of conservative management and fertility outcome in women with borderline tumors of the ovary. *Fertil Steril* 2003;79:1216–21

37. Ward RM, Bristow RE. Cancer and pregnancy: recent developments. *Curr Opin Obstet Gynecol* 2002;14:613–17

38. Serkies K, Wysocka B, Emerich J, *et al.* Salvage hemipelvis radiotherapy with fertility preservation in an adolescent with recurrent vulvar carcinoma. *Gynecol Oncol* 2002;85:381–3

39. Azem F, Yovel I, Wagman I, *et al.* Surrogate pregnancy in a patient who underwent radical hysterectomy and bilateral transposition of ovaries. *Fertil Steril* 2003;79:1229–30

40. Mikami M, Ono A, Sakaiya N, *et al.* Case report of serous ovarian tumour of borderline malignancy (Stage 1c) in a pregnant woman. *Eur J Obstet Gynecol Reprod Biol* 2001;98:237–9

41. Kuczyk M, Machtens S, Bokemeyer C, *et al.* Sexual function and fertility after treatment of testicular cancer. *Curr Opin Urol* 2000;10:473–7

42. Thaler-DeMers D. Intimacy issues: sexuality, fertility, and relationships. *Semin Oncol Nurs* 2001;17:255–62

43. Cleeland CS, Mendoza TR, Wang XS, *et al.* Assessing symptom distress in cancer patients. *Cancer* 2000;89:1634–46

44. Soothill K, Morris SM, Harman J, *et al.* The significant unmet needs of cancer patients: probing psychological concerns. *Support Care Cancer* 2001;9:597–605

45. Bahadur, G. Death and conception. *Hum Reprod* 2002;17:2769–75

46. De Sutter P. Gender reassignment and assisted reproduction. *Hum Reprod* 2001;16:612–14

47. Human Fertilisation and Embryology Act 1990. London: HMSO, 1990

48. Crockin S. Legally speaking: New Jersey Supreme Court to hear frozen embryo appeal (J.B. v. M.B.). *Am Soc Reprod Med News* 2000; 34:23–5

49. Mason JK, McCall Smith RA. *Law and Medical Ethics.* London: Butterworths, 1999

50. Singer P. *Practical Ethics.* Cambridge: Cambridge University Press, 1993

51. Bahadur G, Whelan J, Ralph D, *et al.* Gaining consent to freeze spermatozoa from adolescents with cancer: legal, ethical and practical aspects. *Hum Reprod* 2001;16:188–93

52. Bahadur G. The Human Rights Act (1998) and its impact on human reproductive issues. *Hum Reprod* 2001;16:785–9

53. *R v. Human Fertilisation and Embryology Authority,* exp Blood, 1997. 2 All ER 687, (1997) 35 BMLR 1, CA

54. Bahadur G, Whelan J, Davies MC, *et al.* Cancer patients, gametes, gonadal tissue and the UK legal status. *Reprod Biomed Online* 2001;2:8–10

55. Husain FA. Reproductive issues from the Islamic perspective. *Hum Fertil* 2000;3:124–8

56. Hirsh AV. Infertility in Jewish couples, biblical and rabbinic law. *Hum Fertil* 1998;1:14–19

57. Bahadur G. The moral status of the embryo: the human embryo in the UK Human Fertilisation and Embryology (Research Purposes) Regulation 2001 debate. *Reprod Biomed Online* 2003;7:10–14

58. Verlinsky Y, Rechitsky S, Schoolcraft W, *et al.* Preimplantation diagnosis for Fanconi anemia combined with HLA matching. *J Am Med Assoc* 2001;285:3130–3

59. Dyer C. Couple at centre of IVF controversy begin treatment. *Br Med J* 2003;326:1106

60. Boyle RJ, Savulescu J. Ethics of using preimplantation genetic diagnosis to select a stem cell donor for an existing person. *Br Med J* 2001;323:1240–3

61. Turner BC, Glazer PM, Haffty BG. *BRCA-1/BRCA-2* in breast conserving therapy. *J Clin Oncol* 1999;17:3689

62. Lancaster JM, Wiseman RW, Berchuck A. An inevitable dilemma: prenatal testing for mutations in *BRCA-1* breast–ovarian cancer susceptibility gene. *Obstet Gynecol* 1996;87: 306–9

63. ASRM, Ethics Committee of the American Society for Reproductive Medicine. Human immunodeficiency virus and infertility treatment. *Fertil Steril* 2002;77:218–22

64. Englert Y, Van Vooren JP, Place I, *et al.* ART in HIV infected couples. Has the time come for a change of attitude? *Hum Reprod* 2001;16: 1309–15

65. Dworkin G. *Taking Rights Seriously.* London: Gerald Duckworth & Co Ltd, 1991:205

66. Scott G. *Making Ethical Choices: Resolving Ethical Dilemmas.* Paragon House, 1998

67. Mason JK, McCall Smith RA. *Law and Medical Ethics.* London: Butterworths, 1999

68. Roy DJ, Williams JR, Dickens BM. *Bioethics in Canada.* Scarborough, Ontario: Prentice Hall, 1994:37–8

69. Stern JE, Cramer CP, Green RM, *et al.* Determining access to reproductive technology: reactions of clinic directors to ethically complex case scenarios. *Hum Reprod* 2003;18: 1343–52

70. Leavitt F. Hospital ethics committees may discourage staff from making their own decisions. *Br Med J* 2000;321:1414

71. Schmidt KLT, Byskov AG, Nyboe Andersen A, *et al.* Density and distribution of follicles in single pieces of cortex from 21 patients and in individual pieces of cortex from three entire human ovaries. *Hum Reprod* 2003;18:1158–64

72. Ahuja KK, Simons EG. Cancer of the colon in an egg donor: policy repercussions for donor recruitment. *Hum Reprod* 1998;12:2230–4

73. Kovalevsky G, Rinaudo P, Coutifaris C. Do assisted reproductive technologies cause adverse fetal outcomes? *Fertil Steril* 2003;79:1270–2

Index

hormone replacement 259
ovarian follicle pool 7
menstrual cycle 40–2
'metabolic shift' 194
methotrexate 30, 43, 55, 227–8
MHC-1 (major histocompatibility complex-1)
    proteins 129–30
mice
  ovarian follicle culture 197–9, 201
  ovarian tissue xenografts 181–2, 185
  spermatogonial transplantation 127
  testicular tissue transplantation 171
microtubules 146
microvascular endothelial cells 70–1
minimal residual disease, detection 163
miscarriage 2–3, 4, 49–50, 56, 117, 225, 230
mitochondria 8–9, 67
mitochondrial DNA (MtDNA) 9
mitoxantrone 30
MOPP protocol 25, 55, 79, 226
morality 107, 261, 262, 266
  see also ethics
mortality, childhood cancer survivors 238–9
multiple fetuses 220, 263, 267
mutation induction 230–2
MVPP protocol 25, 28, 29, 52, 79

National Cancer Institute, North America 209
National Wilms' Tumor Study Group
    (NWTSG) 218
negligence 254
nephroblastoma 46
neuroblastoma, retroperitoneal 213
New Jersey, laws 249
non-Hodgkin's lymphoma (NHL)
  female fertility 29–30, 84, 185
  incidence 38
  male fertility 25, 52–3, 77
  survival 22, 23
non-maleficence 262
NOVP protocol 231–2
nulliparity 259

older women 4, 17
oligospermia
  after chemotherapy 25–6, 77, 226
  testicular cancer 22–3
oocyte cryopreservation 85–6, 105
  biology 145–8
  current status 143–5
  ethical issues 259, 261
  limitations 105, 157–8, 178, 239
  methods 142, 145, 149–50

  potential advantages 141, 181
  storage of preserved oocytes 145
oocytes
  decline with age 3, 8–13, 67–8, 258
  development *in vivo* 191–2
  'limited oocyte model' 10
  maturation *in vitro* (IVM) 104–5, 141, 201
  radiation sensitivity 207–8
oogenesis 39–40
oogonia 39
oophorectomy
  ovarian cancer 91
  ovarian transplantation 86
  prophylactic 180
'open-pulled straws' (OPS) 150
oral contraceptives 1
osmotic buffers 146, 165
osmotic stress 115, 146, 161
osteosarcoma 179, 184
ovarian cancer 90–3, 243, 259
  epithelial cell 92–3
  fertility options 92–3
  fertility-sparing surgery 90–2, 259
  germ cell 30, 92
  radiation-induced 85
'ovarian concept' 2–3
ovarian cyst
  benign 168, 183
  radiation-induced 85
ovarian cystectomy 91, 92
ovarian failure
  after chemotherapy 28–34, 53–5, 177
  after radiotherapy 27–8
  impacts on patient 27
  non-germline cells 70–1
  partial 31–3
  radiotherapy 46–7
ovarian follicle culture 192–7
  culture environment 192–4
  future priorities 199–201
  large animals 199, 200
  preantral follicles 195–7
  primordial follicles 194–5, 196
  small animals 197–9
ovarian follicles
  decline 2, 3, 7–10, 11, 167, 258
    factors influencing 12–13
  development *in vivo* 5–6, 12,
      39–40, 191–2
  in vitro maturation 170
  resting pool 6–7
  somatic cells 192
ovarian metastases 106, 168, 184–5

stem cell transplantation (SCT) 44, 47, 51, 56, 57
 graft-versus-host disease 44, 49
 indications 168, 179
 pregnancy after 50
 see also spermatogonial stem cells, transplantation
stillbirth 225, 227, 228, 229
sucrose 149
superoxide radical 119
surgery
 female cancers 90–2, 259–60
 male cancers 24
 ovarian transplantation 86–7, 182, 183
 ovarian transposition 83–5, 186
surrogacy 186, 253, 261, 267
survival, cancer 21, 22, 23, 177, 178, 217, 237
Sweden 260–1
systemic lupus erythematosus 30–1, 54–5, 106, 179

tamoxifen 104, 178, 180, 242
targeted drugs 43, 44
taxanes 33–4, 241
taxol 33–4
teratoma 79
testicular cancer 45, 46, 51, 52, 77
 germ cell tumors 238
 impact on fertility 22–3
 incidence 38
testicular function
 after chemotherapy 24–6, 50–3
 after radiotherapy 24, 45–6, 226
 in cancer 22–3, 51
 suppression 77–81
testicular germ cell harvesting 238
testicular sperm extraction (TESE) 233, 238
testicular tissue cryopreservation 163, 170–1
 transplantation 171
testis 42
 irradiation 45–6
testis tissue, implantation 128–9
testosterone 42
 intratesticular levels 133, 135
 radiotherapy 46
 and spermatogenesis recovery 78–9
thawing, sperm 116, 117
theca cells 192, 199
therapeutic insemination (TI) 111–12
 history 112–13
 success rates 117–20
 synchronization with ovulation 120
therapeutic donor insemination (TDI) 112
thyroid stimulating hormone 48
tobacco smoking 12, 68
total body irradiation (TBI)
 female fertility 46, 47, 49, 209–10

male fertility 26
 pregnancy after 50
trachelectomy, abdominal radical 95, 243
transforming growth factors (TGF) 162
transmission electron microscopy 171
trehalose 151
tubal pregnancy 56
tubulin 148
tumor markers, ovarian cancer 91
twin studies 13

ultrasonography 94, 220–1
unethical practices 266–7
Uniform Parentage Act (2002) 251
United Kingdom, ethical and legal issues
 250, 260, 262–3, 264
United States
 ethical issues 261
 legal issues 248–50, 253
urogenital problems 49
uterus
 radiation injury 48–9, 209–11
 transplantation 95–6
utilitarianism 262

VACOP-B protocol 25, 30
vaginal changes 49, 57–8
vaginitis, radiation 212
vascular endothelial growth factor
 (VEGF) 162
vinblastine 25, 30, 43, 51, 79, 80
Vinca alkaloids 30, 43, 51, 79, 80
vincristine 25, 30, 43, 79
vitamin E 162
vitrification 103–4, 160, 171
 oocytes 105, 145, 149, 150–1
 solutions 149
vulvar cancer 259

Wilms' tumor 22, 49, 184, 208, 213, 238, 239
 children of survivors 228
Woodward v. Commissioner of Social
 Security 249–50
'wrongful birth' 255
'wrongful life' 255

X chromosome 13
xenotransplantation 163
 ovarian tissue 169–70, 181–2, 185
 spermatogonial stem cells 134–5
 testicular tissue 171

Zoladex 77–8
zona pellucida 191–2